Practical Forensic Psychiatry

Edited by Tom Clark and
Dharjinder Singh Rooprai

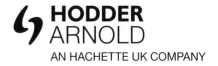

HODDER
ARNOLD

AN HACHETTE UK COMPANY

First published in Great Britain in 2011 by
Hodder Arnold, an imprint of Hodder Education, Hodder and Stoughton Ltd, a division of Hachette UK
338 Euston Road, London NW1 3BH

http://www.hodderarnold.com

[Environmental statement to be inserted on all biblio pages and deleted by Production if using printers where statement is NOT true]
Hachette UK's policy is to use papers that are natural, renewable and recyclable products and made from wood grown in sustainable forests. The logging and manufacturing processes are expected to conform to the environmental regulations of the country of origin.

Whilst the advice and information in this book are believed to be true and accurate at the date of going to press, neither the author[s] nor the publisher can accept any legal responsibility or liability for any errors or omissions that may be made. In particular, (but without limiting the generality of the preceding disclaimer) every effort has been made to check drug dosages; however it is still possible that errors have been missed. Furthermore, dosage schedules are constantly being revised and new side-effects recognized. For these reasons the reader is strongly urged to consult the drug companies' printed instructions, and their websites, before administering any of the drugs recommended in this book.

British Library Cataloguing in Publication Data
A catalogue record for this book is available from the British Library

Library of Congress Cataloging-in-Publication Data
A catalog record for this book is available from the Library of Congress

ISBN-13   978-1-444-12063-9

1 2 3 4 5 6 7 8 9 10

Commissioning Editor: Caroline Makepeace
Project Editors: Jo Silman and Mischa Barrett
Production Controller: Joanna Walker
Cover Design: Helen Townson

Typeset in 10 on 12pt Goudy Old Style by Phoenix Photosetting, Chatham, Kent
Printed and bound in the UK by CPI Group (UK) Ltd., Croydon, CR0 4YY

What do you think about this book? Or any other Hodder Arnold title?
Please visit our website: www.hodderarnold.com

Contents

Contributors

Rebekah Bourne MBChB MRCPsych DipMedEd
specialty registrar in forensic psychiatry, Birmingham & Solihull Mental Health NHS Foundation Trust; honorary clinical teacher to the Birmingham MRCPsych Course

Tom Clark MBChB LLM MRCPsych
consultant forensic psychiatrist, Reaside Clinic, Birmingham & Solihull Mental Health NHS Trust; honorary senior clinical lecturer in forensic psychiatry, University of Birmingham training programme director for forensic psychiatry, West Midlands School of Psychiatry; visiting forensic psychiatrist, HMP Birmingham

John Croft MBChB MRCPysch
consultant forensic psychiatrist, Ardenleigh Womens Forensic Mental health Service, Birmingham & Solihull Mental Health NHS Foundation Trust

Muthusamy Natarajan MBBS MRCPsych
consultant forensic psychiatrist, William Wake House, St Andrew's Healthcare, Billing Road, Northampton

Clare Oakley MBChB MRCPsych
clinical research worker, St Andrew's Academic Centre, Institute of Psychiatry, King's College London

James Reed MBChB BMedSci LLM MRCPsych
locum consultant forensic psychiatrist, Reaside Clinic, Birmingham & Solihull Mental Health NHS Foundation Trust

Dharjinder Singh Rooprai MBBS LLM MRCPsych
consultant forensic psychiatrist (forensic LD, ASD and ABI), Fromeside, Avon and Wiltshire Mental Health Partnership NHS Trust, West of England Forensic Mental Health Service

Renarta Rowe MBChB MSc MRCPsych
consultant forensic psychiatrist, Reaside Clinic, Birmingham & Solihull Mental Health NHS Foundation Trust

Leela Sivaprasad MBBS DPM MRCPsych
consultant forensic psychiatrist, Reaside Clinic, Birmingham & Solihull Mental Health NHS Foundation Trust

Helen Whitworth MBChB MSc MRCPsych Cert MHS
clinical lecturer, Keele University, visiting lecturer, Coventry University; consultant forensic psychiatrist, Hatherton Centre, South Staffordshire and Shropshire Healthcare NHS Foundation Trust

Preface

We conceived this book with two broad aims in mind. Firstly, we wanted to present key factual information in a concise, readily retrievable format, with a relative absence of opinion and debate. Of course the occasional opinion has crept in, and we think that the book is more interesting and thought provoking for that, but it remains a densely factual book. Secondly, as a 'jobbing' consultant and, at the time, higher trainee respectively, we wanted to provide practical guidance on the day-to-day tasks that a forensic psychiatrist is required to deal with. This is particularly aimed at forensic trainees and psychiatrists working in other fields, for whom forensic matters are so often relevant.

The book is unashamedly aimed at psychiatrists. While forensic psychiatric services are necessarily multidisciplinary, we think that there is value in focusing on the role of the psychiatrist, allowing a more pithy and direct approach, and enabling the role of the psychiatrist to be set more clearly within its proper place as but one part of the team. At the risk of appearing to try to eat our cake, we hope that those working in other disciplines and in other types of mental health services will also find the information and clinical guidance presented here useful. Most forensic patients used to be general psychiatric patients and will be so again, and much of the interface between the criminal justice system and mental health services is served by general rather than forensic psychiatry, and often by nurses rather than doctors.

We are aware of gaps and areas of clinical practice that might have warranted more space than we have been able to give. In particular we have not tried to cover the law in jurisdictions other than England and Wales. More weighty and comprehensive textbooks are available; our book is conceived more as a vade mecum. We have tried to point the reader in the direction of further reading that might fill some of these gaps. Those references that we consider to be particularly important are marked with an asterisk. Our view would be that a higher trainee in forensic psychiatry should read all of these key references during the course of their training, though it is by no means an exhaustive list.

Preparing a rather stylized yet multiple author book is a harder task than we imagined. We are very grateful to our contributors, each chosen for their particular experience or knowledge in relation to some aspect or other of forensic clinical practice, for producing such valuable chapters while tolerating our editorial interference in the pursuit of a consistent style.

TC & DSR

Abbreviations

AC	approved clinician
ACCT	assessment, care in custody and teamwork
ADOS	Autism Diagnostic Observation Schedule
AESOP	Aetiology and Ethnicity of Schizophrenia and Other Psychoses
AMHP	approved mental health professional
AOT	assertive outreach team
ARA(I)	actuarial risk assessment (instrument)
ASBO	antisocial behaviour order
ASD	autistic spectrum disorder
AUC	area under the curve
AWOL	absent without leave (from MHA detention) or absent without official leave
BCS	British Crime Survey
BME	black and minority ethnic
CAMHS	Child and Adolescent Mental Health Services
CAMCOG	Cambridge Cognitive Exam
CANFOR	Camberwell Assessment of Needs – forensic version
CARATS	counselling assessment referral advice and throughcare Service
CATIE	Clinical Antipsychotic Trials of Intervention Effectiveness
CBT	cognitive–behavioural therapy
CCRC	Criminal Cases Review Commission
CIS-R	Clinical Interview Schedule – Revised
CJA 2003	Criminal Justice Act 2003
CJA 2009	Coroners and Justice Act 2009
CJCSA 2000	Criminal Justice and Court Service Act 2000
CJS	criminal justice system
CLDT	community learning disability team
CMHT	community mental health team
CPS	Crown Prosecution Service
CoP	Code of Practice to the Mental Health Act 1983
CPA	care programme approach
CPIA	Criminal Procedure (Insanity) Act 1969
CPN	community psychiatric nurse
CrimPR	Criminal Procedure Rules
CSA	childhood sexual abuse
CTO	community treatment order
DCR	discretionary conditional release
DH	Department of Health
DHSS	Department of Health and Society Security
DPP	detention for public protection

DSH	deliberate self-harm
DSM	*Diagnostic and Statistical Manual of Mental Disorders*
DSPD	dangerous and severe personality disorder
DTO	Detention and Training Order
DVCVA 2004	Domestic Violence, Crime and Victims Act 2004
ECA	Epidemiological Catchment Area Survey
ECHR	European Convention on Human Rights
ERASOR	estimate of risk of adolescent sexual offence recidivism
FME	forensic medical examiner
GDP	gross domestic product
HCR-20	Historical Clinical Risk-20
HMIP	Her Majesty's Inspectorate of Prisons
HoNOS	Health of the Nation Outcome Scales
ICD	International Classification of Diseases
ICT	iterative classification tree
IMB	independent monitoring board
IMCA	independent mental capacity advocate
IPDE	international personality disorder examination
IPP	imprisonment for public protection or indeterminate sentence for public protection
LD	learning disability
LHRH	luteinizing hormone-releasing hormone
LSC	Legal Services Commission
MAPPA	multi-agency public protection arrangement
MAPPP	multi-agency public protection panel
MCA 2005	Mental Capacity Act 2005
MDT	multidisciplinary team
MDO	mentally disordered offender
MEAMS	Middlesex Elderly Assessment of Mental State
MHA 1983	Mental Health Act 1983
MHA 2007	Mental Health Act 2007
MHU	Mental Health Unit (of the MoJ)
MMSE	Mini-Mental State Examination
MoJ	Ministry of Justice
MSU	medium secure unit
NGBROI	not guilty by reason of insanity
NICE	National Institute for Health and Clinical Excellence
NOMS	National Offender Management Service
OABH	occasioning actual bodily harm
OASys	Offender Assessment System
OBP	offending behaviour programme
OCD	obsessive–compulsive disorder
OGP	OASys General reoffending Predictor
OGRS	Offender Group Reconviction Scale
OM	offender manager
OR	odds ratio
OT	occupational therapy

OVP	OASys Violence Predictor
PACE 1984	Police and Criminal Evidence Act 1984
PANSS	Positive and Negative Syndrome Scale (for schizophrenia)
PAR	population attributable risk
PCCA	Powers of Criminal Courts Act 2000
PCL-R	Psychopathy Checklist – Revised
PCL-SV	Psychopathy Checklist – Screening Version
PCL-YV	Psychopathy Checklist – Youth Version
PCT	primary care trust
PD	personality disorder
PED	parole eligibility date
PICU	psychiatric intensive care unit
PIPES	psychologically informed planned environment
PPG	penile plethysmography
PSR	pre-sentence report
PTSD	post-traumatic stress disorder
RC	responsible clinician
RCP	Royal College of Physicians
RCPsych	Royal College of Psychiatrists
RM2000	Risk Matrix 2000
RMO	responsible medical officer
RMP	registered medical practitioner
ROC	receiver operator characteristics
ROSH	risk of serious harm (according to OASys)
RRASOR	rapid risk assessment for sex offender recidivism
RSU	regional secure unit
RSVP	Risk of Sexual Violence Protocol
SAPROF	Structured Assessment of Protective Factors for violence risk
SAVRY	Structured Assessment of Violence Risk in Youth
SCA	structured clinical assessment
SCAN	Schedules for Clinical Assessment in Neuropsychiatry
SCID-II	Structured Clinical Interview for DSM-IV axis II diagnoses
SCMH	Sainsbury Centre for Mental Health
SCT	supervised community treatment
SHA	strategic health authority
SI	statutory instrument
SMB	strategic management board (for MAPPA)
SNASA	Salford Needs Assessment Schedule for Adolescents
SOPO	sex offender prevention order
SORAG	sex offender risk appraisal guide
SOTP	sex offender treatment programme
SPJ	structured professional judgement
SSRI	selective serotonin reuptake inhibitor
START	short-term assessment of risk and treatability
TC	therapeutic community
TCO	threat control over-ride
ViSOR	Violent and Sexual Offenders Register

VLU	victim liaison unit
VORAS	Violent Offender Risk Assessment Scale
VRAG	Violence Risk Appraisal Guide
WAIS	Weschler Adult Intelligence Scale
WHO	World Health Organization
wte	whole-time equivalent
YJB	Youth Justice Board
YOI	young offenders' institution
YOT	Youth Offending Team

1

The Development of Forensic Psychiatric Services

● Historical Background

Offenders with mental illness have always posed unique difficulties for the criminal justice system and psychiatrists. Prior to the nineteenth century there were no specific facilities for dealing with them, although in practice they were usually compulsorily committed to hospital by the courts.

The need for secure hospitals

In 1800 James Hadfield tried to kill King George III and was found not guilty by reason of insanity:

- He was transferred to Bethlem Hospital from prison, but escaped in 1802 before being recaptured and sent back to prison.
- The 'Report from the Select Committee Appointed to Enquire into the State of Lunatics' criticized the practice of admitting 'criminal lunatics' to 'a common gaol':
  - inadequate security of asylums and uncertainties about funding were both cited as significant problems
  - recommended 'separate confinement' for 'insane offenders' funded by parishes.
- 'Criminal wings' were constructed at the Government's expense at Bethlem Hospital in 1816:
  - 60 beds (45 male, 15 female), extended in 1837 by 30 male beds.
- Patients with less serious offences were routinely detained in county asylums.

The development of criminal asylums

- Dundrum Central Criminal Asylum in Ireland opened in 1850 (120 beds)
- Broadmoor Criminal Lunatic Asylum in Berkshire opened in 1863 (500 beds):
  - repeatedly extended due to overcrowding and demand
- Rampton Criminal Lunatic Asylum in Nottinghamshire opened in 1912
- Ashworth Hospital was created in 1989 by merging two adjacent high secure hospitals:
  - Moss Side Hospital had opened in 1914
  - Park Lane Hospital had opened in 1974.

These were known collectively as 'special hospitals' and later 'high secure services'. They became part of the NHS in 1948 but remained geographically and professionally isolated from general psychiatric services.

The birth of forensic psychiatry

A series of reports beginning in the early 1960s heralded the emergence of forensic psychiatry and began to foresee possibilities for secure services on a more local footing. The large special hospitals remained remote, and there were concerns about the numbers of beds and the conditions within the hospitals.

The Emery Report (Ministry of Health, 1961)

- The Mental Health Act 1959 began a trend of reducing restrictive practices and security in general psychiatric hospitals:
  - led to a reduction in mentally disordered offenders admitted.
- A working party on special hospitals was set up to consider the role of special hospitals in managing these patients.
- Proposed provision of secure beds by regional health bodies to relieve pressure on special hospitals.
- No resources were provided and there was little tangible result.

The Gwynne Report (Ministry of Health, 1964)

- Examined the state of medical services in prisons (then separate from the NHS).
- Recommended appointing 'forensic psychiatrists' jointly between prison medical services and the NHS as a response to the clear lack of psychiatric expertise within prisons.
- Seven consultant posts founded between 1966 and 1975.
- Worked in prisons and with liaison and assessment, but had no secure hospital beds available.

The Glancy Report (DHSS, 1974)

- Lack of secure beds as proposed by Emery was causing great difficulties:
  - ongoing problems of managing those with mental disorder within the prison system
  - special hospitals overcrowded, although Park Lane Hospital in development at that time.
- Working party commissioned to revisit the issues raised by Emery, and consider existing security provisions and make recommendations for future provision.
- Recommended that regional health authorities provide secure beds on a regional level:
  - 1000 beds for England and Wales proposed.

The Butler Committee on mentally abnormal offenders

By the early 1970s there was serious overcrowding in the special hospitals, an increasing awareness of the difficulties posed in attempting to manage the mentally ill in prison and a general downgrading of the security provided in general psychiatric hospitals.

The Butler Committee was established in 1972 following the conviction of Graham Young, who had poisoned a large number of people (killing three) after discharge from Broadmoor Hospital (see Bowden, 1996, for a full account of the case). The committee was charged with considering the criminal law relating to mentally disordered offenders, and making recommendations about facilities and treatment provided.

An interim report was published (Home Office and DHSS, 1974) given the urgency of the problem of a lack of secure beds:

- Set a framework for the development and expansion of forensic psychiatry:

- increasing numbers of consultant appointments
- all psychiatric trainees to have experience in the specialty.
- Recommended immediate construction of 'regional secure units' (RSUs):
  - to be financed by direct allocation of Government money
  - proposed initially 1000 beds, rising to 2000 over time
  - not to be used for long-stay admissions – suggested indicative admissions of 18 months
  - interim secure units (ISUs) to be opened while RSUs constructed.

The final report (DHSS, 1975) was presented to Parliament in October 1975 and made numerous recommendations:

- Reiterated the need for secure accommodation and noted that little progress had yet been made.

The Butler Report set the agenda for forensic psychiatry to be provided outside of custodial settings and in purpose-built hospitals. Contemporaneously, some (Scott, 1974) argued that it would be better to develop facilities within the prison system, rather than invest in new provision which would inevitably leave prison health care as a poor relation.

The development of regional secure units

Interim secure units were set up within general hospitals while regional health authorities developed plans for constructing RSUs.

The RSU programme was subject to considerable delays (Snowden, 1985):

- Reluctance among health authorities to proceed, despite money being available.
- Concerns about the cost of staffing and running the units long term, after construction costs met.
- Had to combat significant opposition from unions, local residents, lobbyists, MPs, etc.:
  - a review of reports into serious untoward incidents from four RSUs over 4 years found no measurable effect on serious crime rates in the local community (Gradillas *et al.*, 2007).
- Problems with staffing and running costs.
- Forensic psychiatrists were often not involved in construction or service development until late stages.
- Ideas about models of care provision changed with experience, but often too late to change plans that were already in the late stages of development.

The first RSU opened in Middlesbrough in 1980, followed by units in Devon, Trent and Mersey in 1983:

- By 1990, 600 of the 1000 proposed had been opened.

Eventually RSUs became established, and regional forensic psychiatry services built up around them, providing a broad range of services:

- Psychiatric input in prisons.
- Court liaison and diversion schemes.
- Providing management advice to general psychiatry.
- Community follow-up in some cases.

The Reed Review

The broad remit for the Reed Review was to examine the health and social services provided to mentally disordered offenders (MDOs) and those non-offenders with similar needs. This was in the context of changes in the structure of the NHS, along with ongoing concerns about the difficulties in dealing with such offenders.

The review proposed important guiding principles to underpin care of these patients:

- Patients should be cared for as far as possible in the community, rather than institutional settings.
- Conditions of security should be no greater than could be justified by the danger posed to themselves or to others.
- Care should be provided as near as possible to the patient's home or family.

The final report (Department of Health and Home Office, 1992) made nearly 300 recommendations:

- Formal arrangements for cooperation between the various agencies involved (health, social care, criminal justice) should be put in place.
- Specialized teams for dealing with mentally disordered offenders should be established, with a broad multidisciplinary staff.
- The application of the care programme approach (CPA) to mentally disordered offenders, including those released from prison and those returned to prison after hospital treatment.
- Effort should be made to address the over-representation of ethnic minorities among MDOs.
- A new national target of 1500 medium secure beds proposed, with expansion in training and recruitment of forensic psychiatrists and related professions.

Impact of the Reed recommendations

- Raised awareness of the issue and Government-acknowledged need.
- Some court diversion schemes established at a local level.
- Increased funding for medium secure beds:
  - Butler target of 1000 beds was met in 1996
  - approximately 2000 beds by 1999, 500 of which were provided outside the NHS (Coid *et al.*, 2001).

● Principles of Security

The Reed Report described three domains of security:

- Physical security:
  - aspects of environment and building design that support containment and safety
  - includes the secure perimeter, design and management of the entry point, locking of doors, window design, alarm systems, etc.
- Relational security:
  - the quality of the relationship between patient and carers, enabling a detailed and in-depth knowledge of patients, their history, their reason for admission and progress to date
  - allows early detection of alterations in presentation which might herald increased risk
  - security and treatment closely linked.
- Procedural security:
  - 'The methodology or systems by which patients are managed and safe security maintained' (Exworthy and Gunn, 2003)
  - policies and practices governing patient movement and observation, such as maintaining a list of contraband items, restricting access to potential weapons ('sharps'), screening and approving visitors, searching patients before and after leave, routine searches of wards for contraband items
  - also includes higher level clinical and professional governance arrangements, major incident planning, investigation of serious incidents, communication of lessons learned, etc.

The distinction between levels of security is shown in Table 1.1 and discussed further in Kennedy (2002) and Crichton (2009).

Table 1.1 Security characteristics at different levels of security

	Low	Medium	High
Physical	National Standards Guidance gives considerable latitude depending on the population served, but all security measures should be discreet	Traditionally designed to be 'escape-retardant'; current expectations are to deter all but the most determined escapers	Equivalent to a category B prison – designed to be escape-proof
	Standard hospital perimeter, with enclosed garden	5.2 m high perimeter – close-mesh fence or connecting buildings Daily checks of the perimeter	6 m high wall
	Dedicated entry point, not through rest of hospital; airlock is recommended	Entry through an 'air lock', controlled by reception	Entry through dedicated gate lodge, including X-ray machine and metal detector
	Clear lines of sight, and appropriate space/door size for physical interventions	Staff electronic keys may allow monitoring of movement. May have some CCTV	CCTV covering entire site
	Solid-core, outward opening doors, mostly lockable. Window opening restricted to less than 125 mm	Doors secured with standard locks or magnetic locking device	All doors secured with prison specification locks
	Wall-mounted alarms and/or personal alarms for staff	Individual personal alarms provided for all staff	
Procedural	Dedicated security staff unlikely	Some units have a dedicated security team	Dedicated security team supporting clinical teams
	Rub down searching may take place on return from community leave, otherwise not used routinely		Routine use of rub-down searches
	No routine monitoring of telephone calls and no Mental Health Act (MHA) power to interfere with mail		Routine monitoring of patient telephone calls and mail
	Fewer restrictions on items and those with a specific purpose in rehabilitation (e.g. access to computers or mobile phones) may be permitted	Tight restrictions on items allowed in the hospital (potential weapons, communication devices, etc.). There may be some flexibility for staff and in non-clinical areas	Tight restrictions on items allowed within the secure perimeter
	Visiting controlled as in general hospital-locked wards	Visitors subject to approval process, but generally less rigorous than high security. Visits supervised by nursing staff	Visiting restricted with careful vetting beforehand. Visits are closely supervised by security staff
	Depending on the nature of the unit, patients may have considerable access to community	Many patients will have regular leave outside the hospital, either escorted or unescorted	Relatively few patients have leave outside the hospital perimeter except for essential visits (e.g. hospital appointments)
Relational	Lower nursing numbers than medium and high security	Increased nurse : patient ratio	
	Detailed documentation and regular meetings of all clinical team members to discuss cases	Relatively long admissions allow more detailed knowledge of patients over time to be accrued The range of environment within medium security, from acute or intensive care wards to rehab wards with extensive community leave, provides a particularly rich knowledge	Dedicated security team collects security-related data and information Long admissions allow detailed knowledge of a patient to be gathered, albeit only within a highly controlled environment

The differential impact of 'security creep'

The last 10 years has seen an incremental increase in the level of security provided in secure hospitals, together with, for medium secure units, a reduction in the level of political/managerial tolerance for escapes and absconds. In particular:

- The Tilt Report (Tilt *et al.*, 2000) made recommendations to increase the physical and procedural security at the three high secure hospitals.
- The national specification for medium secure services (Department of Health, 2007) has increased the physical security requirements for medium secure services.

This inexorable shift in the direction of increased security should be seen in the context of the changing socio-political climate, with increased risk-aversion, more punitive sentencing, and the political drive to increase rates of MHA detention for those deemed dangerous.

Reports, inquiries and managers tend to give greater emphasis to physical and procedural than to relational security measures. Physical and procedural security measures are:

- conceptually simpler and more tangible
- easier to articulate and therefore recommend
- easier to achieve
- easier to measure, audit and demonstrate.

Increasing physical and procedural security risks less effective relational security, because:

- the range of environments in which the patient is managed is more limited
- there are fewer opportunities for therapeutic risk taking and testing out
- an over-emphasis on demonstrating readily auditable physical and procedural security reduces the attention given to relational security.

Consequently, medium secure care environments have become more restrictive and less like the community. The gap that must be bridged by rehabilitation has become wider.

- Low secure units, originally conceived as providing primarily long-term care, have begun to seek to fill that rehabilitative gap.
- This forensic version of functionalization in itself has important implications for continuity of care and relational security.

● Current Secure Hospital Provision

Recent figures for the size of the forensic population/secure bed provision include:

- Forensic patient population increased from 2650 in 1997 to nearly 4000 in July 2007.
- In 2005, 2886 NHS beds and 1827 independent sector secure beds (Rutherford and Duggan, 2007).
- In 2007, 3022 NHS and 1913 independent sector secure beds (BBC, 2008).
- In 2009 there were a daily average of 3438 secure NHS beds available across all three levels of security (figures available at http://www.dh.gov.uk/en/Publicationsandstatistics/Statistics/Performancedataandstatistics/Beds/DH_083781).

High secure services

The three high secure hospitals are:

- Ashworth Hospital, Maghull, Liverpool; approx 275 beds
- Rampton Hospital, Retford, Nottinghamshire; approx 370 beds:
  - includes the national high secure services for women, learning disability and the deaf.

- Broadmoor Hospital, Crowthorne, Berkshire; 260 beds.

Patients are admitted to high security when they are considered to pose a 'grave and immediate danger' to the public. This decision may be based on:

- having been charged with or convicted of a grave offence, including those with sadistic or sexual motive
- the immediacy of risk to others if they were at large
- evidence of a capacity to coordinate an organized escape attempt, or engage in subversion of staff.

Cases with a high national profile are also likely to be admitted to high security, on the basis that an 'abscond from hospital would seriously undermine confidence in the criminal justice system'.

In previous years the high secure hospitals were subjected to much criticism, the problems perhaps resulting in part from the nature of the patient group and the professional and managerial isolation from other parts of the NHS. In particular, at Ashworth Hospital:

- The Blom-Cooper Report in 1992 (Blom-Cooper *et al.*, 1992) was highly critical of the culture and abusive practices that were uncovered. It found evidence of systematic mistreatment and abuse of patients, and failures of management throughout the organization.
- The Fallon Inquiry report in 1994 (Department of Health, 1994) identified severe shortcomings in the running of the personality disorder service. Patients were discovered to have been dealing in drugs, alcohol and pornography and security had been compromised to a large extent. There was also evidence of widespread corruption. The report again strongly criticized the management of the service and the hospital and recommended its complete closure, although this did not take place.

Since then, the management of each high secure hospital has been brought into that of the local NHS provider; the high secure services are managed as one part of a range of secure services in that region. There has also been significant retraction in services since 2000 (Abbott *et al.*, 2005):

- due to projections of reduced need for high secure care as a result of increased provision in medium security
- high secure beds reduced from 1276 in 2000 to 879 in 2009 (Hansard, 2010)
- movement of patients into regional services for long-term care
- rehabilitation of patients through medium and low secure services where appropriate.

Medium secure services

There are currently in the region of 3500 medium secure beds across NHS and independent sector providers. Medium secure units provide the mainstay of forensic psychiatric inpatient care, and are often the regional centres in which other forensic outreach, prison inreach and liaison services are based.

The original expectation that admissions would be for 18 months to 2 years is no longer valid:

- Long-term medium secure beds have been provided for those patients who require long-term care in such conditions, including some previously housed in high security.
- For others the duration of admission has increased significantly beyond this.

The Department of Health has issued a formal specification for medium secure services (Department of Health, 2007):

- Seven key domains – safety, clinical and cost-effectiveness, governance, patient focus, accessible and responsive care, care environment and amenities, public health.
- For each domain a number of specific quality principles, with specified measures of performance and evidence required.
- Used as a basis for the evaluation of quality of care provided in medium secure services.

The Royal College of Psychiatrists has established a 'Quality Network for Forensic Mental Health Services' which provides a peer review process based on the Department of Health standards (http://www.rcpsych.ac.uk/quality/quality,accreditationaudit/forensicmentalhealth.aspx)

Bed numbers have continued to increase and more specialized services developed:

- Provided by a mixture of NHS and independent sector providers.
- Specialized services for women, forensic CAMHS, older adults, autistic spectrum disorder (ASD), etc.

Low secure services

In contrast to medium secure units, low secure provision has developed organically, without any clear statement of need or policy, mostly over the last 10–15 years.

- There are no reliable data on numbers, and the services provided in low security are diverse.

National minimum standards for psychiatric intensive care units (PICUs) and low security developed by the Department of Health (2002):

- Defined as services delivering 'intensive, comprehensive and multidisciplinary treatment and care by qualified staff for patients who demonstrate disturbed behaviour in the context of a serious mental disorder and who require the provision of security'.
- Set standards for all aspects of the units including physical design and layout, service structure, involvement of patients and carers, policies and procedures, clinical audit, etc.
- Envisioned to provide longer-term care (around 2 years) as compared with 8 weeks for PICUs.

Low secure services have evolved into a combination of active rehabilitation and long-term facilities, providing

- a step-down from medium security into the community, allowing for extended community rehabilitation
- long-term care for those in medium security who are unlikely to be successfully discharged into the community due to the nature of their illness and ongoing risks
- a sideways move from PICUs for those who require longer-term care in such conditions.

Recent papers have suggested that a large expansion in low secure bed numbers is needed to match the expansion in medium security and provide suitable pathways into the community (Beer, 2008; O'Grady, 2008; Turner and Salter, 2008).

● Forensic Community Services

The Reed Report recommended the development of forensic community services but generally this lagged behind the RSU programme.

In contrast to general, psychiatric, functionalized community teams there are no agreed standards for forensic community teams, and there is considerable variation in service model between forensic services:

- No community service, all inpatients passing from secure care to general psychiatric teams for community follow-up, either with or without an intervening period of general psychiatric inpatient care.
- Parallel model, in which a distinct forensic community team carries care programme approach (CPA) responsibility for a defined case load of patients. This provides the clearest demarcation of roles and responsibilities.
- Integrated model, in which the forensic community team works within general psychiatric community teams, supporting them in managing their 'forensic' patients:
  - may reduce stigma associated with being a forensic patient
  - encourages development of skills in general psychiatric teams (Whittle and Scally, 1998).
- Consultation and liaison models. Most forensic services provide this service to general psychiatric colleagues either on a traditional medical referral basis, or in the form of a distinct and specifically commissioned forensic liaison service:
  - the development of such services was given renewed impetus by the Bradley Report (Department of Health, 2009).

● Commissioning Arrangements and the Independent Sector

Commissioning is the process by which most services in the NHS are developed and funded:

- Defined by the Audit Commission as 'the process of securing and monitoring services to meet individuals' needs at a strategic level'.
- 'Purchasers' are given control of money.
- Services for patients are purchased from 'providers' (usually NHS organizations, but also includes independent sector).

Up until 2011, the purchasers for most services were primary care trusts (PCTs). However, most secure services were classed as specialist services:

- Regional Specialized Commissioning Teams, based within strategic health authorities (SHAs), negotiated with all the purchasers within the region to commission a regional service.
- This means that the provider does not have to negotiate with a series of different purchasers at once.
- In most cases the 'preferred provider' is the NHS service, but where necessary due to capacity issues or a particular clinical need, the commissioning teams also negotiate and agree contracts with independent sector providers.
- The commissioning team has a responsibility to ensure that the services provided to the patients of that region is of high quality.

Some particularly specialist services, were commissioned nationally due to the relatively small demand and high complexity:

- The National Commissioning Group (NCG) was responsible for this (http://www.ncg.nhs.uk).
- Mostly complex medical and surgical problems (pancreas transplants, amyloidosis, etc.).
- Secure forensic mental health services for young people (otherwise known as forensic CAMHS) were commissioned on this basis by the NCG.

Reorganizations are frequent, mostly varying the nature of the purchasers:

- The 2011 reforms (Department of Health, 2010) proposed abolition of PCTs, which had previously commissioned most services, and SHAs which had commissioned specialist services such as secure psychiatric care:

– establishment of GP consortia to take over as the main commissioners
– secure psychiatric care would continue to be commissioned regionally, through the central NHS Commissioning Board.

The relationship between the NHS and independent sector

According to Murphy and Sugarman (2010) the independent sector now provides more than half of the medium secure beds nationally:

- Mostly generic secure mental illness services, but also include services for personality disorder and some other specialist needs.

The regional NHS service usually provides a 'gate-keeping' service to the commissioning team, carrying out clinical assessments of the needs of patients referred for secure care. Where the NHS service either lacks capacity, or cannot address some particular need, an alternative independent provider is sought. Historically, independent sector placements tended to be more expensive than the NHS, but this difference has declined in recent years.

NHS services continue, generally, to provide a more comprehensive service than independent providers, who tend to concentrate just on inpatient care. For some, the establishment of the independent sector as providing a major contribution to forensic psychiatric services in the UK is a matter of political or economic concern. See Murphy and Sugarman (2010) and Pollock (2010).

References

Abbott P, Davenport S, Davies S, Nimmagadda SR, O'Halloran A, Tattan T. (2005) Potential effects of retractions of the high-security hospitals. *Psychiatric Bulletin* **29**, 403–6

BBC. (2008) Today Program, 'Mental Health Care Escapes "horrifying"', 9 September 2008

Beer D. (2008) Psychiatric intensive care and low secure units: where are we now? *Psychiatric Bulletin* **32**(12), 441–3

Blom-Cooper L, Brown M, Dolan R, Murphy E. (1992) *Report of the Committee of Inquiry into complaints about Ashworth Hospital. Cmnd 202*. London: HMSO

Bowden P. (1996) Graham Young (1947–90); the St Albans poisoner: his life and times. *Criminal Behaviour and Mental Health* **6**, 17–24

Coid J, Nadji K, Gault S, Cook A, Jarman B. (2001) Medium secure forensic psychiatry services. Comparison of seven English health regions. *British Journal of Psychiatry* **178**, 55–61

*Crichton JHM. (2009) Defining high, medium, and low security in forensic mental healthcare: the development of the Matrix of Security in Scotland. *Journal of Forensic Psychiatry and Psychology* **20**(3), 333–53

Department of Health. (1994) *Report of the Committee of Inquiry into the Personality Disorder Unit, Ashworth Special Hospital (The Fallon Inquiry)*. London: The Stationery Office

Department of Health. (2002) *Mental Health Policy Implementation Guide. National Minimum Standards for General Adult Services in Psychiatric Intensive Care Units (PICU) and Low Secure Environments*. London: Department of Health

*Department of Health. (2007) *Best Practice Guidance: Specification for adult medium-secure services*. London: Department of Health

Department of Health. (2009) *The Bradley Report: Lord Bradley's review of people with mental health problems or learning disabilities in the Criminal Justice System*. London: Department of Health

Department of Health. (2010) *Equity and Excellence: Liberating the NHS.* London: The Stationery Office

*Department of Health and the Home Office. (1992) *Review of Health and Social Services for Mentally Disordered Offenders and Others Requiring Similar Services (The Reed Report). Cm 2088.* London: HMSO

Department of Health and Social Security. (1974) *Revised Report of the Working Party of Security in NHS Psychiatric Hospitals (Glancy Report).* London: HMSO

Department of Health and Social Security. (1975) *Report of the Committee of Mentally Abnormal Offenders (Butler Report).* London: HMSO

Exworthy T, Gunn J. (2003) Taking another tilt at high security hospitals. *British Journal of Psychiatry* **182**, 469–71

Gradillas V, Williams A, Walsh E, Fahy T. (2007) Do forensic inpatient units pose a risk to local communities? *Journal of Forensic Psychiatry and Psychology* **18**(2), 261–5

Hansard. (2010) HC vol 505 col 1046W, 10 February 2010

Home Office and DHSS. (1974) *Interim Report of the Committee on Mentally Abnormal Offenders (Butler Report).* London: HMSO

Kennedy HG. (2002) Therapeutic uses of security: mapping forensic mental health services by stratifying risk. *Advances in Psychiatric Treatment* **8**, 433–43

Ministry of Health. (1961) *Special Hospitals: Report of a Working Party (Emery Report).* London: Ministry of Health.

Ministry of Health. (1964) *Report of the Working Party on the Organisation of the Prison Medical Service (Gwynne Report).* London: Ministry of Health.

Murphy E, Sugarman P. (2010) Should mental health services fear the independent sector: no. *British Medical Journal* **341**, 5385

O'Grady J. (2008) Time to talk. Commentary on … forensic psychiatry and general psychiatry. *Psychiatric Bulletin* **32**(1), 6–7

Pollock A. (2010) Should mental health services fear the independent sector: yes. *British Medical Journal* **341**, c5382

Rutherford M, Duggan S. (2007) *'Forensic Factfile 2007': Forensic Mental Health Services: Facts and figures on current provision.* Sainsbury Centre for Mental Health. Available at: http://www.centreformentalhealth.org.uk/publications/forensic.aspx?ID=526

Scott P. (1974) Solutions to the problem of the dangerous offender. *British Medical Journal* **4**(5495), 640–1

Snowden P. (1985) A survey of the Regional Secure Unit Programme. *British Journal of Psychiatry* **147**, 499–507

Tilt R, Perry B, Martin C. (2000) *Report of the Review of Security at the High Security Hospitals.* London: Department of Health.

Turner T, Salter M. (2008) Forensic psychiatry and general psychiatry: re-examining the relationship. *Psychiatric Bulletin* **32**(1), 2–6.

Whittle M, Scally M. (1998) Model of forensic community care. *Psychiatric Bulletin* **22**, 748–50

2

Entry into Secure Care

Mental health problems are common, and offending is common:

- In 2006, 15 % of people (24 % of males, 6 % of females) between 10 and 52 years had at least one conviction.
- Of males born in 1973, 29 % had been convicted before the age of 30 (Ministry of Justice, 2010a).

Overlap is inevitable.

There is no agreed definition of a 'forensic patient', the specialty having developed pragmatically, driven by clinicians and public policy, rather than from a cohesive body of research, a treatment approach or a defining pathology. Movement between forensic and general psychiatric services is fluid, and often dependent on local provision and organization:

- Assertive outreach team (AOT) patients have many criminogenic needs in terms of socio-economic disadvantage, substance misuse and a history of offending (Priebe *et al.*, 2003).
- In a small European study Hodgins *et al.* (2006) found no difference between discharged forensic and general psychiatric patients on HCR-20 or PCL-R scores. A history of serious physical violence towards others, including violent crimes and physical violence which had not resulted in legal sanction, seemed to distinguish the forensic group.

● Sources of Referrals

Referrals to forensic services may be:

- for diversion from the criminal justice system (CJS) (prisons, courts, police stations)
- to consider movement between levels of security:
  - up, usually from general psychiatric wards
  - down, from high security or medium security, or
  - sideways between services to address some specific need
- for 'gate-keeping' assessments for specialist services within or outside of the NHS
- for a second opinion on diagnosis/risk/management.

Admission rates to high and medium secure hospitals demonstrate a linear correlation with levels of socio-economic deprivation in patients' catchment areas of origin (Coid, 1998):

- So demands on urban forensic services will be higher.

Most patients entering secure care are diverted from a custodial setting:

- Coid and Kahtan (2001) described a sample of 2608 admissions to 7 regional secure units (RSUs) between 1988 and 1994. The pre-admission locations were:

- 39–65 % from prison
- 11–26 % from psychiatric hospitals
- 3–40 % from community, including police stations
- 6–19 % from high secure hospitals.

- It is likely that there has been some change in these patterns in the intervening years. Anecdotally, the proportion of patients admitted to medium security from prison is higher now than it was then.
- Jamieson *et al.* (2000) looked at high secure admissions between 1986 and 1995. Women were more likely than men to be admitted from other hospitals than as prison transfers:

Source of referral	Male (%)	Female (%)
Prison	41	21
Courts	35	37
Hospital	21	40

Table 2.1 Some factors relevant to deciding the appropriate level of security (adapted from Department of Health, 2007; Kennedy, 2002)

High secure	Medium secure	Low secure/psychiatric intensive care unit (PICU)
Grave offence, especially sadistic or sexual	Serious offence or past failed placements at lower level	History of non-violent offending behaviour
Immediate danger to others if in community	Danger to others would be less immediate	
Risk is predominantly to others		Mix of risk to others/challenging behaviour/deliberate self-harm
Significant capacity to coordinate outside help for an escape attempt or absconding would undermine confidence in the criminal justice system	Significant risk of escape or absconding, or Pre-sentence for serious charge	Low risk of absconding
Unpredictable relationship between risk and mental state	Recovery likely to be prolonged, some risks remain even when well	Acute illness, likely to respond promptly to treatment
Previously unmanageable in medium security	Previously unmanageable in low security/PICU	Previously unmanageable on open ward

● Diversion from CJS

The policy objective of diversion from custody encourages the removal of people with mental disorders from the CJS to a suitable hospital or community placement where they can receive treatment:

- This reflects a social consensus that sick people should be treated rather than punished (James *et al.*, 2002).

Contemporary diversion policy began with Home Office Circular 66/90:

- Set out the Government's policy to divert mentally disordered persons from the CJS in cases where the public interest did not require a prosecution.
- Non-penal disposals were encouraged where a prosecution was necessary.

Subsequently:

- The Reed Report (Department of Health and Home Office, 1992):
  - recommended nationwide provision of court diversion schemes
  - recommended alternative community provisions for mentally disordered offenders
  - led to an increase in the number of prisoner transfers to hospital.

Box 2.1 Assessment of referrals for admission from a setting of lower security or CJS

Before the assessment it is important to ensure that the funding stream is established and allocation of the case is correct. Establishing the relevant commissioner is explained for prison transfers in Department of Health (2007), and is based on, in order:

- the patient's GP or their address if unregistered
- the area in which their offence occurred if they had no address/GP
- the area in which the prison is located if usually resident outside the UK.

Ensure that you know what the referrer wants:

- It is common for a referral letter to seek a general 'forensic opinion', without explicating what the referring team is really hoping for. This is especially likely to be true where a trainee has written the letter.
- Speak to the referring consultant, so that you know what the real issues are and understand the urgency of the referral.

Consider:

- Whether there is additional information that needs to be supplied in advance of the assessment.
- Who should carry out the assessment and whether more than one discipline is required.
- The need for a collateral history and facilitate this if possible – for example, by asking the patient to bring a carer to an outpatient appointment, or ensuring that their keyworker will be present when you assess an inpatient.

Before seeing the patient:

- Review the case notes, noting in particular incidents and precipitants of violence/aggression, apparent changes in mental state, periods of leave, use of drugs/alcohol, medication changes, level of engagement in treatment, subversive behaviours.
- Discuss these areas of inquiry with nursing staff, and understand any dynamic issues with particular staff, with other individual patients, or relating to the current mix of patients on the ward as a whole.
- Consider safety issues relating to interviewing this patient, and the interview room itself. Make any adjustments that you consider necessary.

The interview needs to be flexible and adaptable according to the presentation/mental state of the patient and the desired outcome:

- For assessments already in secure services, make use of existing detailed reports for background history and concentrate on current clinical and dynamic factors important to your decision-making.
- Particularly concentrate on the level of insight and understanding of mental illness and offending, the level of engagement in treatment and likely motivations, their aims for the future and their conceptualization of a pathway to achieve these.
- Assessments of patients in the CJS are more likely to require a full background history from the patient and other informants.

Always remember to make an entry in the case notes to record your assessment and ensure that any immediate concerns , either related to mental state or risk, are effectively communicated to those with ongoing responsibility for the patient's care.

After the assessment take your time to assimilate all the information and discuss within the multidisciplinary team. You need to consider:

- The patient's diagnosis, the likely effectiveness of treatment in the current setting and the impact that this will have on risk behaviours.
- Risks of violence to others (see Chapter 6) but also to self, of absconding/escaping and perhaps other idiosyncratic risks.
- What enhanced measures might be employed in the current setting to manage these risks.
- Whether they are manageable within the current setting until treatment is likely to have been effective.
- The likely effectiveness of treatment within the proposed setting.
- Any idiosyncratic treatment needs that would require specific planning or referral to a specialist service.

Deciding on whether a patient (1) should be admitted and (2) if no to what level of security are complex clinical judgements with no simple determining factors:

- therefore your opinion should be circumspect, open-minded and, where appropriate, should specify the circumstances in which you would want to review the case.

Assessing a referral for transfer from higher security

This follows the same principles as described above and many of the same issues are relevant. In relation to incidents of violence, other risk behaviours and subversion, you need to make a judgement about whether an apparent decline or cessation is due to positive clinical change or simply due to the highly restricted environment:

- A period of testing at lower security may still be appropriate if it seems to be the latter, but you are likely to proceed more cautiously.

You need particularly to consider the likely cost of escape or absconding, which will become considerably more possible with a move down to medium or low security:

- You must understand how much leave they have had and how restrictive this has been.

There should be adequate background history already available. Use your assessment to:

- clarify any gaps or queries in their background, or changes in how they see their history consequent to therapy in hospital
- understand exactly what therapy they have engaged in, and what impact this has had
- understand their current clinical state, particularly their level of engagement and degree of insight into their disorder and offending
- formulate any change in risk behaviours that is evident
- think about and specify outstanding rehabilitative needs.

- The All-Party Parliamentary Group on Prison Health (2006) concluded that 'a fundamental shift in thinking' was required to decriminalize the mentally ill, transferring their care from the CJS to health.
- The Bradley Report (Department of Health, 2009) recommended nationwide provision of court diversion schemes and the establishment of Criminal Justice Mental Health Teams (CJMHTs) to:
  - ensure continuity of care for individuals in contact with CJS
  - identify and divert mentally disordered offenders (MDOs) as early as possible.
- The policy drive of the 2010 Coalition Government to reduce overcrowding in prisons was often justified by the need to divert the mentally disordered out of the CJS.

The evidence is that the 'organizational embedding' of diversion and liaison schemes is often poor, leading to doubts about the sustainability of individual schemes (Pakes and Winstone, 2010).

There has sometimes been a tendency to dichotomize the ill and the criminals, such that psychiatric treatment and prosecution are seen as mutually exclusive. This is discussed further in relation to prosecuting inpatient violence in Chapter 16.

- Always remember that diversion does not require the discontinuation of criminal proceedings.
- Very often both treatment and prosecution should proceed in parallel.

Diversion in practice

An MDO may be diverted from:

- the police station (at the point of arrest)
- the magistrates' court
- prison.

Diversion from the police station is discussed in Chapter 16. Most such cases will not require secure care and will be admitted to PICUs or open wards.

Court diversion schemes

Magistrates' courts are a good point for diversion because they are a filter through which all charged cases must pass at an early stage (James, 1999):

- On the recommendation of the Reed Report a number of schemes were set up locally, but without any central commissioning or framework.
- So nationwide coverage has not been achieved and services have developed in a piecemeal and haphazard way (Sainsbury Centre for Mental Health, 2009).
- The Bradley Report (Department of Health, 2009) provided a further impetus, again without provision of funds.

Potential effects of a court diversion scheme include:

- reduced reoffending and improved mental health outcomes:
  - savings of >£20 000 per case in reduced CJS costs and reduction in reoffending (Sainsbury Centre for Mental Health, 2009)
- reduced delay in receiving treatment:
  - identification at court reduced the mean time between arrest and admission from 50 days to 8 days (James and Hamilton, 1992)
- increased admissions to hospital from court (four-fold for James and Hamilton, 1992), leading to an increased demand for beds.

According to Joseph (1994), psychiatric assessment at court has other advantages:

- More information is available to the psychiatrist.
- There is greater liaison with other professionals (e.g. solicitors and probation officers).
- There is the opportunity to discuss the possibility of discontinuance with the CPS where a seriously mentally ill individual has been charged with a relatively minor offence.

Most patients diverted from court do not require a secure service. Kingham and Corfe (2005) reported that the need for a secure bed led to an 8- to 12-week delay in hospitalization.

An early court diversion scheme in central London was described by Joseph and Potter (1990, 1993). They reported that, of 201 psychiatric examinations:

- 75% had previously been detained in hospital
- 77% had a previous criminal record, more than half of whom had previously been imprisoned
- Schizophrenia was the most common diagnosis (39%)
- 34% were considered unfit to plead
- 65 patients were admitted to hospital, 1 to an RSU and the rest to unlocked wards, from where 46% absconded.

They concluded that:

- admissions should generally be to locked wards
- psychotic patients benefitted most from diversion.

Although they are often conflated, diversion should be distinguished from liaison:

- Diversion schemes require the active participation of at least one psychiatrist (and an approval mental health professional [AMHP] for civil detention)
- Liaison schemes are often nurse-led and aim to:
  - identify offenders who require diversion, and
  - liaise with secondary mental health providers who will undertake diversion.

Prison transfers

The provision of mental health care in prisons is discussed in Chapter 19. Despite the great improvements in prison health care over the last 10 years, prisoners with severe mental illness generally require to be transferred out to a hospital setting.

- According to the Sainsbury Centre for Mental Health (2009) 97% of restricted transferred prisoners are admitted to medium or high security.
- The increased frequency of transfers reported by Hotopf *et al.* (2000) may have been due to:
  - increasing size of the prison population
  - more psychiatrists visiting prisons
  - limited availability making it is easier to coordinate admissions to secure beds from prison than court (Birmingham, 2001).

As a result of these pressures, waiting times for admission have increased:

- 42 prisoners per quarter waited more than 3 months for transfer from prison to hospital in England in 2006 (Sainsbury Centre for Mental Health, 2009).
- A pilot study investigating the feasibility of a 14-day transfer standard (Royal College of Psychiatrists, 2010) found:
  - the mean waiting time for transfer was 29 days; the median was 18 days.
- An observational study at HMP Brixton (Forrester *et al.*, 2009) found:
  - mean wait of 102 days
  - 20% were referred, assessed and transferred within a month.

The Bradley Report (Department of Health, 2009) recommended a minimum target of 14 days for the transfer of prisoners with severe mental illness.

Transfers late in sentence

It is common for professionals in prison to become concerned about a prisoner's mental health or risk close to the point at which they are to be released:

- The prospect of release sensitizes professionals to risk.
- Pre-release assessments may uncover a previously undetected problem.
- The prospect of release may be a stressor for some, leading to deterioration in mental health.

Clinically, detention close to expected release is undesirable, because it is likely negatively to affect initial engagement with treatment.

Transfers to hospital should not be sought in order to prolong an individual's time in detention on risk grounds:

- In *R (on the application of TF) v Secretary of State for Justice* [2008] EWCA Civ 1457, the Court of Appeal held, in relation to a young offender with personality disorder, that:

  if the decision is being taken ... right at the end of sentence ... a decision to direct transfer cannot simply be taken on the grounds that a convicted person will be a danger to the public if released ... but can only be taken on the grounds that his medical condition & its treatability ... justify the decision.

- In response to this judgment, the Mental Health Unit will turn down requests for transfers late in sentence unless there is good evidence that hospital treatment will be of benefit to the prisoner and there are good reasons why transfer could not have been achieved earlier in sentence (e.g. recent deterioration in a patient's condition or recent onset of serious mental illness).

- Such cases may be dealt with by detention under s2 or s3:
  - the papers may be completed in advance of release from prison
  - the prison authority is able to transfer to hospital.

● Admissions Under Part 3 of the Mental Health Act 1983

Amendments introduced by the Mental Health Act 2007

Part 3 of the Act was not significantly amended itself, but some changes impact upon the detention of those concerned in criminal proceedings or under sentence. In particular:

- A single definition of mental disorder replaces the previous four categories, and removes the exclusion of sexual deviance.
- Mental disorder means 'any disorder or disability of mind', but:
  - dependence on alcohol or drugs is not considered a mental disorder
  - a learning-disabled person is not mentally disordered unless their disability is associated with 'abnormally aggressive or seriously irresponsible conduct'.
- Abolition of the 'treatability' test:
  - The introduction of the 'appropriate medical treatment' test, together with the broad definition of medical treatment in ss3(4) and 145(4), which preserves existing case law, means that this change is of limited impact.
- The responsible medical officer (RMO) is replaced by the responsible clinician (RC), who need no longer be a registered medical practitioner (RMP).

Admissions by court order prior to sentencing

Section 35 – Remand to hospital for report

A defendant convicted of or awaiting trial for an offence punishable with imprisonment (unless convicted of murder).

Magistrates' or Crown court:

- is satisfied on the written or oral evidence of one s12(2) approved RMP that there is 'reason to suspect that the accused person is suffering from mental disorder'
- 'It would be impracticable for a report … to be made … on bail'
- is satisfied on the evidence of the RC or representative of the managers of the hospital that the patient will be admitted within 7 days

Duration of 28 days, renewable on the evidence of the RC, up to maximum of 12 weeks. Not subject to consent to treatment, so there is no power to treat compulsorily.

Section 36 – Remand to hospital for treatment

A defendant in custody awaiting trial or sentencing for an offence punishable with imprisonment (other than murder).

A Crown court is satisfied:

- on the written or oral evidence of two RMPs, one s12(2) approved:
  - that 'he is suffering from mental disorder of a nature or degree which makes it appropriate for him to be detained in a hospital for medical treatment', and
  - appropriate medical treatment is available
- on the evidence of the RC or representative of the managers of the hospital that they will be admitted within 7 days.

Duration of 28 days, renewable on the evidence of the RC, up to maximum of 12 weeks. Subject to consent to treatment provisions of the Act.

Section 38 – interim hospital order

A defendant who has been convicted of an offence punishable with imprisonment (other than murder).

A Crown court is satisfied:

- on the written or oral evidence of two RMPs, one s12(2) approved, one of whom is employed in the admitting hospital:
  - 'that the offender is suffering from mental disorder', and
  - there is reason to suppose that it 'is such that it may be appropriate for a hospital order to be made'
- on the evidence of the RC or representative of the managers of the hospital that they will be admitted within 28 days.

Maximum initial duration of 12 weeks, renewable for 28-day periods, on the evidence of the RC, to maximum of 1 year. Subject to consent to treatment.

> For ss35, 36 and 38:
>
> - patients are not required to attend court for renewal hearings, so long as they are legally represented
> - the court may direct that the person be taken to a place of safety, pending admission within the statutory period.

Section 44 – Committal to hospital under section 43 hospital order

Where a magistrates' court refers a case to the Crown court for the purpose of making a restriction order, and is satisfied that the criteria for a hospital order are in place, the court may direct the offender to be admitted until the Crown court deals with the case.

The patient is treated as though detained under s37/41.

MHA sentences available to criminal courts

Section 37 – Hospital order

A defendant convicted of an offence punishable with imprisonment, other than murder:

- Note s37(3), which provides that a magistrates' court may make such an order without convicting him, if it is satisfied that he 'did the act or made the omission charged'.

A magistrates' or Crown court:

- is satisfied on the written or oral evidence of two RMPs, one s12(2) approved:
  - 'that the offender is suffering from mental disorder'
  - 'of a nature or degree which makes it appropriate for him to be detained in a hospital for medical treatment, and
  - appropriate medical treatment is available for him'
- 'is of the opinion, having regard to all the circumstances including the nature of the offence and the character and antecedents of the offender … that the most suitable method of disposing of the case' is a hospital order
- is satisfied on the evidence of the RC or representative of the managers of the hospital that he will be admitted within 28 days.

A restriction order under s41 may or may not be added. Once it has been made, an unrestricted hospital order operates much as a section 3, except that there is no right of appeal to the first tier tribunal in the first 6 months and the nearest relative has no power to discharge.

- It may be renewed for 6 months in the first instance, and then annually.

Section 45A – Hospital direction and limitation direction

A defendant convicted of an offence punishable with imprisonment, other than murder.

Where a Crown court 'considers making a hospital order ... before deciding to impose a sentence of imprisonment', and:

- is satisfied on the written or oral evidence of two RMPs, one s12(2) approved, and one of whom gives oral evidence:
  - 'that the offender is suffering from mental disorder'
  - 'of a nature or degree which makes it appropriate for him to be detained in hospital for medical treatment' and
  - appropriate treatment is available for him
- is satisfied on the evidence of the RC or representative of the managers of the hospital that they will be admitted within 28 days.

A hospital direction cannot be given without a limitation direction, which has much the same effect as a restriction order under s41.

For both s37 and s45A, if it appears not practicable for them to be admitted to the specified hospital, the Secretary of State may vary the hospital to which they will be admitted.

Transfers from custody by warrant

Sentenced prisoners, or remand prisoners who require hospital treatment urgently, may be transferred by warrant of the Secretary of State for Justice.

Section 47 – Removal to hospital of a sentenced prisoner

If the Secretary of State:

- is satisfied by reports from two RMPs, one s12(2) approved:
  - that the offender is suffering from mental disorder
  - 'of a nature or degree which makes it appropriate for him to be detained in hospital for medical treatment', and
  - appropriate treatment is available for him
- they may issue a transfer direction, which expires after 14 days.

If a restriction direction is made, it ends automatically on the day that the patient would have been entitled to be released from custody:

- If the patient remains detained under a 'notional s37', which operates in the same way as an s3, the patient may still be liable to detention in hospital under s47 of the MHA. This is equivalent to being detained under s37 of the Act and is known as a 'notional s37 hospital order'.

Section 48 – Removal to hospital of an unsentenced prisoner

Applicable to prisoners on remand from magistrates' or Crown courts, immigration detainees, and civil prisoners.

If the Secretary of State:

- is satisfied by reports from two RMPs, one s12(2) approved:
  - that the offender is suffering from mental disorder
  - 'of a nature or degree which makes it appropriate for him to be detained in hospital for medical treatment'
  - he is in urgent need of such treatment
  - appropriate treatment is available for him
- they may issue a transfer direction, which expires after 14 days.

A restriction direction (s49) must be made in the case of a remand prisoner, and may be made for civil or immigration detainees.

The transfer direction ends automatically when the case is disposed of by the court

- If there is concern that an s48 patient may be released by the court, they may be made subject to an s3 concurrently and prophylactically.

For both ss47 and 48:

- warrants under ss47 and 48 each expire after 14 days – admission must be completed within that time or a fresh warrant will be required
- if a restriction direction is made, the transfer direction can specify that the patient be admitted to a particular unit of a hospital
- the Ministry of Justice requires that:
  - the warrant is issued within 2 months of the date of the medical reports, and
  - the reports are dated within 2 weeks of the examination of the patient.

Restriction orders and restriction directions

Section 41 – Restriction order

A Crown court may add a restriction order to a hospital order:

- where 'It appears to the court … that it is necessary for the "protection of the public from serious harm"'
- after hearing oral evidence from one of the RMPs who recommended the hospital order.

A magistrates' court may not make a restriction order, but it may commit a case to Crown court where it is of the opinion that a restriction order should be made (s43 of the MHA 1983). The criteria for making a restriction order are considered in Chapter 20, in the context of providing oral evidence.

The effect of the restriction order is that:

- the Part 2 rules relating to duration, renewal and expiration of the authority to detain do not apply
- provisions relating to SCT do not apply
- there are no nearest relatives powers
- leave of absence, transfer or discharge may only be granted by the RC or the hospital managers with the consent of the Secretary of State
- the RC must provide at least annual reports to the Secretary of State.

Section 49 – Restriction direction

This has the same effect as s41, and is attached to an s47 or s48.

Limitation direction

A limitation direction (under s45A) is different from a restriction order in three respects:

- It ends when the patient would have been entitled to be released from prison (the hospital direction may continue).
- While a limitation direction is in force, the offender may be removed to prison (criteria as for remission of s47/48 – see Chapter 5).
- While a limitation direction is in force, discharge by the tribunal requires the consent of the Secretary of State.

● Mental Health Act Statistics

The NHS Information Centre (2009) reported on rates of admissions to NHS and independent sector beds in England for 2008–9. There were 28673 admissions under the MHA, 2138 of which were under Part 3:

Section	s35	s36	s37	s37/41	s45A	s47	s47/49	s48	s48/49
Number	119	19	392	565	3	74	433	4	341

Use of part 3 of the MHA has been increasing in recent years, as shown in Figures 2.1 and 2.2.

The rate of increase in the prevalence of detained restricted patients has been greater than in new admissions, implying that restricted patients are staying in hospital for longer.

In the calendar year 2008:

- there were 1501 new restricted admissions to hospital, of which 110 (7%) were to high secure hospital
- these included 442 under s47, 484 under s48, 343 under s37/41, 2 under s45A, and 190 recalled patients.

On 31 December 2008 there were a total of 3937 restricted patients in hospital:

- 88% were male
- including 703 under s47, 234 under s48, 2678 under s37/41, and 13 under s45A
- 3% were under 21, 49% were 21–39, 40% were 40–59, 8% were 60 years and above.

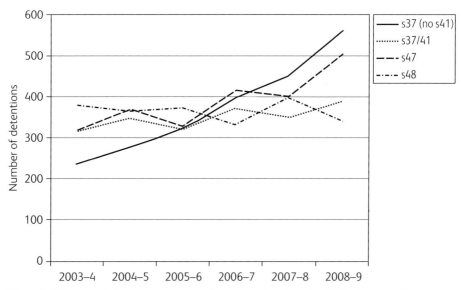

Figure 2.1 Numbers of detentions under part 3 per year (data from the NHS Information Centre, 2009)

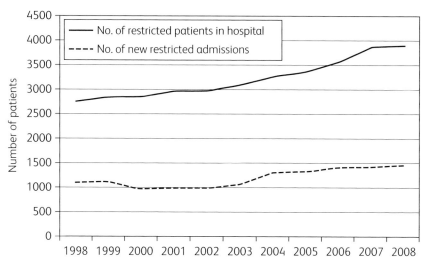

Figure 2.2 Restricted patients detained in hospital (Ministry of Justice, 2010b)

References

All-Party Parliamentary Group on Prison Health. (2006) *The Mental Health Problem in UK HM Prisons*. London: House of Commons. Available at: http://nacro.org.uk/data/files/nacro-2006110801-352.pdf

Birmingham L. (2001) Diversion from custody. *Advances in Psychiatric Treatment* **7**,198–207

Coid JW. (1998) Socio-economic deprivation and admission rates to secure forensic services *Psychiatric Bulletin* **22**, 294–7

Coid J, Kahtan N. (2001) Medium secure forensic psychiatry services; comparison of seven English health regions. *British Journal of Psychiatry* **178**, 55–61

*Department of Health. (2007) *Procedure for Transferring Prisoners to and from Hospital under Sections 47 & 48 of the Mental Health Act (1983)*. Available at: http://www.dh.gov.uk/prod_consum_dh/groups/dh_digitalassets/documents/digitalasset/dh_081262.pdf

Department of Health. (2009) *The Bradley Report: Lord Bradley's review of people with mental health problems or learning disabilities in the Criminal Justice System*. London: Department of Health

Department of Health and the Home Office. (1992) *Review of Health and Social Services for Mentally Disordered Offenders and Others Requiring Similar Services (Reed Report)*. London: HMSO

Forrester A, Henderson C, Wilson S, Cumming I, Spyrou M, Parrott J. (2009) A suitable waiting room? Hospital transfer outcomes & delays from two London prisons. *Psychiatric Bulletin* B, 409–12

Hodgins S, Muller-Isberner R, Allaire J-F. (2006) Attempting to understand the increase in numbers of forensic beds in Europe: a multi-site study of patients in forensic and general psychiatric services. *International Journal of Forensic Mental Health* **5**(2), 173–84

Hotopf M, Wall S, Buchanan A, Wessely S, Churchill R. (2000) Changing patterns in the use of the Mental Health Act 1983 in England, 1984–1996. *British Journal of Psychiatry* **176**, 479–84

James D. (1999) Court diversion at 10 years: can it work, does it work and has it a future? *Journal of Forensic Psychiatry* **10**, 507–24

James DV, Hamilton LW. (1992) Setting up psychiatric liaison schemes to magistrates' courts: problems and practicalities. *Medicine Science & the Law* **32**,167–76

James D, Farnham F, Moorey H, Lloyd H, Hill K, Blizard R, Barnes TRE. (2002) *Outcomes of Psychiatric Admissions through the Courts*. Home Office RDS Occasional paper 79. London: Home Office

Jamieson E, Butwell M, Taylor P, Leese M. (2000) Trends in special (high secure) hospitals: referrals and admissions. *British Journal of Psychiatry*, **176**, 253–9

Joseph P. (1994) Psychiatric assessment at the magistrates' court: early intervention is needed in the remand process. *British Journal of Psychiatry* **164**, 722–4

Joseph P, Potter M. (1990) Mentally disordered homeless offenders – diversion from custody. *Health Trends* **22**, 51–3

Joseph P, Potter M. (1993) Diversion from custody II: effect on hospital and prison resources. *British Journal of Psychiatry* **162**, 330–4

Kennedy HG. (2002) Therapeutic uses of security: mapping forensic mental health services by stratifying risk. *Advances in Psychiatric Treatment* **8**, 433–43

Kingham M, Corfe M. (2005) Experiences of a mixed court diversion and liaison scheme. *Psychiatric Bulletin* **29**, 137–40

Ministry of Justice. (2010a) *Conviction Histories of Offenders between the Ages of 10 and 52*. Available at: http://www.justice.gov.uk/criminal-histories-bulletin.pdf

Ministry of Justice. (2010b) *Statistics of Mentally Disordered Offenders 2008 England and Wales*. Available at: http://www.justice.gov.uk/publications/mentally-disordered-offenders.htm

NHS Information Centre. (2009) *In-patients Formally Detained in Hospitals under the Mental Health Act 1983 and Patients Subject to Supervised Community Treatment: 1998–99 to 2008–09*. Available at: http://www.ic.nhs.uk

Pakes F, Winstone J. (2010) A site visit of 101 mental health liaison and diversion schemes in England. *Journal of Forensic Psychiatry and Psychology* **21**(6), 873–86

Priebe S, Fakhoury W, Watts J, Bebbington P, Burns T, Johnson S, *et al.* (2003) Assertive outreach teams in London: patient characteristics and outcomes. *British Journal of Psychiatry* **183**, 148–54

Royal College of Psychiatrists. (2010) *Briefing Note: Consultation on Clinicians' Experiences of Prison Transfers*. London: RCPsych.

Sainsbury Centre for Mental Health. (2009) *Diversion: a better way for criminal justice & mental health*. Available at: http://www.centreformentalhealth.org.uk/criminal_justice/a_better_way.aspx

3

Treatment and Outcomes in Secure Care

The principles of providing psychiatric treatment in secure hospitals are no different from providing psychiatric treatment in general psychiatric services.

Differences in emphasis in forensic services include:

- the patients tend to have a multiplicity of interdependent needs
- a greater awareness of risk of harm to others
- a greater prominence of legal issues, with more external restrictions on the patient
- inpatient treatment tends to be longer term, including both acute treatment and prolonged rehabilitation
- progress is made in small graduated steps, with testing out at each one
- an emphasis on continuity of care rather than functionalization of care
- greater availability of psychological treatment
- more prominent security, which has a complex relationship with therapy
- greater need to work with other agencies (particularly MAPPA agencies and the Ministry of Justice), which demands an acute sensitivity to confidentiality and medical ethics
- staff may require different forms of support because of the complexities of:
  - the patients
  - combining both a therapeutic and a custodian role.

● The Needs and Characteristics of Patients in Secure Settings

Secure settings have an overwhelmingly male population:

- overall 88% of patients in secure hospitals are male (Rutherford and Duggan, 2007)
- 88% of restricted patients in 2008 were male (Ministry of Justice, 2010).

BME populations are over-represented in secure services (Rutherford and Duggan, 2007):

	Patients in forensic services (%)			Prison population (%)	General population (%)
	s37	s47	s48		
Non-white British ethnic origin	33	29	56	25	7.9
Black or black British	18	12	20	15	2
Asian or Asian British	4	4	7	6	4

The distribution of legal classification among all restricted patients prior to the Mental Health Act (MHA) 2007 was (Rutherford and Duggan, 2007):

- mental illness 76%
- psychopathic disorder 12%
- mental impairment 5%
- unclassified/other 7%.

It is often argued that these figures underestimate the rate of personality disorder (PD), because many of those detained for mental illness will have co-morbid PDs.

Structured and standardized assessments of need (or measures of outcome) sometimes used in forensic services include:

- Camberwell Assessment of Needs – forensic version (CANFOR – Thomas *et al.*, 2003):
  - the forensic version of the Cambridge Assessment of Needs
  - separate staff and patient ratings in 25 domains
- Health of the Nation Outcome Scores (HoNOS) secure:
  - required as part of the minimum data set for services
  - quick and easy to use, but uncertain validity and reliability (Dickens *et al.*, 2007)
- Recovery-Star (see http://www.mhpf.org.uk):
  - 10 domains are rated collaboratively by patient and a professional.

Surveys of patients in medium security

A survey of patients from one inner London health authority found that of 183 patients in secure psychiatric care (Lelliot *et al.*, 2001):

- 87% were men
- mean age 36 (range 17–64)
- 93% were unemployed prior to admission
- 93% had psychosis or bipolar affective disorder
- 10% had a primary or secondary diagnosis of PD
- half the patients had multiple previous admissions over many years.

In 2007, a similar picture was found in a cross-sectional survey of the inpatient population at Reaside Clinic medium secure unit (MSU), Birmingham. Of 80 male patients:

- the mean age was 37 years (range 21–71)
- 65% were admitted from prison, 15% from community, 10% from another secure setting, 10% from a general psychiatric setting
- most were subject to MHA detention:
  - 56% were detained under s37/41
  - 14% under a civil section
  - 4% s37
  - 12.5% s47/49
  - 6.3% s48/49
- index offences included:
  - 25% homicide/attempted murder
  - 29% wounding
  - 20% assault
  - 10% sexual offence
  - 7.5% arson
- most suffered from a severe mental illness:
  - 86% schizophrenia or schizoaffective disorder
  - 5% bipolar affective disorder

- — 1% persistent delusional disorder
- 85% had a history of problematic use of alcohol or drugs:
  - — most commonly alcohol or cannabis
- the mean number of years since first psychiatric contact was 14:
  - — 56% had a history of disengagement from follow-up
  - — 70% had a history of non-adherence to pharmacological treatment.

There is a group of patients in medium security who require secure care for considerably longer than the original expectation of up to 2 years (see Chapter 1). Jacques *et al.* (2010) found that 21% of men in their medium secure service had been in hospital for more than 5 years and separated them into two groups based on needs identified by the CANFOR:

- Chronic challenging behaviour, treatment-resistant mental illness and considerable daily support needs.
- A more able group who were dependent on the hospital.

Surveys of patients in high security

A survey of 1255 patients in high security found that 85% were men (Harty *et al.*, 2004):

- The men had a mean age of 40 (range 19–84) and a mean duration of admission of 9.8 years (range 0–54).
- The women were younger, with a mean age of 37.
- 57% were classified under the MHA category of mental illness, 25% under psychopathic disorder and 10% were dually classified:
  - — 61% had schizophrenia
  - — 45% had a personality disorder
  - — 10% had learning disability.
- CANFOR needs domains that were commonly unmet included daytime activities, sexual offending (especially among men), arson (especially among women), drugs and alcohol.

● The Multidisciplinary Team

For forensic services in particular, the multidisciplinary team (MDT) is the cornerstone on which effective and safe clinical care is founded:

- Most clinical decisions will be made at the MDT clinical meeting.

The patient sits at the centre of a complex arrangement of multiple agencies (Figure 3.1):

- These agencies have differing agendas and approaches, which commonly overlap but occasionally conflict.
- This is particularly important in forensic services because of the practical and ethical complexities of the therapy/risk dynamic.
- The MDT as a whole, and the RC in particular, must be able to manage the interagency dynamics in a properly balanced way, and bearing in mind issues of confidentiality.

The role of a forensic psychiatrist

While there may be occasional variation, in most services at present, leadership of the MDT is provided by the responsible clinician (RC), who is usually a psychiatrist:

- For the patient, their detention and the associated parameters of restriction are often paramount. So the patient tends to see the RC as being 'in charge'.
- As yet there has not been a wholesale expansion of the RC role to other disciplines following the MHA 2007. Forensic services tend to be relatively conservative, so, if this change happens, it is likely to happen gradually.

Core roles of the forensic psychiatrist (variously delegated to juniors) in an inpatient setting include:

- providing leadership to the MDT, and accepting responsibility for the governance of team functioning
- holding overall responsibility for each patient's detention, care and treatment
- assessing psychopathology, using appropriate medical investigations and arriving at diagnoses
- deciding on pharmacological and other medical interventions
- ensuring that the physical health needs of patients are addressed
- carrying out the statutory functions required by the MHA:
  - renewal of detention
  - consent to treatment
  - providing evidence to courts or tribunals
  - reporting to the MoJ on restricted patients.

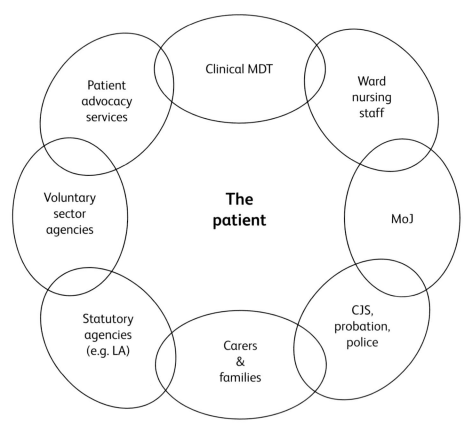

Figure 3.1 Agencies working with patients in secure services (CJS = criminal justice system, LA = local authority, MDT = multidisciplinary team, MoJ = Ministry of Justice)

Other key roles within forensic MDTs

Other key roles within forensic MDTs are described in Table 3.1.

Table 3.1 Key roles within forensic multidisciplinary teams (MDTs)

Psychologist	Clinical and forensic psychologists have differing professional backgrounds, the former tending to have trained in a health environment and the latter more likely to have trained in a penal environment Conducting psychometric assessments relating to intellectual function and personality style Delivering group and individual psychological interventions (see below) Developing individual formulations of risk and mental disorder Providing a psychologically informed perspective to MDT functioning
Nurses	Manage the day-to-day care of the patient within the ward environment, and liaise with the MDT when necessary Includes both traditional therapeutic nursing roles and security roles such as searching of patients, rooms and possessions, drug testing and maintaining ward security Managing observations, leave, visits and other patient activities Managing incidents of aggression and violence or of self-harm Managing the ward environment, patient interactions, and observing for changes in mental state, conduct and risk
Social workers	Statutory functions relating to the Mental Health Act Family and carer liaison Liaison with local authority, may lead on child protection or adult safeguarding issues, including child visitors May lead on liaison with probation, victim liaison unit and multi-agency public protection arrangement Providing a sociological or situational perspective to the MDT
Occupational therapists	Providing assessments and interventions aimed at potentiating an individual's occupational function Standardized assessments such as the Model of Human Occupation Screening Tool (Parkinson *et al.*, 2005) provide consistency Providing and encouraging participation in activities, to enable assessment and foster ability to structure time Assessing and developing independent living skills Supporting and facilitating access to educational, vocational or leisure activities Delivering cognitive–behavioural therapy-based interventions
Pharmacists	Patients often have long histories of pharmacological treatment and complex treatment-resistant illnesses Compiling reviews of a patient's medication history Providing information to patients on their treatment

Conflict within teams

Individuals working in MDTs have loyalties both to the team and to their profession (Mason and Vivian-Byrne, 2002).

- In an effective team these are balanced, bringing a creative tension to team discussions, in which the eclectic richness of approach and practice is used productively.
- Where there is too great an identification with the team, that creative tension may be lost.
- Where there is too great an identification with profession, the intra-team conflict may become obstructive.

It might be that, in forensic MDTs, conflict is heightened by:

- the complexities of the patient's psychopathology, leading to conflicting formulations
- the particular psychopathology of some patients, especially those with damaged attachment styles, leading to splitting within teams

> ### Box 3.1 The psychiatrist, the patient and the Ministry of Justice (MoJ)
>
> Traditionally, forensic services have tended to adopt a paternalistic approach, founded on a predominantly medical model of treating illness and the authority of clinicians:
> - In some cases this fosters dependence on the part of patients, and it is sometimes through a dependent relationship that risk is effectively managed.
> - Reducing offending was often a welcome consequence of establishing mental health, rather than an end in its own right.
>
> More recently risk reduction has come to occupy equal billing in the prioritized aims of forensic clinicians, leading to a more explicit focus on criminogenic needs themselves.
> - Interestingly criminal justice system (CJS) offending behaviour programmes (OBPs) have begun to recognize and emphasize the importance of collaboration with the offender in risk reduction, adopting engagement strategies from health.
>
> The MoJ carries a yet more explicit authority than the clinicians, creating a complex triangle of care/control.
> - For the clinician, it is sometimes useful to locate the controlling aspect of the therapeutic relationship in the MoJ, enabling the development of a collaboration with the patient to satisfy the MoJ.
> - The risk of this approach lies in disingenuously, or seemingly, denying the clinician's custodian/public protection/authoritarian role, leading to the patient feeling cheated or let down when it reappears.
>
> In recent years, the patient advocacy movement and a trend in emphasis away from curing illness to enhancing strengths, well-being and self-acceptance have begun to change the way in which forensic services work with their patients.
> - This improves the degree to which forensic services are patient-centred, and benefits are likely.
> - There may be costs too, because some patients have done well with a traditional forensic approach.
> - Mezey *et al.* (2010) describe some of the obstacles to embracing a recovery approach in forensic services.

- the primacy of risk, requiring formulation, management and therapeutic risk taking.

While all clinical teams work differently, in principle effective team functioning can be maintained by:

- regular multidisciplinary meetings and good communication within teams
- engaging in debate and discussion within the team, while presenting a coherent team approach to patients and carers
- respecting individual team members' roles
- involving the team in most decisions – few issues cannot wait until the next team meeting
- developing an agreed formulation of the patient's engagement with the team
- ensuring effective intra-discipline support
- consciously acknowledging the challenges of MDT working in secure environments
- regular team awaydays/practice development days, perhaps with external facilitation
- acknowledging problems relating to particular patients and accessing psychotherapeutic supervision or assessment to understand the psychopathology/dynamics further.

● The Patient Journey in Secure Care

The characteristics of treatment within secure services vary greatly among different levels of security and different patient groups. In general terms, patients should move in the direction shown in Figure 3.2.

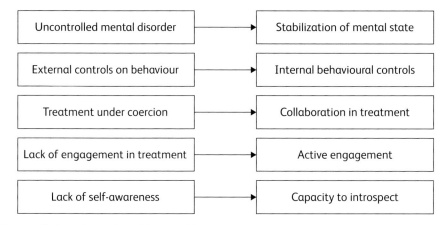

Figure 3.2 General objectives of treatment in secure care

Admission to secure care

Prior to admission:

- the responsible clinician, clinical team and care coordinator should be identified
- an initial care plan and risk assessment with immediate and short-term plans and goals is agreed
- the patient's room is searched and cleaned.

On admission, according to local policies and procedures:

- an effective handover from escorting staff to ward staff is essential
- the patient is greeted and searched:
  - belongings are recorded on a property list
  - the list of contraband items may vary among units and security levels
- detention papers are checked by medical records staff
- the patient is orientated to the ward and provided with:
  - written and/or oral information about the ward routine, basic policies and procedures (particularly meal times, smoking arrangements, visits, etc.)
  - the patient is informed of their MHA rights
- an initial nursing assessment is followed by formal medical clerking
- nursing staff will complete a patient profile including:
  - a physical description and perhaps a photograph
  - individuals at risk and to be contacted in the event of the patient being absent without leave.
- the initial care plan will at least include:
  - observation level
  - mental and physical state
  - keyworker sessions
  - leave and visitors
  - initial medication, both regular and as required sedative medication where necessary.

The acute phase of treatment

The key aims for the acute phase of treatment are:

- to carry out initial assessments and risk management
- to confirm the diagnoses

- to stabilize the mental state
- to decide on the initial care pathway and work through the criminal justice process.

At the ward level, this phase is characterized by:

- close observation levels ranging from constant observation by one or more staff to intermittent observations at a frequency of between 5 minutes to an hour
- close observation of mental state, behaviour and interactions with other patients and staff
- regular physical observations including weight checks and drug testing
- regular and random searches of a patient's personal and living environment
- facilitating and monitoring personal and professional visits
- gradually reducing restrictions, contingent on risk behaviours and mental state:
  - reducing observation level
  - increasing leave within the building
  - access to kitchen (e.g. for hot drinks), use of sharps on the ward (e.g. for shaving) and other freedoms according to local policies and practice.

At the team level:

- building a therapeutic relationship with the patient
- frequent mental state examination to document current psychopathology
- detailed history taking and collation of information from other sources
- engagement of carers and relatives
- establishment of initial pharmacological treatment
- specific standard initial assessments of, for example, problematic substance use, IQ, personality style, occupational needs
- liaison with courts and solicitors over ongoing legal proceedings and provision of reports
- dealing with issues relating to previous accommodation, benefits and debts.

Rehabilitation in secure care

A patient may move to the rehabilitation phase once:

- there is some stability of their mental state
- there is a relatively sustained cessation of risk behaviours, indicating improved internal controls
- they are showing some positive engagement and collaboration in their care.

The key aims are:

- to maintain mental state stability, enabling psychosocial rehabilitation
- to provide further psychological assessment and treatment
- to develop a shared formulation of the mental disorder, risk behaviours and the relationship between them, encompassing where relevant:
  - problematic substance use
  - interpersonal relationships
  - situational factors
- to develop a shared relapse prevention plan
- systematic assessment of psychosocial needs, perhaps using a structured instrument, and tailored interventions to meet them
- to reintroduce the patient to a community setting gradually, allowing assessment at each step.

This phase is characterized by:

- some relaxation of procedural security, though not relational security:
  - generally reduced frequency of observations and searching

- more permitted possessions
- increased freedom to move around within the hospital
- ongoing assessment and treatment in more varied settings:
  - including individual and group work, in the occupational therapy department and social activities
  - progression to leave within the hospital grounds and then the community
- greater responsibility for treatment:
  - self-medication regimes
- development of relationships with families, relatives, carers and friends
- increased emphasis on occupational and educational as well as leisure activity, developing the patient's ability to structure time
- ongoing formulation of mental disorder and risk, and development of a relapse prevention plan:
  - sharing this with other agencies or carers as and when appropriate
- establishing accommodation needs and options
- preparation for a tribunal, or other discharge mechanism.

● Pharmacological Treatment in Secure Care

Pharmacological treatment for mental disorder is no different in forensic services from that in other settings. The association of serious risk with mental ill-health brings an added impetus to preventing relapse or detecting relapse early, thus enabling intervention.

For Patel and David (2005) long-acting injectable antipsychotics have advantages over oral preparations in the treatment of schizophrenia.

- improved treatment adherence
- abolition of covert treatment non-adherence:
  - probably the most important pragmatic advantage among high-risk patients
  - non-adherence may be both a cause and a consequence of relapse
- improved global outcome and reduced rate of hospitalization (Robert and Geppert, 2004)
- more predictable and consistent pharmacodynamics and pharmacokinetics
- dose changes are more gradual, reducing risk of sudden relapse
- reduced risk of overdose.

They consider that many of the disadvantages of depots may be construed as perception problems:

- stigmatizing and disempowering/coercive:
  - there is no intrinsic reason why this should be so
- reduced patient acceptability:
  - often an individual matter – some patients prefer depots; many do not
- potential for increased side effects:
  - specific side effects may include pain and local inflammation at the injection site
  - otherwise there is little evidence for greater side effects with depots, when comparing like drugs
  - improved pharmacodynamics may lead to a better side-effect profile for depots
- dose changes are more gradual, reducing the ability to respond promptly to side effects or patient choice.

● Treating Aggression

The literature on the pharmacological treatment of violence is small and the evidence is conflicting. A Cochrane Review of the use of antiepileptics in treating aggression and associated impulsivity (Huban *et al.*, 2010) identified 14 studies involving 672 subjects:

- The subjects differed between studies, and there were both positive and negative findings.
- No firm conclusions could be drawn on effectiveness.

Recent structured reviews (Volavka and Citrome, 2008; Topiwala and Fazel, 2011) of the available evidence for treating aggression in patients with schizophrenia have reached the following conclusions:

- There is good evidence that clozapine reduces levels of aggression, and that this effect is independent of impact on psychotic symptoms.
- Otherwise, there is no convincing evidence that any specific antipsychotic confers added benefit in comparison to the others.
- The evidence on mood stabilizers is inconsistent:
  - controlled studies do not support efficacy of valproate
  - carbamazepine may reduce agitation, but little anti-aggression effect
  - no evidence to support the use of lithium or lamotrigine.
- There is limited evidence for the use of adjunctive beta blockers, but they may not be well tolerated.

● Physical Health of Patients in Secure Care

The standardized mortality ratio is 1.5 for those with mental disorder generally, and 3–4 for those with schizophrenia. Being an inpatient in secure care may be associated with:

- a generally sedentary lifestyle
- reduced opportunities for exercise
- effects of psychotropic medication
- boredom, leading to compensatory behaviours such as snacking and smoking cigarettes
- reduced motivation for self-care.

Psychiatrists must accept responsibility for the physical health of their patients, but the evidence suggests that dedicated primary care services offer benefits within long-term inpatient settings (Cormac *et al.*, 2004). Practice, supported by policy, should address (Royal College of Psychiatrists, 2009):

- schedules for physical monitoring, with reference to prescribed medication and other risk factors:
  - including especially weight/body mass index (BMI), blood pressure (BP), smoking status, lipids, random/fasting glucose, electrocardiogram (ECG)
- health promotion and education
- encouragement of healthy exercise
- diet and nutrition
- weight management
- infectious diseases and sexual health
- addictions and alcohol use:
  - including particularly tobacco use, secure units increasingly becoming smoke-free environments.

● Management of Disturbed/Violent Behaviour

The short-term management of disturbed/violent behaviour may be considered in three stages (National Institute for Health and Clinical Excellence, 2005):

- Prediction:
  - including risk assessment and searching.
- Prevention:
  - using de-escalation techniques and observations

  – managing the environment to reduce stimulation, consider use of designated room for 'time out'; this should not routinely be the seclusion room
  – discussing issues in calm manner, aiming to develop rapport while maintaining an awareness of cues and body language.
- Interventions for continued management:
  – rapid tranquillization (see National Institute for Health and Clinical Excellence, 2005, and local policies)
  – seclusion
  – physical intervention.

There is little empirical evidence that seclusion or any other form of physical intervention is more effective than the other. The relative use of different types of intervention varies greatly internationally, due to cultural and historical practice issues rather than an evidence base. Bowers *et al.* (2005) compared methods of containment of disturbed behaviour between the UK, Greece and Italy, and showed more use of seclusion in the UK, and more use of physical restraints on the Continent.

NICE guidelines (2005) recommend that teams should work with patients to prepare advance directives of preferences for interventions in the event of violent or disturbed behaviour. This practice is widely used in intensive care units in all levels of security.

Seclusion

There is no definitive international definition of seclusion. For example:

- the UK MHA CoP (Department of Health, 2008) defines seclusion as:
  – 'The supervised confinement of a patient in a room, which may be locked. Its sole aim is to contain severely disturbed behaviour which is likely to cause harm to others'
- mental health legislation of the Australian State of Victoria uses:
  – 'sole confinement of a person at any hour of the day or night in a room of which the doors and windows are locked from the outside'.

Seclusion areas should be specially built and designed to be a safe and secure, low-stimulus environment. However, seclusion is not defined by the area in which it occurs. If a patient is confined elsewhere, their bedroom, for example, this is still seclusion.

Each unit will have its own policies and procedures regarding the seclusion of patients. Generally these will include the following factors:

- The decision to seclude a patient should be made by a senior clinician or the professional in charge of the ward.
- There should be a regular review of the need for seclusion to continue, including regular multidisciplinary review.
- There should be a suitably trained professional within sight of the seclusion room at all times.

Ching *et al.* (2010) discuss the negative aspects of seclusion, which should be seen as a measure of last resort. They describe a successful strategy to reduce the use of seclusion within a forensic service.

Physical intervention

All physical interventions should be seen as a last resort, to be avoided if possible and de-escalation techniques should be used continuously throughout a period of restraint. Such interventions carry a risk of injury to patient and to staff.

Manual holding

- The most commonly used method in the UK.
- Requires specific training and uses a team approach, each individual having a particular responsibility, one person having responsibility for protecting the patient's head and neck.

There have been incidents of patient deaths occurring while in restraint, the most well-known case being that of David Bennett, who was manually restrained for over half an hour in the prone position. NICE guidelines state that during physical restraint at no time should pressure be applied to the patient's neck, thorax, back, abdomen or pelvic area. They also recommend that cardiopulmonary resuscitation equipment be available within 3 minutes of the setting where these interventions are being used.

Mechanical restraints

Restraints such as body belts, straps or straitjackets are rarely used in the UK but are more widely used in other countries (including continental Europe and the USA). There are some circumstances where mechanical restraints are used in this country:

- Handcuffs are used routinely by prisons, including when transferring prisoners to hospital. Use of handcuffs has become more common in secure psychiatric hospitals in recent years, for transporting high-risk patients to attend court or general hospitals.
  - There is no clinical evidence base to support this, and handcuffs may be extremely stigmatizing, particularly in a general health-care setting.
- The use of some mechanical restraints in high secure hospitals. This is generally for short periods, at times of extremely disturbed behaviour when transferring patients from one care area to another.
- The use of mechanical restraints in prisons. Again these are used for short periods of time when other interventions would not be appropriate.

● Psychological Treatment in Secure Care

Traditionally, forensic services tended to take an individualistic approach to treatment:

- An individual formulation was key.
- Interventions tended to be delivered on an individual basis to reflect this individual formulation, the effects of psychosis in particular being seen as too idiosyncratic to allow a more programmatic approach.
- Individual interventions adopted a variety of approaches, including both treatments based on cognitive–behavioural therapy and more dynamically orientated approaches.
- Often the chosen approach was dependent primarily on the professional background of the therapist.

In more recent years:

- psychological interventions have tended to become more programmatic and group-based
- forensic psychotherapy has begun to create a more defined role within mental illness-dominated medium secure units (MSUs).

Individual assessment, formulation and treatment remain crucial for effective clinical care and risk management because:

- group interventions cannot provide sufficient responsivity, to take account of the patient's individual needs, particularly the idiosyncratic effects of psychosis
- it is necessary to engage difficult-to-engage patients, and sometimes this is best done individually

- relapse prevention plans and risk management plans are necessarily individual
- confidentiality issues may obstruct group work for some.

The approach used in individual treatment is flexible, and may be determined by both professional and patient factors.

Group-based interventions may be:

- traditionally delivered psychoeducation or CBT-based interventions, targeting mental health needs, such as:
  - mental health awareness
  - problematic substance use
  - hearing voices
  - recovering from psychosis
- interventions targeting criminogenic needs, often based on accredited offending behaviour programmes, such as:
  - reasoning and rehabilitation
  - anger management
  - fire setting groups
  - sex offender treatment programmes.

Howells *et al.* (2004) discuss the application of the 'What Works' principles (Risk, Needs, Responsivity) to psychiatric settings. The recently developing literature about group-based interventions in forensic settings is nevertheless limited:

- It has not yet moved beyond parochial descriptions of individual interventions in single units.
- Such interventions generally have high face validity.
- Demonstrating positive outcomes consequent to a particular intervention that is delivered within the context of a much wider care package in a secure setting is a considerable challenge (see, for example, Swain *et al.*, 2010).

In reporting the results of an audit of psychology provision in a forensic service, Gudjonsson and Young (2007):

- draw attention to the tendency for direct treatment to be subordinated to assessment and indirect patient care
- contrast risk management models with strength-based models
- describe the service model for psychological intervention that their service has adopted.

Forensic psychotherapy

Psychotherapy within secure settings and prisons has a long history, and is established in:

- high security, where treatment for PD is also established
- the small number of MSUs which specifically provide treatment for those with PD
- a few prisons, notably HMP Gendon (see Chapter 18)
- some outpatient services, notably the Portman Clinic, London.

Current provision within mental illness-focused MSUs is limited and variable. McGauley and Humphrey (2003) describe the role of forensic psychotherapy in secure units:

- Direct clinical work:
  - providing assessments to inform understanding of the patient
  - providing treatment, individual or group.
- Supervisory work:
  - either of other professionals doing direct clinical work, or

    – regarding psychodynamic processes of an institution.
- Clinical meetings:
  - case conferences, clinical team meetings and patient reviews.
- Consultation or institutional supervision:
  - provided to an institution from outside.

Through reflective practice groups, supervisory work may particularly seek to improve staff's awareness of the unconscious dynamics among the triad of:

- the patient
- the staff
- the institution.

For further reading see Cordess and Cox (1998) and, particularly, Bartlett and McGauley (2009).

● Leave for Restricted Patients

Restricted patients may only be given leave of absence (LOA) under s17 MHA with the permission of the Secretary of State for Justice. Three standard types of LOA may be considered, a patient generally being expected to move through them sequentially prior to discharge:

- escorted community leave (ECL)
- unescorted community leave (UCL)
- overnight leave (ONL):
  - usually to a proposed discharge address.

Other types of leave include:

- compassionate leave:
  - a leave required at short notice, usually due to serious illness or death in a close relative
  - specific permission should be sought even where the patient has already been granted ECL or UCL
- leave to attend hospital:
  - MoJ permission is not required for escorted leave to attend hospital for medical examination or other urgent treatment
  - The MoJ should be informed in advance if possible for s48 patients, and immediately afterwards for all others.
- leave to attend court:
  - permission is not required for escorted leave to attend criminal court in relation to alleged offences.

For patients transferring between hospitals, leave status:

- does not usually transfer with a patient moving from high security
- may or may not transfer from medium to low security
- usually does transfer between hospitals of the same level of security.

Section 48 patients are not normally granted s17 leave. For s47 patients:

- UCL will usually only be considered within 2 years of their parole eligibility date (PED), or once they have served half their custodial sentence, whichever is the later.
- ONL will be considered within 3 months of their PED.
- For life sentenced prisoners, ECL will be considered on its merits, and UCL may be considered within 3 years of the tariff date.

Box 3.2 Liaising with the Ministry of Justice (MoJ) in relation to leave

Each type of leave requires a separate application:

- The responsible clinician (RC) must apply using a standardized form available on the MoJ website.
- The MoJ aims to respond to leave requests within 3 weeks.

Leave is usually granted at the discretion of the RC, with a report required after 3 months:

- The RC may decide upon the duration and destination of each leave.
- Occasionally restrictions will be added, relating to restriction zones, for example.
- It is usual for the next stage of leave not to be considered until such a report has been made.

A small naturalistic study suggested that clinical leave decisions are often based on implicit shared knowledge which may not be voiced, and may be less focused on risk than on humanity (Lyall and Bartlett, 2010):

- The risk of absconding should be considered explicitly in terms of both likelihood and likely cost.

Remember that the presence of a nursing escort does not prevent a determined absconder. The escort can only:

- try to dissuade the patient from absconding
- try to keep an absconding patient in sight
- raise the alarm promptly.

The MoJ should always be informed immediately if changes are made to leave status at a clinical level. Where the RC has rescinded leave, the MoJ will inform the RC if further permission is required to reinstate it.

Outcomes of Treatment in Secure Care

Reconviction rates are the most commonly used outcome measure for research, probably because reconviction may be detected reliably. But:

- official rates are likely to underestimate the true rate of offending, particularly among the mentally disordered
- patients may be institutionalized for significant periods after discharge from secure care, limiting the opportunity for offending
- reconviction rates may not be a good measure of mental health outcomes.

For restricted patients, rates of reoffending within 2 years of first discharge are (Ministry of Justice, 2010):

- all offences 7%
- sexual or violent offence 2%
- grave offence 1%:
  - homicide, serious wounding, rape, buggery, arson, robbery, aggravated burglary.

Reconviction following discharge from high security

Buchanan (1998) studied a cohort of 425 consecutive discharges from all UK high secure hospitals in 1982–83, without accounting for post-discharge setting.

	Prevalence of reoffending (%)	
	5½ years	10½ years
Violent offence	9	7.5
Sexual offence	5	15
Any offence	26	34

Jamieson and Taylor (2004) followed up 204 patients discharged from one high security hospital in 1984 for 12 years, reporting an overall reconviction rate of 38%:

- 86% of reoffenders did so after having begun to live in the community
- reconviction was associated with MHA classification of psychopathic disorder and younger age
- those with mental impairment were as likely to be re-convicted as those with psychopathic disorder.

Reconviction following discharge from medium security

Maden *et al.* (2004) studied a national cohort of 959 discharges and gave a 2-year reconviction rate of 15%. Davies *et al.* (2007) (n = 550, from 1 MSU over 20 years, mean follow-up 9.4 years) reported 49% reconvicted with mean time to reconviction of 3 years. Reconviction rates are shown in Table 3.2.

Table 3.2 Reconviction rates from Davies *et al.* (2007)

	2 years (%)	5 years (%)
Standard list	26	42
Grave offence	7	12

Coid *et al.* (2007) (n = 1344, from seven regions) reported differing reconviction rates (mean 6.2 years follow-up) for men and women as shown in Table 3.3.

Table 3.3 Reconviction rates from Coid *et al.* (2007)

	Men (%)	Women (%)
Acquisitive offence	20	7
Violent offence	18	5
Sexual offence	2	–
Arson	1	4.5
Any offence	34	15

These studies suggest that factors associated with increased risk of reoffending are:

- male gender
- younger age
- early age of onset of offending
- number of previous convictions
- diagnosis of PD
- history of alcohol or drug problems
- history of sexual abuse
- having lost contact with services
- longer period of detention prior to discharge
- restriction order.

Davies *et al.* (2007) also reported:

- 10% of their sample had died
- 38% had been readmitted to secure care
- a six-fold increase in mortality compared with general population:
  - the standard mortality rate was highest for suicide, followed by unnatural death, followed by natural death.

References

*Bartlett A, McGauley G (2009) *Forensic Mental Health: Concepts, systems and practice.* Oxford: Oxford University Press

Bowers L, Douzenis A, Galeazzi GM, Forghieri M, Tsopelas M, Simpson A, Allan T. (2005) Disruptive and dangerous behaviour by patients on acute psychiatric wards in three European centres. *Social Psychiatry and Psychiatric Epidemiology* **40**, 822–8

Buchanan A. (1998) Criminal conviction after discharge from special (high security) hospital. Incidence in the first 10 years. *The British Journal of Psychiatry* **172**, 472–6

Ching H, Daffern M, Martin T, Thomas S. (2010) Reducing the use of seclusion in a forensic psychiatric hospital: assessing the impact on aggression, therapeutic climate and staff confidence. *Journal of Forensic Psychiatry and Psychology* **21**(5),737–60

Coid J, Hickey N, Kahtan N, Zhang T, Yang M. (2007) Patients discharged from medium secure forensic psychiatry services: reconvictions and risk factors. *British Journal of Psychiatry* **190**, 223–9

Cordess C, Cox M. (1998) *Forensic Psychotherapy: Crime, psychodynamics and the offender patient.* London: Jessica Kingsley

Cormac I, Martin D, Ferriter M. (2004) Improving the physical health of long-stay psychiatric in-patients. *Advances in Psychiatric Treatment* **10**(2), 107–15

*Davies S, Clarke M, Hollin C, Duggan C. (2007) Long-term outcomes after discharge from medium secure care: a cause for concern. *British Journal of Psychiatry* **191**(1), 70–4

Department of Health. (2008) *Mental Health Act 1983 Code of Practice.* London: The Stationery Office

Dickens G, Sugarman P, Walker L. (2007) HoNOS-secure: a reliable outcome measure for users of secure and forensic mental health services. *Journal of Forensic Psychiatry and Psychology* **18**(4), 507–14

*Gudjonsson G, Young S. (2007) The role and scope of forensic clinical psychology in secure unit provisions: a proposed service model for psychological therapies. *Journal of Forensic Psychiatry and Psychology* **18**(4), 534–56

Harty M-A, Shaw J, Thomas S, Dolan M, Davies L, Thornicroft G, *et al.* (2004) The security, clinical and social needs of patients in high secure psychiatric hospitals in England. *Journal of Forensic Psychiatry and Psychology* **15**(2), 208–21

Howells K, Day A, Thomas-Peter B. (2004) Changing violent behaviour: forensic mental health and criminological models compared. *Journal of Forensic Psychiatry and Psychology* **15**(3), 391–406

Huban N, Ferriter M, Nathan R, Jones H. (2010) Antiepileptics for aggression and associated impulsivity. *Cochrane Database of Systematic Reviews* 2010(2): Art.No:CD003499. DOI:10.1002/14651858. CD003499.pub3

Jamieson L. Taylor PJ. (2004) A reconviction study of special (high security) hospital patients. *British Journal of Criminology* **44**(5), 783–802

Jacques J, Spencer S-J, Gilluley P. (2010) Long-term care needs in male medium security. *British Journal of Forensic Practice* **12**(3), 37–44

Lelliot P, Audini B, Duffett R. (2001) Survey of patients from an inner-London Health Authority in medium secure psychiatric care. *British Journal of Psychiatry* **178**(1), 62–6

Lyall M, Bartlett A. (2010) Decision making in medium security: can he have leave? *Journal of Forensic Psychiatry and Psychology* **21**(6), 887–901

Maden A, Scott F, Burnett R, Lewis G, Skapinakis P. (2004) Offending in psychiatric patients after discharge from medium secure units: prospective national cohort study. *British Medical Journal* **328**, 1534

Mason T, Vivian-Byrne S. (2002) Multi-disciplinary working in a forensic mental health setting: ethical codes of reference. *Journal of Psychiatric and Mental Health Nursing* **9**(5), 563–72

McGauley G, Humphrey M. (2003) Contribution of forensic psychotherapy to the care of forensic patients. *Advances in Psychiatric Treatment* **9**, 117–24

Mezey G, Kavuma M, Turton P, Demetriou A, Wright C. (2010) Perceptions, experiences and meanings of recovery in forensic psychiatric patients. *Journal of Forensic Psychiatry and Psychology* **21**(5), 683–96

Ministry of Justice. (2010) *Statistics of Mentally Disordered Offenders 2008*. Available at: http://www.justice.gov.uk/publications/

National Institute for Health and Clinical Excellence. (2005) *Guidelines for the Short-term Management of Disturbed/Violent Behaviour*. Accessed using: http://guidance.nice.org.uk/CG25

Parkinson S, Forsyth K, Kielhofner G. (2005) *The Model of Human Occupation Screening Tool (Version 2.0)*. Chicago, IL: MOHO Clearinghouse

Patel M, David A. (2005) Why aren't depot antipsychotics prescribed more often and what can be done about it? *Advances in Psychiatric Treatment* **11**, 203–11

Robert LW, Geppert CMA. (2004) Ethical use of long-acting injections in the treatment of severe and persistent mental illness. *Comprehensive Psychiatry* **45**, 161–7

Royal College of Psychiatrists. (2009) *OP67 Physical Health in Mental Health: Final report of scoping group*. Available at http://www.rcpsych.ac.uk/files/pdfversion/OP67.pdf

*Rutherford M, Duggan S. (2007) *Forensic Mental Health Services: Facts and figures on current provision*. Sainsbury Centre for Mental Health. Available at: http://www.centreformentalhealth.org.uk/pdfs/scmh_forensic_factfile_2007.pdf

Swain E, Boulter S, Piek N. (2010) Overcoming the challenges of evaluating dual diagnosis interventions in medium secure units. *British Journal of Forensic Practice* **12**(1), 33–7

Thomas S, Harty MA, Parrott J, McCrone P, Slade M, Thornicroft G. (2003) *CANFOR: Camberwell Assessment of Need – Forensic Version. A needs assessment for forensic mental health service users*. London: Gaskell

Topiwala A, Fazel S. (2011) The pharmacological management of violence in schizophrenia: a structured review. *Expert Review of Neurotherapeutics* **11**(1), 53–63

*Volavka J, Citrome L. (2008) Heterogeneity of violence in schizophrenia and implications for long term treatment. *International Journal of Clinical Practice* **62**(8), 1237–45

4

Challenging Issues in Secure Care

Working in a secure setting is particularly challenging because:

- the patient group has high levels of co-morbidity, particularly personality disorder (PD) and substance misuse
- there is an increased risk of violence or assault
- professionals must reconcile conflicting roles of clinician and custodian
- legal issues, whether criminal, Mental Health Act (MHA), immigration or other, may incentivize patients to modify their presentation.

This chapter highlights some of these challenges and outlines some of the ways forensic services work to meet them.

● The Relationship Between Security and Therapy

The Code of Practice to the Mental Health Act 1983 (Department of Health, 2008), establishes the 'least restriction principle':

People taking action without a patient's consent must attempt to keep to a minimum the restrictions they impose on the patient's liberty, having regard to the purpose to which the restrictions are imposed.

Secure services seek a balance between:

- restrictions aimed at containment and prevention of harm, and
- the provision of an adequate environment and opportunities for effective rehabilitation.

Dual loyalties or symbiosis

For some, mental health professionals working in secure settings have conflicting 'dual loyalties', to treatment in the patient's interest and to security in the state's interest (Weinstein, 2002):

- The distinction between these nursing and security roles varies among countries:
  - In the UK a dual role model dominates, certain security procedures such as searches being the responsibility of nursing staff.
  - In North America it is more common for specific security personnel to undertake these tasks.
- A Swedish study of forensic nurses highlighted the conflict that many feel in their dual role in providing therapy while also being a custodian (Rask and Halberg, 2000).

- This distinction between the European model (integrated care and toleration of dual roles) and the American model (separation of care and security roles) is reflected in medico-legal expert witness work (see Chapter 21).

For others, security and therapy have a closer, less conflicting and even symbiotic relationship:

- Crichton (2009) has defined the purpose of security as:
  - 'to provide a safe and secure environment for patients, staff and visitors which facilitates appropriate treatment for patients and appropriately protects the wider community'.
- For Gournay *et al.* (2008):
  - care and control should not be viewed as two separate, competing entities, but as lying on one continuum
  - improved levels of care (intensity, quality and evidence base) in collaboration with the patient actually lower the need for control using security measures.

So, for some patients, the enforced stability and restrictions inherent in secure care are necessary to enable them to benefit from treatment.

● Escapes and Absconding

Exworthy and Wilson (2010) gave the following definitions:

- Escape involves a breach of the physical perimeter of the facility, be that prison or hospital. It can be seen as a breach of both physical and procedural security measures.
- Absconding refers to breaking the conditions of leave of absence from the hospital or prison; this may be while escorted or unescorted. This is a breach of relational and procedural security measures.

Reports that 116 people had 'escaped' from medium and low secure units in 2007 (*The Times*, 2008) reflected a society characterized by risk aversion and sensationalist media scrutiny. The consequent reduced tolerance of escape/absconding reflects contemporary political managerialism and media sensitivity:

- The development of national minimum standards for security for both medium and low secure units has tended to increase the level of security from previous standards.
- A political imperative that escape by a transferred prisoner from a medium secure hospital should never occur (National Patient Safety Agency, 2010).

Although no reliable national figures are currently available, absconds are much more common than escapes:

- Gradillas *et al.* (2007) found 178 incidents of absconding at four medium secure units over a period of 5 years.
- The 2009 annual report of the National Confidential Inquiry (2009) gave the following figures in relation to general psychiatric care:
  - in the period 1997–2006 there were 469 suicides after inpatients had absconded (25 % of in-patient suicides); only 1 % had absconded from a secure unit
  - between 1997 and 2005 there were 21 homicides committed by psychiatric in-patients, 17 of which occurred off the ward
  - of the homicides committed off the ward 41 % had absconded; none had absconded from a secure unit.

Box 4.1 Assessing and managing risk of escape and absconding

This is a task for the entire multidisciplinary team; there should be particular attention paid to the patient's history and any previous attempts. It is important to be aware of factors that may make the risk higher:

- immediately following admission
- remand prisoners
- around the time of tribunals or court appearances
- around significant dates (bereavements, date of index offence, etc.)
- when there has been a reduction in level of supervision/escort level during leave
- psychosocial stress/family issues
- when mental state has deteriorated
- high level of impulsivity
- poor collaboration in care and treatment.

The clinical team are all responsible for taking part in discussions about risk of escape or absconding. In order to reduce the risk, the following measures are usually taken:

- Decisions made regarding changing leave or escort levels should be made by experienced staff who know the patient well.
- Clinical teams should be aware of any dates significant to the patient.
- Each patient should have an established care plan to cover any need to leave the unit in an emergency, such as for physical health treatment.
- Before any patient goes on agreed leave there is an assessment of mental state documented by nursing staff.
- If patient going on unescorted leave, there is a record made of the clothing worn on leaving the unit.

Each unit will have its own procedures to follow in the event of a patient escaping or absconding. When working in secure settings it is important to be familiar with these. General points will be:

- contacting the local police and providing appropriate information (see section on confidentiality)
- if the patient is restricted or a transferred prisoner contact the Ministry of Justice (there is a 24-hour telephone number)
- informing the Care Quality Commission
- all on-call staff (including the community team) should be informed
- each patient should have a specific care plan addressing risks in the event of absconding, including known likely risk behaviours, likely sanctuaries or destinations, specific potential victims, people who should be informed.

● Managing Substance Misuse

The prevalence of problematic substance use among psychiatric patients is between 30 and 50% (Swartz *et al.*, 2006; Weaver *et al.*, 2003). In forensic psychiatric populations it is at the upper end of this range at least (Isherwood and Brooke, 2001; Maden *et al.*, 1999).

Substance misuse leads to offending (McMurran, 2002):

- by exacerbating dispositional impulsivity and aggression
- through a direct effect on reasoning and problem-solving skills
- by causing economic hardship
- by leading to an association with a criminal peer group
- by interfering with therapeutic interventions.

Substance misuse exacerbates schizophrenia by:

- a direct effect upon the illness in terms of earlier age of onset, increased frequency of episodes of psychosis, increased symptom severity, higher rates of anxiety and depression

- association with poor adherence to pharmacological treatment and poor concordance with other aspects of care
- causing additional disability through homelessness, lack of economic independence, impaired occupational functioning, criminality, poorer relationships with family/carers
- adverse effects upon physical health.

Although patients with schizophrenia use substances for the same range of reasons as the non-mentally disordered, patients:

- are more likely to use to alleviate dysphoria
- are relatively less likely to use for pleasure enhancement or social reasons.

There is little evidence to support the notion that patients use substances as 'self-medication' for psychosis. See Gregg *et al.* (2007) for further discussion of reasons for use.

Substance use within secure psychiatric hospitals

A review of NHS medium secure units in 2005 (Durand *et al.*, 2006) found that:

- all units reported problems with substance misuse over the previous year
- all units had written policies about substance misuse or used a variety of security measures to limit availability of drugs
- there was a dearth of comprehensive treatment programmes for inpatients with problematic substance use.

Alcohol and drug use among inpatients:

- worsens symptoms of mental illness and reduces the efficacy of treatment
- may result in disinhibition, increased impulsivity and increased likelihood of risk behaviours
- undermines the procedural security of the unit:
  - a history of substance misuse was the single factor that best distinguished rule breakers from non-rule breakers in a medium secure unit (Main and Gudjonsson, 2006).

The distribution of contraband goods (including drugs and alcohol) is associated with bullying and victimization.

Treatment of problematic substance use in secure inpatient settings

The National Institute for Health and Clinical Excellence (NICE) guidelines (Kendall *et al.*, 2011) on treating psychosis and substance misuse are based exclusively on opinion and low-quality evidence, and offer little guidance on treatment approaches.

In secure settings there may be an issue of culture:

- Health professionals generally hold negative stereotypical views about drug users, and nurses working in forensic settings are particularly likely to hold such moralizing and stereotypical views (Foster and Onyeukwu, 2003).
- Durand *et al.* (2006) found little consensus on the most appropriate treatment philosophy in terms of:
  - parallel, serial or integrated care
  - abstinence or harm minimization.

The treatment approach should mirror that in the community and follow national guidelines (National Institute for Health and Clinical Excellence, 2007a,b). Treatment should:

- be integrated – that is delivered by the same staff who are treating the patient's other mental health needs
- be long term, seeing problematic substance use as a chronic, relapsing condition
- be appropriate to the patient's motivational stage, building hope and readiness to change
- include relapse prevention to help patients manage high-risk situations.

The stages of treatment will include elements of (Luty, 2003):

- detection and assessment of use
- detoxification if necessary
- engagement in treatment programme, using techniques such as motivational interviewing
- pharmacological treatment (either replacement for opiates or to treat withdrawal symptoms)
- psychological interventions:
  - motivational enhancement therapy
  - cognitive–behavioural therapy and relapse prevention.

Treatment in secure settings must also take account of the stage that the patient is at in their rehabilitation:

- Assessment, engagement and some motivational work may be done early in an admission.
- Relapse prevention work should be tied into further progression of rehabilitation and the increased freedom that this entails.

Specialist advice or joint working with substance misuse services may be appropriate, particularly for those with alcohol dependence, or problematic heroin or cocaine use. However:

- this requires active engagement on the part of the patient, which may not be consistent for some with severe mental illness who nevertheless require treatment
- there is limited assistance for those with problematic cannabis use, which is the most common problem among those with schizophrenia.

There is some evidence, from a post-hoc analysis of data collected for another purpose (Drake *et al.*, 2000), that among patients with schizophrenia, treatment with clozapine may be associated with greater improvement in substance use than other antipsychotics.

Limiting the availability of drugs within secure hospitals

It is very difficult for a unit that rehabilitates patients using community leave to maintain a drug-free environment. Security techniques commonly used in secure hospitals to limit drug availability, the extent varying among units, include:

- physical security, such as fences to prevent items being thrown or passed into the unit
- searches:
  - of patients on return from leave
  - of visitors, staff and their belongings
- staff observation of visits to prevent passing of illicit substances
- checking gifts or food sent into the unit
- the use of sniffer dogs to detect drugs
- effective relational security, to identify patients involved in drug distribution.

Although the availability of drugs must be limited as far as possible, the therapeutic opportunities offered by drug use and temptation to use must not be missed:

- All staff should be trained to recognize and use such opportunities.

Drug testing of inpatients

Testing patients for the presence of drugs is important both therapeutically and from a security perspective. Testing may be point-of-care, or laboratory based.

The immediacy of point-of-care testing may be seen as an advantage, but it carries the risk that too much weight will be placed on the outcome of a single test – nursing staff may tend to manage the drug test result rather than the patient. Laboratory-based testing brings greater reliability and quality assurance, as well as the promise of a mutually beneficial working relationship between a responsive laboratory and the clinical service.

There are three samples commonly used for testing:

- Urine testing is the most well established and commonly used. In secure settings the procedure for collecting samples should be strictly prescribed to reduce the likelihood of fraudulent samples being provided.
- Oral fluid testing is useful for cocaine and opiates, but cannabinoids are not released into saliva from the blood. Oral fluid testing will therefore only detect cannabinoids left in the mouth during smoking.
- Hair testing is used uncommonly and is currently relatively expensive. It offers a very different time window of detection.

Detection periods (Table 4.1) show considerable variation depending on the test and individual factors, particularly the amount used:

- In an inpatient setting, the time window for detection of cannabis in urine may be just a few hours, because use is often intermittent and the amount taken small.

Table 4.1 Detection periods for drug testing after cessation of use

	Urine	Oral fluid	Blood	Hair
Casual cannabis use	1–2 days	18–24 hours	24–48 hours	Up to 90 days, depending on length of sample
Chronic cannabis use	1–28 days			
Amphetamines	1–2 days	12 hours	12 hours	
Cocaine	1–3 days	24 hours	24 hours	
Opiates	1–3 days	6 hours	6 hours	

● Malingering

Neither ICD-10 nor DSM-IV categorizes malingering as a mental or behavioural disorder. ICD-10 (World Health Organization, 1992) categorizes 'persons feigning illness with obvious motivation' under factors influencing health status and contact with health services. The DSM-IV (American Psychiatric Association, 1994) definition describes malingering as:

> … the intentional production of false or grossly exaggerated physical or psychological problems, motivated by external incentives such as avoiding military duty, avoiding work, obtaining financial compensation, evading criminal prosecution, or obtaining drugs.

This must be distinguished from:

- factitious disorders – the intentional production of symptoms without apparent external incentive or gain, perhaps in order to assume a patient role
- conversion disorders – in which the symptoms are produced unconsciously, without deliberate intent.

There are two dimensions to consider:

- The degree to which the production of symptoms is conscious and deliberate.
- The degree to which the presented symptoms are an exaggeration of true symptoms.

Relatively few cases fall at either extreme of either dimension:

- For example, 64% of US personal injury cases showed atypical performance on psychological testing, suggesting exaggeration if not pure malingering (Heaton *et al.*, 1978).
  - Hay (1983) identified five patients who were diagnosed as malingering out of approximately 12 000 consecutive general psychiatric admissions in Manchester. Four of them went on to develop schizophrenia.
- The number of successful feigners will never be known.

The motivations for malingering are complex, but may involve the wish:

- to mitigate offences and avoid punishment
- to avoid military conscription
- to seek financial gain either through benefits or through civil courts for psychological injury
- to obtain medication or to engineer transfer from prison to hospital
- to avoid repatriation.

In clinical practice the most common reason for exaggeration of symptoms is to gain effective care and treatment. It is best to distinguish this from malingering for other gains.

Resnick (1997) contrasted the typical presentations of malingering and conversion disorder, as shown in Table 4.2.

Table 4.2 Differential diagnosis of malingering and conversion disorder following trauma (Resnick, 1997)

Malingering	Conversion disorder
Suspicious, uncooperative and resentful	Highly cooperative, clinging and dependent
Tries to avoid examination and investigation	Eager for intervention and anxious to be cured
Likely to refuse adapted employment	More likely to accept adapted employment
Likely to give detailed account of the accident and consequences	More likely to give an inaccurate account, with gaps and vague or generalized complaints

Clues to malingered insanity defence (Resnick, 2003) are:

- a non-psychotic, alternative rational motive for the crime
- suspicious or atypical hallucinations or delusions
- current crime fits an established pattern of prior criminal conduct
- absence of active or subtle signs of psychosis during evaluation
- presence of a partner in the crime
- double denial of responsibility (denying crime and also denying responsibility due to psychosis)
- alleged intellectual deficit coupled with alleged psychosis
- alleged illness inconsistent with documented level of functioning.

'Compensation neurosis' is:

- A term introduced to refer to the reported increase in reports of disability following railway accidents in Germany after introduction of compensation laws in 1871.

A commonly quoted paper (Miller, 1961) reported that 48 of 50 patients who had been diagnosed with 'accident neurosis' after head injury recovered without treatment within 2 years of settlement of claim. Many subsequent authors have disputed the implied pejorative conclusion, and many follow-up studies fail to support the hypothesis that clinical outcome is predicted by financial settlement (Resnick, 1997).

Box 4.2 Clinical assessment of the malingering patient
(adapted from Malone and Lange, 2007)

The initial suspicion of malingering is intuitive; clinicians are often reluctant to diagnose malingering, so assessment should be thorough and well documented:

- The key is a very detailed history and mental state examination.
- Use as much collateral information as possible. Sources may include relatives and carers, witness statements, observations of behaviour by nursing staff in hospital, or reports from health-care or custodial staff in prison.

Document in detail an account of any psychopathology, including cognitive assessment if necessary. Use open-ended questions and allow the patient to talk fluently without interruptions. Clarify outstanding issues or details later:

- In malingering, approximate answers are more common, as are 'I don't know' responses, or use of phrases such as 'probably', 'it may have been', 'I'm not sure'.
- The account of symptoms may be exaggerated, or internally inconsistent.
- Look for errors of omission (not having expected cardinal symptoms of the disorder) or errors of commission (symptoms not usually seen in people with the diagnosed condition), or unusual constellations of symptoms.
- Observed presentation or behaviour may not be consistent with the reported symptoms. For example, a person who scores very badly on cognitive testing, but has no observed difficulties in daily activities.
- Look for inconsistencies in presentation over time, adoption of symptoms/signs that other patients report/show and suggestibility of symptoms.
- Look for the source of the malingered symptoms – friend or relative with mental illness, copying of other patient's symptoms.
- Look for suggestibility, by suggesting unlikely symptoms.

Clinical assessment may be supported by structured psychometric tests such as:

- the validity scales of the Multiphasic Personality Inventory-2 (MMPI-2)
- Structured Interview of Reported Symptoms (SIRS), which looks for rare symptoms and unusual clusters of symptoms
- Test of Memory Malingering (TOMM), a test of memory that only appears to be difficult.

The overall aim of assessment should be to gather a detailed picture of the patient, exclude the genuine diagnosis and attempt to ascertain the primary gain sought by the malingerer.

● Confidentiality and Disclosure

Maintaining the confidentiality of a patient's personal information is a legal and ethical duty of all health professionals. So, it seems, is sharing of information. According to the General Medical Council (2009):

> Without assurances of confidentiality patients may be reluctant to seek medical attention or give doctors the information they need to provide good care. But appropriate information sharing is essential to the efficient provision of safe and effective care, both for the individual patient and the wider community of patients.

Disclosure of information without a patient's consent is sometimes necessary:

- When there is a legal obligation to disclose the information.
- When a court orders that the information be shared.
- Disclosure to regulatory bodies (such as the General Medical Council, GMC), tribunals and inquiries.
- When disclosure is in the public interest.

Disclosure in the public interest requires a professional judgement as to whether the benefit or prevention of harm brought by the disclosure outweighs the duty to maintain confidentiality (Box 4.3). Such circumstances include (Royal College of Psychiatrists, 2006):

- where serious harm may come to a third party
- where a doctor believes the patient is a victim of neglect or emotional or physical abuse and disclosure is in the best interests of the patient
- where a doctor is acting in the best interests of a child or young person who is their patient
- where without disclosure the prevention, detection or prosecution of a serious crime would be prejudiced or delayed
- when the doctor's patient is a health professional and they have concerns about fitness to practise
- where a doctor has concerns about a patient's fitness to drive.

In all of the above circumstances there must also be a decision made as to how much information to disclose and to whom. There should always be fully documented evidence of the decision including the balancing exercise that has taken place. It is always best to seek legal advice from your hospital, trust or medical defence organization when making such decisions.

Box 4.3 Disclosure when working with the criminal justice system (CJS)

In working closely with the CJS, the forensic practitioner will regularly encounter situations where they are requested to provide information that is confidential to the patient. These include:

- In court: when preparing a medico-legal report and giving evidence under oath, there is no confidentiality of patient information. Therefore when seeing a defendant for a report this should be clearly explained to them and documented (see Chapter 21).

Otherwise, including at MAPPPs, you must consider whether or not to disclose information in the usual way. Consider the available professional guidance:

- *Confidentiality Guidance for Doctors* (General Medical Council, 2009)
- *Confidentiality and Disclosure of Health Information* (British Medical Association, 1999)
- *Good Psychiatric Practice; Confidentiality and information sharing* (Royal College of Psychiatrists, 2010)
- *Confidentiality: NHS Code of Practice* (Department of Health, 2003).

When in doubt:

- discuss the case with colleagues
- seek legal advice from trust solicitor
- seek advice from your medical defence organization.

Disclosure of third party information

In the process of risk assessment, collateral information is often sought from carers and family members. Such information can be essential for the assessment of the patient's clinical condition and assessment of risk.

As patients and their legal representatives will potentially have access to their notes and any reports prepared, it is essential that any third party information is treated with confidentiality unless the party has consented for it to be disclosed to the patient.

The disclosure of third party information to the patient may:

- put the third party at risk
- damage their relationship with the patient (especially in the case of family members)
- damage the engagement of carers and relatives with the clinical team
- prevent further disclosure of important information.

In all clinical notes and reports such information should be included in a separate section, clearly marked 'third party not for disclosure to the patient'.

● Immigration and Asylum

Around the world migration between countries is growing. The control and social conse-quences of migration are high on the political agenda in many countries. In England and Wales there have been five major Acts of Parliament relating to immigration over the last 10 years (Bacon *et al.*, 2010).

Definitions

Legal immigrants include:

- Refugee: a person who flees their country due to a well-founded belief that they would suffer persecution and who is unwilling or unable to return, so seeks formal refugee status in another country.
- Asylum seekers: someone who has left their country and is seeking formal refugee status, but this has not yet been granted.
- Economic migrants: a person who enters a country for the purpose of employment, with the permission of that country.

Illegal immigrants

- Those who have entered the country without permission.
- Those who breach the conditions under which they have been allowed to stay (such as working on a student visa).
- Those who have committed a criminal offence which means that they no longer have a legal right to remain in the country.

Mental health and the immigrant population

The rate of mental illness is higher among immigrant populations worldwide (Bhugra and Jones, 2001), particularly of anxiety, depression, post-traumatic stress disorder (PTSD), sui-cide and self-harm in refugees and asylum seekers. Porter and Haslam (2005) conducted a meta-analysis of studies comparing refugee populations and control groups, finding that there was an overall increase in psychopathology.

The adversities listed in Table 4.3 are associated with immigration and may be important in leading to increased rates of mental illness (McColl *et al.*, 2008).

Table 4.3 Adversities associated with immigration

Pre-migration adversities	Post-migration adversities
War	Discrimination
Imprisonment	Detention
Genocide	Dispersal destitution
Suffering or witnessing physical and sexual violence	Denial of the right to work
Traumatic bereavement	Denial of health care
Starvation and homelessness	Delayed decisions on asylum applications
Lack of health care	

Implications for forensic services

This population comes into contact with forensic services in the following ways (Bacon *et al.*, 2010):

- *Section 86 repatriation*:
  - Under s86 of the Mental Health Act ('Removal of alien patients'), patients who are detained under either part 2 or 3 of the Act who do not have the right to remain in the UK are repatriated.
  - This is granted by the Secretary of State and it must be deemed to be in the patient's best interests, with the agreement of a mental health tribunal.
- *Restricted hospital order patients*:
  - Those detained under s37/41 may be liable to be deported once they have been granted a conditional discharge.
  - This is in line with Government policy to remove from the country those foreign nationals who may 'cause harm' (whatever their legal status to remain is).
- Prisoners transferred under s48:
  - When people detained (either in prison or detention centres) under immigration legislation become mentally unwell, they may be transferred to a secure hospital under s48.
  - Once recovered, they will be liable to be returned to the place of detention and deported. The process of deportation is slow and health-care facilities in detention centres tend to be poor.

Challenges for forensic services

Assessing and treating patients whose first language is not English can be complicated and prolonged, and requires the use of interpreters who may not be readily available.

Planning the rehabilitation and discharge for a patient whose future in this country is uncertain is difficult. Many failed asylum seekers will have no right to housing or benefits, making community resettlement virtually impossible.

Making the decision that discharge is appropriate with the knowledge of the stress that they may face during the process of detention and deportation poses an ethical dilemma. This means that many patients in this situation are in hospital for prolonged periods.

Liaison with the UK Borders Agency can be difficult. Decisions regarding deportation may be made at the last minute, leaving both the patient and clinical team with uncertainty.

Arranging follow-up for patients who are being returned to their country of origin is problematic. In many counties mental health care is not well structured and the availability of certain drugs such as atypical antipsychotics cannot be assured.

References

American Psychiatric Association. (1994) *Diagnostic and Statistical Manual of Mental Disorders*, 4th edn. Washington DC: APA

Bacon L, Bourne R, Oakley C, Humphreys M. (2010) Immigration policy: implications for mental health services. *Advances in Psychiatric Treatment* **16**, 124–32

Bhugra D, Jones P. (2001) Migration and mental illness. *Advances in Psychiatric Treatment* **7**, 216–23

British Medical Association. (1999) *Confidentiality & Disclosures of Health Information*. London: British Medical Association

Crichton JHM. (2009) Defining high, medium, and low security in forensic mental healthcare: the development of the Matrix of Security in Scotland. *Journal of Forensic Psychiatry and Psychology* **3**, 333–53

*Department of Health. (2003) *Confidentiality: NHS Code of Practice*. London: DH

Department of Health (2008) *Code of Practice. Mental Health Act 1983*. London: The Stationery Office

Drake RE, Xie H, McHugo GJ, Green AI. (2000) The effects of clozapine on alcohol and drug use disorders among patients with schizophrenia. *Schizophrenia Bulletin* **26**(2), 441–9

Durand MA, Lelliott P, Coyle N. (2006) Availability of treatment for substance misuse in medium secure psychiatric care in England. A national survey. *Journal of Forensic Psychiatry and Psychology* **17**(4), 611–25

Exworthy T, Wilson S. (2010) Escapes and absconding from secure psychiatric units. *The Psychiatrist* **34**, 81–2

Foster JH, Onyeukwu C. (2003) The attitudes of forensic nurses to substance using service users. *Journal of Psychiatric and Mental Health Nursing* **10**, 578–84

*General Medical Council. (2009) *Confidentiality*. London: General Medical Council

Gournay K, Benson R, Rogers P. (2008) Inpatient care and management. In: Soothill K, Rogers P, Dolan M (eds), *Handbook of Forensic Mental Health*. Cullompton: Willan Publishing

Gradillas V, Williams A, Walsh E, Fahy T. (2007) Do forensic psychiatric inpatient units pose a risk to local communities? *Journal of Forensic Psychiatry & Psychology* **18**(2), 261–5

Gregg L, Barrowclough C, Haddock G. (2007) Reasons for increased substance use in psychosis. *Clinical Psychology Review* **27**(4), 494–510

Hay GG. (1983) Feigned psychosis – a review of the simulation of mental illness. *British Journal of Psychiatry* **143**, 8–10

Heaton RK, Smith HH, Lehman RAW, Vogt AT. (1978) Prospects for faking believable deficits on neuropsychological testing. *Journal of Clinical and Consulting Psychology* **46**, 892–900

Isherwood S, Brooke D. (2001) Prevalence and severity of substance misuse among referrals to a local forensic service. *Journal of Forensic Psychiatry* **12**, 446–54

Kendall T, Tyrer P, Whittington C, Taylor C. (2011) Assessment and management of psychosis with coexisting substance misuse: summary of NICE guidelines. *British Medical Journal* **342**, d1351

Luty J. (2003) What works in drug addiction? *Advances in Psychiatric Treatment* **9**, 280–8

Maden A, Rutter S, McClintock T, Friendship C, Gunn J. (1999) Outcome of admission to a medium secure psychiatric unit: short and long term outcome. *British Journal of Psychiatry* **175**, 313–16

Main N, Gudjonsson G. (2006) An investigation into the factors that are associated with non-compliance in a mediums secure unit. *Journal of Forensic Psychiatry and Psychology* **17**(2), 171–81

Malone RD, Lange CL. (2007) A clinical approach to the malingering patient. *Journal of the American Academy of Psychoanalysis and Dynamic Psychiatry* **35**(1), 13–21

McColl H, McKenzie K, Bhui K. (2008) Mental healthcare of asylum-seekers and refugees. *Advances in Psychiatric Treatment* **14**, 452–9

McMurran M. (2002) *Dual Diagnosis of Mental Disorder and Substance Misuse*. NHS National Programme on Forensic Mental Health Research and Development

Miller H. (1961) Accident neurosis. *British Medical Journal* **i**, 919–25

National Confidential Inquiry (2009) National Confidential Inquiry into suicide and homicide by people with mental illness, Annual Report July 2009. Available at: http://www.medicine.manchester.ac.uk/psychiatry/research/suicide/prevention/nci/inquiry_reports/

National Institute for Health and Clinical Excellence. (2007a) *Drug Misuse: Psychosocial interventions*. Accessed using: http://guidance.nice.org.uk/CG51

National Institute for Health and Clinical Excellence. (2007b) *Drug Misuse: Opioid detoxification*. Accessed using: http://guidance.nice.org.uk/CG52

National Patient Safety Agency. (2010) *National Reporting and Learning Service. Never Events Framework: Update for 2010/11.* Available at: http://www.nrls.npsa.nhs.uk

Porter M, Haslam N. (2005) Pre-displacement and post-displacement factors associated with the mental health of refugees and internally displaced persons: a meta-analysis. *Journal of the American Medical Association* **294**, 602–12

Rask M, Halberg IR (2000) Forensic psychiatric nursing care: nurses apprehension of their responsibility and work content. *Journal of Psychiatric and Mental Health Nursing* **7**(2), 163–77

Resnick PJ. (1997) Malingering of post traumatic disorders. In: Rogers R (ed.) *Clinical Assessment of Malingering and Deception.* New York: Guilford Press

Resnick PJ. (2003) Malingering. In: Rosner R (ed), *Principles and Practice of Forensic Psychiatry,* 2nd edn. London: Hodder Arnold

Royal College of Psychiatrists. (2006) *Good Psychiatric Practice: Confidentiality and information sharing.* London: Royal College of Psychiatrists

*Royal College of Psychiatrists (2010) *Good Psychiatric Practice: Confidentiality and information sharing,* 2nd edn. College Report CR160. London: Royal College of Psychiatrists

Swartz MS, Wagner HR, Swanson JW, Stroup TS, McEvoy JP, Canive JM *et al.* (2006) Substance misuse in persons with schizophrenia: baseline prevalence and correlates from the NIMH CATIE study. *Journal of Nervous and Mental Disease* **194**, 164–72

Times, The. (2008) Security fears as 116 mentally ill criminals escape in a year. Available at: http://www.thetimes.co.uk/tto/health/article1882360.ece

Weaver T, Madden P, Charles V, Stimson G, Renton A, Tyrer P *et al.* (2003) Comorbidity of substance misuse and mental illness in community mental health and substance misuse services. *British Journal of Psychiatry* **183**, 304–13

Weinstein HC. (2002) Ethics issues in security hospitals. *Behaviour Science and the Law* **20**, 443–61

World Health Organization. (1992) *International Classification of Diseases (ICD-10),* 10th revision. Geneva: WHO

5

Leaving Secure Care and Community Follow-up

The care pathway for patients in secure care varies according to the clinical needs of the patient and the local configuration of services:

- Patients in high security rarely move directly out of secure care.
- Patients in medium security often move directly into the community or to non-secure hospital placements:
  - some move into low security, and it may be that the proportion who do so will increase over the coming years as commissioners increasingly focus on throughput, at the expense of continuity of care.
- Patients in low security generally move directly into community placements.

● Who Can Discharge a Detained Patient?

There are five bodies that can discharge a detained patient, depending on the patient's status (Table 5.1):

- responsible clinician (RC)
- nearest relative (NR):
  - defined by s26 of the Mental Health Act (MHA), but the MHA 2007 enables patients to apply to the county court to specify who should act as NR

Table 5.1 Rights to discharge detained patients

Section	Who can discharge?
Section 3	RC at any time, by order made in writing NR must give 72 hours notice of intention to discharge. This is blocked if the RC provides a report to the hospital managers certifying that if discharged the patient 'would be likely to act in a manner dangerous to other persons or himself' (s25) An application to the tribunal or the hospital managers may be made by the patient or the NR
Section 37	As section 3 except: – the NR has no power to discharge – the patient or the NR may apply to the tribunal, but not during the first period (6 months) of detention
Restricted patients	The power to discharge, either conditionally or absolutely, lies with the Secretary of State for Justice (SoSJ) or the tribunal The SoSJ may also revoke a s41, leaving the patient detained under an unrestricted s37. For transferred prisoners, discharge from detention under the MHA generally leads to remission to prison (see Box 5.2 in relation to rehabilitation of indeterminate prisoners)

Box 5.1 Returning a patient to prison

See http://www.justice.gov.uk/guidance/mentally-disordered-offenders.htm for guidance.

To satisfy s50 or s51 MHA, the RC (or a Tribunal) must notify the Secretary of State that:

- the patient 'no longer requires treatment in hospital for mental disorder', or
- '... no effective treatment for his disorder can be given in the hospital to which he has been removed'.

Under usual circumstances a transferred prisoner is returned to the same prison from which they came. The Ministry of Justice (MoJ) requires:

- a s117 meeting to have been held with the prison mental health team, unless there are exceptional circumstances, usually related to risk or serious management problems
- the name and contact details of someone in the prison who can confirm that the prison is prepared to accept the patient.

In most cases remission to prison can be arranged in collaboration with the patient:

- This allows the patient to organize final visits and deal with those belongings that they will not be able to take back to prison.
- Some patients may need greater support during this period, and there may be an increased risk of self-harm, non-compliance with care and attempted escape.
- Occasionally, where these risks are very significant, it is necessary to arrange remission to prison without informing the patient.

- hospital managers:
    - the managers' panel must consist of at least three individuals appointed by the board, none of whom are employees or executives of the trust
- First Tier Tribunal (see below)
    - the most common route for restricted patients
- Secretary of State for Justice (SoSJ).

In contrast to a tribunal, the RC or SoSJ have no statutory criteria to consider when discharging a patient.

While the MoJ seeks to encourage applications for discharge of restricted patients, and

Box 5.2 Discharging an indeterminate sentenced prisoner to the community

Not infrequently it is decided that, because of an individual's mental health needs, it is not appropriate for them to return to prison:

- A patient serving a determinate sentence usually must wait until their parole eligibility date (PED), when the restrictions will automatically end and they are detained under a 'notional section 37'. Then the RC may discharge them when clinically appropriate.
- For an indeterminate sentenced prisoner there is no equivalent date on which their restrictions end, so a discharge by the tribunal would lead to remission to prison.

In these latter cases, the prisoner must first apply to the tribunal, and then if they are successful the Parole Board will consider releasing them on licence:

- The tribunal decides whether the patient would be entitled to discharge if they were subject to a restriction order (rather than a restriction direction) and notifies the SoSJ of this (see s74 MHA).
- The tribunal may recommend that if he is not discharged by the SoSJ, then he should remain in hospital rather than be remitted to prison.
- On the strength of this, the prisoner may apply to the Parole Board to be released on life licence.
- Navigating the bureaucracies of first the tribunal and then the Parole Board tends to take many months.

The patient is then supervised by the probation service on life licence, the MHA restrictions having ended with the end of their prison sentence or hospital admission.

there has been some recent increase in discharges, the majority are still dealt with by the tribunal. Data for 2008 showed that, of a total of 1255 discharges of restricted patients (Ministry of Justice, 2010):

- 74 patients were conditionally discharged by the SoSJ
- 333 patients were conditionally discharged by the tribunal
- 14 patients were given an absolute discharge without first being conditionally discharged
- 357 s48 patients were disposed of by the court to prison (296) or the community (61)
- 186 remained in hospital without restrictions
- 233 were remitted to prison as sentenced (167) or unsentenced (66) prisoners
- 34 died.

The clinical process of discharging a patient to the community is no different from other inpatient settings:

- S117 places a statutory duty on health agencies and social services authorities to provide aftercare to all patients who have been detained under ss3, 37, 45A, 47 and 48.

● The First Tier Tribunal (Mental Health)

The Tribunals, Courts and Enforcement Act 2007 abolished most existing tribunals, combining them into a single generic First Tier Tribunal:

Box 5.3 Some issues to consider at a 'section 117 meeting'

Clinical matters:
- Ensure that accommodation is secure, utilities are turned on, and necessary furniture and appliances are present and functional.
- Ensure that benefits are in place.
- Clarify weekly structure of activities, social network and personal support.
- Supply of medication prescribed and/or dispensed.
- Ensure that patient has contact numbers for hospital or care team.
- Have they registered with a GP?

Future care:
- Ensure that risk assessment and management plan are up to date.
- Ensure that relapse prevention plan is agreed.
- Has the patient made an advance directive in relation to future treatment?
- Identify the hospital to which they should be recalled.

Care programme approach and legal matters:
- Identification of care coordinator.
- Identification of social supervisor and clinical supervisor for restricted patients.
- Dates of first appointments, and initial frequency of contact with each mental health professional.
- Clarification of the conditions of a conditional discharge or of supervised community treatment (SCT).
- Is there any requirement to register with the police (as a sex offender, for example)?
- Completion of clinical discharge paperwork.

Notification of other agencies:
- community care team
- GP
- Ministry of Justice
- probation or multi-agency public protection arrangement
- accommodation provider.

- The First Tier Tribunal is itself separated into six chambers.
- The First Tier Tribunal (Mental Health) sits within the Health, Education and Social Care Chamber.
- Appeals from the First Tier Tribunal are heard by the Upper Tribunal.

Procedure is governed by the Tribunal Procedure (First Tier Tribunal) (Health, Education and Social Care Chamber) Rules 2008, SI2008/2699.

The First Tier Tribunal hears applications and referrals:

- An application is made by the detained patient, or sometimes by their nearest relative:
  - in general, a patient may appeal once during each period of detention, but
  - for both s37 and s37/41, there is no right of appeal in the first 6 months, so an application may be made in the second 6 months, and then annually
  - a conditionally discharged patient may make an application to the Tribunal (seeking an absolute discharge) within 12 and 24 months after the conditional discharge, and then once in every 2 years.
- The hospital managers or the Secretary of State (depending on whether it is a restricted case) have a duty to refer cases to the tribunal:
  - every 3 years, if no application has otherwise been made
  - as soon as possible after revocation of a community treatment order (CTO)
  - within 1 month of a conditionally discharged patient being admitted to hospital consequent to recall. The hearing must be held between 5 and 8 weeks after receipt of the referral.

The Tribunal has the power:

- to order the discharge of a detained patient or a patient subject to SCT
- to recommend:
  - leave of absence
  - transfer to another hospital
  - that the RC considers SCT (in an unrestricted case), and if no order is made the tribunal may reconvene and reconsider the case.

The First Tier Tribunal does not have the power to:

- vary the conditions of SCT.

Mohan *et al.* (1998) reported that 86% of tribunals considering a restricted patient detained in medium security agreed with the recommendation of the registered medical officer (RMO).

Decisions may be appealed on a point of law. In the first instance the First Tier Tribunal considers whether to review its own decision. It may:

- correct accidental errors
- amend reasons
- set the decision aside, and either re-decide it, or refer to the Upper Tribunal to decide
- if no action is taken and permission to appeal to the Upper Tribunal is denied, then notification of the right to apply for permission to appeal to the Upper Tribunal must be given.

Types of discharge and criteria for discharge by the tribunal

In all cases the tribunal has a discretionary power to discharge the patient, but in addition it must discharge the patient if it is not satisfied as to the statutory criteria provided in s72:

- S72 sets out separate criteria for those detained under s2, those detained under other sections and those subject to SCT.

For patients detained other than under s2, including restricted patients, the criteria are:

- that he is suffering from mental disorder of a nature or degree that makes it appropriate for him to be liable to be detained in a hospital for medical treatment
- that it is necessary for the health or safety of the patient or for the protection of other persons that he should receive such treatment
- that appropriate medical treatment is available for him.

A restricted patient must be absolutely discharged if the tribunal is:

- not satisfied on these criteria, and
- 'satisfied that it is not appropriate for the patient to remain liable to recall to hospital for further treatment'.

Otherwise the patient must be conditionally discharged:

- So the default position is that a restricted patient is conditionally rather than absolutely discharged in the first instance.

The Tribunal cannot comment on the legitimacy of the original detention. The role is limited to the review of the detention criteria at the time of the hearing.
    The effect of a conditional discharge is that:

- the patient may be recalled to hospital by the SoSJ, then becoming detained again under s37/41
- the patient is required to comply with such conditions as are imposed, which may be varied by the SoSJ at any time
- conditions commonly imposed include:
    - to reside at a specified address or where instructed by their social supervisor or RC
    - to allow access to, and/or attend appointments with, mental health professionals
    - to comply with medication and other treatments offered
    - to have no direct or indirect contact with named individuals
    - to abide by a defined exclusion zone
    - to comply with drug testing or not to take drugs.

For restricted patients a tribunal can defer a direction for conditional discharge 'until such arrangements as appear to be necessary to the Tribunal for that purpose have been made':

- In practice, a deferred conditional discharge enables the final pieces of the discharge care plan to be put in place. Then the RC notifies the tribunal in writing, and the tribunal confirms the discharge without any need for a further hearing.
- Deferment cannot be used as a strategy to allow further improvement in mental state or further assessment, on leave, for example.
- If the patient's mental health deteriorates or the necessary arrangements are not made within a reasonable time frame then the tribunal can review or reopen the case.

Section 72(3) provides that a tribunal can delay a discharge to a specified future date, usually for the post-discharge care package to be organized.

The tribunal hearing

The tribunal panel consists of three individuals:

- Legal member:
    - is Chair of the panel
    - ensures proceedings are conducted fairly and clarifies any issues of law
    - may be a solicitor or, in restricted cases, a judge.

Box 5.4 Writing a report for the First Tier Tribunal

Before completing your report ensure that you have discussed the case with the authors of the other statutory reports. In most cases, given that you are working as a team, the reports should be in agreement. If there are areas of disagreement it is best to realize these in advance.

A tribunal is a court-like body operating according to a legal paradigm. So, as with other reports for courts, it is important to adopt a legalistic approach. It is also helpful to explain symptoms in normal English words, though remember that the members of the tribunal generally have considerable experience of mental health, particularly the medical member.

The report for the tribunal hearing should focus on the information that the tribunal requires in order to decide whether or not the patient needs to remain in hospital. So, a good starting point is to use the statutory criteria for discharge.

Mental disorder:

- Give the diagnosis/diagnoses and establish it by reference to the characteristic symptoms and signs.
- What investigations or observations support your diagnosis?
- How certain is the diagnosis? Are there any atypical features?
- Are there any differing opinions now, or in the past?

Nature [of mental disorder] 'refers to the particular mental disorder … its chronicity, its prognosis and the patient's previous response to receiving treatment …' (*R v MHRT for the South Thames Region Ex p. Smith* [1999] C.O.D. 148):

- This is about the characteristics of the disorder: how long they have suffered from it, has it been persistent or remitting and relapsing, what is the future course likely to be, what effect does it have on the individual, what alleviating or exacerbating factors can be identified and what effect are they likely to have?

Degree [of mental disorder] 'refers to the current manifestations of the disorder' (as above):

- The current symptoms, and their intensity and impact on the patient's function. May include consequent likelihood of risk behaviours – especially, but not only, self-harm and harm to others.
- The level of insight that the patient has into their current illness.

Appropriate for him to be liable to be detained in hospital for medical treatment:

- Detention must be proportionate to the risks involved

Treatment in hospital is necessary:

- Why is hospital treatment required? Why can't the treatment be offered on an outpatient basis?
- Why would options other than detention not contain the risks?
- It may be appropriate to refer to past engagement with treatment in the community.

For the health or safety of the patient or for the protection of other persons:

- Consider previous risk behaviours, the impact of current treatment and the likelihood of future high-risk situations.

Appropriate medical treatment is available:

- Defined as 'medical treatment which is appropriate in his case, taking into account the nature and degree of the mental disorder and all other circumstances of his case' [s3(4) MHA].
- Medical treatment 'includes nursing, psychological intervention and specialist mental health habilitation, rehabilitation and care' [s145 (1)]; 'the purpose of which is to alleviate, or prevent a worsening of, the disorder or … its symptoms or manifestations' [s145(4)].
- These sections create a very broad definition, reflecting the approach always taken by the courts.

Particularly for restricted cases there may be a significant delay between preparing a report and the hearing. If so, it is appropriate to prepare an addendum close to the date of the hearing.

- Ensure that this is submitted at least 3 weeks before the hearing, so the MoJ has an opportunity to respond to is contents.

- Medical member:
  - a consultant psychiatrist, who advises the Tribunal on medical matters
  - required, in advance of the hearing, to 'examine the patient … to form an opinion of the patient's mental condition'
  - this leads to a problematic dual role, the medical member perhaps acting as both an expert witness to the tribunal and also a decision-maker (Richardson and Machin, 2000a). The medical member should keep an open mind about detention, and should not give an opinion to the panel prior to the hearing (*R v MHRT, ex p S* [2002] EWHC 2522)
  - however, the evidence is that, in practice, the medical member usually acts according to clinical criteria, that they often give an opinion to the Tribunal in advance of the hearing, and that the Tribunal's decision usually follows the medical member's opinion (Richardson and Machin, 2000a,b).
- Lay member:
  - neither medically nor legally qualified
  - often with experience in social care or welfare.

Tribunal hearings are usually held in private, unless the patient requests a public hearing and the tribunal is satisfied that it would not be contrary to the patient's interests. The victims of those detained under the MHA have a statutory right to make representations to the Tribunal about conditions that should be attached to a discharge (see Chapter 17 for further details).

There are no statutory time limits for holding a hearing, except for s2 (within 7 days of the application) and for referrals following recall of a conditionally discharged patient:

- Adjournments and cancellations are common, adjournments on the day of the hearing having increased from 1% in 2001 to 25% in 2005. Reasons were split equally between availability of reports and attendance:
  - Reports are now required within 21 days of the application.

Box 5.5 Giving oral evidence in the tribunal

Before the hearing:
- Make sure that you have discussed the report with the patient. It is important to assess the patient close to the date of the tribunal – you are likely to be asked when you last saw the patient.
- Ensure that the patient is prepared for the proceedings and supported by nursing staff or advocate.
- Reread your report and the other reports, including any independent reports that have been submitted. Particularly consider any disagreements and how these should be presented or resolved.

Tribunal hearings should have minimal formality, and there is no prescribed procedure, except that the patient should have the last word. A common sequence is:
- for the medical member to summarize their findings on examination
- the evidence of the RC is often taken next, usually by way of being asked to bring the tribunal up to date with the patient's further progress since the written report was prepared
- then each member of the tribunal will have the opportunity to ask questions in turn, followed by the patient (or their representative)
- expect to be asked how long you have known the patient and when you last saw them
- the Chair is likely to be writing notes, so as in other courts speak slowly and clearly and watch.

The social worker's evidence tends to be taken second, followed by the nurse:
- Most often the medical member leads on questioning the RC and the lay member leads on questioning the social worker.

Finally the patient's solicitor takes evidence from the patient, before giving a closing argument setting out exactly what the patient is asking of the tribunal and seeking to justify this. The witnesses and applicant then leave the room to allow the panel to reach a decision.

The decision is usually delivered orally on the day, and must be given in writing within 7 days.

● Forensic Psychiatric Care in the Community

Three service models are often described (Mohan *et al.*, 2004)

- Parallel:
  - Forensic services provide a complete service for forensic patients. On leaving secure care the patient remains under the care of the forensic service, with no involvement from general psychiatric services.
  - In practice all parallel services must pass some patients back to general services before discharge, at discharge or after a period in the community, to avoid becoming overcommitted.
- Integrated:
  - Forensic mental health professionals work within general psychiatric teams, sharing the team base and offering a single point of contact for referrals.
- Hybrid:
  - Some parallel care is provided, but with opportunities for joint working in order to smooth the transition for patients moving from one service to the other.

In practice, services have developed according to local need and preference, with little central direction:

- Judge *et al.* (2004) identified 37 UK community forensic teams: 26 responded to their survey, of which 20 operated a parallel service.
- It is likely that the picture has changed considerably in the years since then, a hybrid model becoming increasingly common.

Advantages of parallel teams include (see also Mohan *et al.*, 2004; Snowden *et al.*, 1999):

- greater continuity of care
- detailed longitudinal knowledge of the patient
- development of expertise in managing forensic patients
- peer support and supervision tailored to managing high-risk patients
- better follow-up across geographical districts
- better links with the criminal justice system (CJS).

Advantages of integrated teams include:

- reduced stigmatization of the patient
- less duplication of services
- general teams that may develop some skills in managing high-risk cases
- easier passage of patient between services
- better access to local community resources.

What characterizes a forensic community service?

Forensic community teams should:

- provide flexibility and responsivity, as opposed to the intensity provided by assertive outreach teams (AOTs)
- use a multidisciplinary teamworking approach
- have a pervasive sensitivity to risk and a detailed understanding of each patient's risk formulation
- work closely with CJS agencies, and be comfortable within a CJS setting.

What are the characteristics of forensic community patients?

In the early days of regional forensic psychiatric services Higgins (1981) distinguished two groups of forensic patient with different care pathways:

- Integrated patients:
  - well known to general psychiatric service, admitted during an acute episode of psychosis, on a civil or unrestricted section
  - to be returned in due course to general psychiatric service.
- Parallel patients:
  - had had fewer contacts with general psychiatric service, were admitted from prison or high security and were usually restricted
  - likely to remain under forensic community care.

An observational study of patients discharged from medium secure care (Coid *et al.*, 2007) reported the following:

- Compared with those discharged to general psychiatric care, forensic community patients were:
  - older
  - had more serious offences
  - were more likely to have a diagnosis of personality disorder
  - had fewer previous hospital admissions
  - were more likely to be subject to restrictions and more likely to adhere to treatment during initial period in community
  - were less likely to die from natural causes (no difference in suicide rate).
- There was no difference in rate of reconviction or rate of rehospitalization, but those managed by forensic services had a shorter time to re-conviction for a violent offence.

Any parallel or hybrid service must have a mechanism to hand patients back to general psychiatric services. Otherwise the forensic caseload will simply continue to increase.

Dowsett (2005) reviewed a forensic community caseload, and considered that:

- some had been stable for a sustained period, and could be handed back to generic services
- others relapsed often but were manageable on a general acute ward
- a third group had paramount criminogenic needs; for Dowsett, this was the group that forensic services should concentrate on.

Others (Turner and Salter, 2005) persuasively argue against attempting to treat criminality as such and question whether there is any role for forensic community teams.

Patients should not be cast as, dispositionally as it were, 'forensic'. Rather, some patients need the particular service provided by a forensic community team at certain times. The most crucial period is following discharge into the community:

- For many, continuity of care with a detailed knowledge of the patient's illness and risk is the essential medium through which risk is effectively managed.

In this context, it may be that Higgin's typology has some value:

- Some patients, previously well known to a general psychiatric team, perhaps with a relatively less serious offence, may be best passed back to general services.
- Patients without previous contact with general psychiatric services, and perhaps with the most serious offences, may be best cared for by the forensic team in the first instance.

Sahota *et al.* (2009) compared patients discharged from medium secure care to general and forensic community teams. They did not demonstrate significant differences in the clinical and criminal characteristics of the two groups. Among those followed up by a forensic service, they found:

- an increased (though statistically not significant) proportion were reconvicted
- a significant reduction in the time to reconviction.

Community follow-up of conditionally discharged patients

The community care of a conditionally discharged patient is overseen by the MoJ. The sole concern of the Mental Health Unit (MHU) is to carry out the Secretary of State's statutory responsibilities:

- To authorize transfer from prison to hospital.
- To consider recommendations from RCs for leave, discharge and transfer of inpatients.
- To prepare the Secretary of State's statements for tribunals.
- To monitor the progress of conditionally discharged patients and to consider:
  - variation of the conditions
  - recall
  - absolute discharge.

The MHU produces guidance documents, all available from www.justice.gov.uk/guidance/mentally-disordered-offenders.htm, in particular the Guidance for Clinical Supervisors.

The MHU maintains oversight primarily through periodic reports provided by clinical and social supervisors at intervals determined by the MHU:

- The standard frequency is within 1 month of discharge, and then every 3 months.
- A clinical supervisor is not expected to submit a report without seeing the patient:
  - so the clinical supervisor is expected to see the patient at least every 3 months.
- All reports should be copied to the social supervisor (and vice versa).
- At least an annual review by both supervisors is expected.

It is expected that the social supervisor has more frequent contact than the clinical supervisor:

- Weekly for 1 month after discharge, reducing to a minimum of monthly as clinically appropriate.

The MoJ has no power to prevent a patient going abroad on holiday, but expects:

- the patient to discuss any such proposal with the clinical team and for it to be put to the MHU in advance
- a careful risk assessment to have taken place.

Recall to hospital

Section 42(3) of the MHA 1983 provides that the Secretary of State 'may at any time … in respect of a patient who has been conditionally discharged … by warrant recall the patient to such hospital as may be specified in the warrant'.

- There are no statutory criteria that must be satisfied.
- Breach of the conditions of a conditional discharge does not automatically trigger a recall:
  - but should lead to a review and consideration of necessary action.
- A deterioration in mental state is not required:
  - deprivation of liberty must be based on 'objective medical evidence' (*Winterwerp* v *Netherlands* [1979] 2 EHRR 387) of mental disorder to avoid engaging Article 5(1), except in emergency cases

---

Box 5.6 Reviewing conditionally discharged patients

It is expected that the patient is seen, at least some of the time, in their own home:

- This provides a better, more naturalistic opportunity to evaluate mental state and functioning, and develop an understanding of their lifestyle and social network.
- It is always helpful to carry out joint reviews with the social supervisor or community psychiatric nurse.
- You must be particularly aware of personal safety issues.
- Try to look around the accommodation.
- Try to gain collateral information from carers.

There is an important balance to be struck between maintaining a therapeutic relationship and policing the patient in the interests of public protection. This is particularly difficult to manage within a patient's own home:

- Always be respectful of the patient's home – ask where to sit, ask if they would be good enough to turn off the television.
- Pay attention to the patient's priorities, particularly social and financial issues.
- You must always adequately cover mental state, asking specifically about early warning signs and idiosyncratic symptoms of mental illness.
- You must always ask about medication and assess their likely concordance/adherence.
- You must ensure that you deal with risk issues, asking about issues relevant to the case such as weapon carrying, incidents of loss temper or frustration, problems in relationships and so on.

Anecdotally, many forensic psychiatrists have had cases of a community patient who has been stable for a long time before committing another offence apparently out of the blue:

- Perhaps the team has started to relax a little.
- Perhaps the patient is always very inviting and hospitable on home visits, which become slightly too comfortable and 'social'.
- It might start to feel wrong to ask important risk questions and the balance between therapeutic relationship and policing is lost.

Issues that must be reported to the Mental Health Unit:

- Withdrawal of cooperation with medication.
- Actual/potential risk to the public.
- Loss of contact or cooperation with supervision.
- Admission of the patient to hospital voluntarily or under a civil section.
- If a patient is accused, charged or convicted of a serious offence.
- If a patient's relatives or carer expresses concern.

- however, the Secretary of State has to balance the rights of the patient along with the need to protect the public (*R* v *Secretary of State for the Home Department, ex p K* [1990] 3 All ER 562)
- therefore the MHU will always seek evidence from the clinical supervisor that the patient is currently mentally disordered, but this is not an absolute requirement.

A conditionally discharged patient may:

- be admitted to hospital voluntarily:
  - recall will usually follow if they are in hospital for 'more than a few weeks' (Ministry of Justice, 2009)
- be detained under a civil section:
  - they will then be recalled.

A conditionally discharged patient who has committed an offence may be dealt with by the CJS. If they are imprisoned, the MoJ usually waits until they are to be released before considering whether to recall to hospital or not.

Box 5.7 Recalling a patient

The MHU runs an on-call system and can be contacted by telephone 24 hours a day to discuss urgent matters such as recall. It is reasonable to discuss a case with the MHU if you are uncertain whether a recall is necessary. The central issues that you will be asked about are whether there is:

- evidence of an increase in risk and
- evidence of a deterioration in mental state – is the patient currently mentally disordered?

A warrant can be issued immediately on the strength of a telephone conversation, which provides sufficient authority for the patient to be detained and brought to hospital under s18 of the MHA:

- The warrant provides authority to the police to assist, though does not impose a duty on them to do so.
- Any such telephone discussion with the MoJ should be followed up in writing at your earliest opportunity.

The patient can be recalled to a different hospital from the one from which they were discharged. It is important always to be clear about which is the appropriate hospital for recall in a particular case.

References

Coid JW, Hickey N, Yang M. (2007) Comparison of outcomes following after-care from forensic and general adult psychiatric services. *British Journal of Psychiatry* **190**(6), 509–14

Dowsett J. (2005) Measurement of risk by a community forensic mental health team. *Psychiatric Bulletin* **29**(1), 9–12

Higgins J. (1981) 'Four years' experience of an interim secure unit. *British Medical Journal* **282**, 889–93

Judge J, Harty MA, Fahy T. (2004) Survey of community forensic psychiatry services in England and Wales. *Journal of Forensic Psychiatry and Psychology* **15**(2), 244–53

*Ministry of Justice. (2009) *Guidance for Clinical Supervisors*. Available at: http://www.justice.gov.uk/guidance/docs/guidance-for-clinical-supervisors-0909.pdf

Ministry of Justice. (2010) *Statistics of Mentally Disordered Offenders 2008 England & Wales*. Available at: http://www.justice.gov.uk/publications/mentally-disordered-offenders.htm

Mohan D, Murray K, Steed P, Mullee M. (1998) Mental Health Review Tribunal decisions in restricted hospital order cases at one medium secure unit, 1992–1996. *Criminal Behaviour and Mental Health* **8**, 57–65

Mohan R, Slade M, Fahy T. (2004) Clinical characteristics of community forensic mental health services. *Psychiatric Services* **55**, 1294–8

Richardson G, Machin M. (2000a) Doctors on tribunals: a confusion of roles. *British Journal of Psychiatry* **176**, 110–15

Richardson G, Machin M. (2000b) Judicial review and tribunal decision making: a study of the Mental Health Review Tribunal. *Public Law* **Autumn**, 494–514

Sahota S, Davies S, Duggan C, Clarke M. (2009) The fate of medium secure patients discharged to generic or specialized services. *Journal of Forensic Psychiatry and Psychology* **20**(1), 74–84

Snowden P, McKenna J, Jasper A. (1999) Management of conditionally discharged patients and others who represent similar risks in the community: integrated or parallel. *Journal of Forensic Psychiatry* **10**(3), 583–96

Turner T, Salter M. (2005) What is the role of a forensic community mental health team? *Psychiatric Bulletin* **29**(9), 352

6

Risk of Violence Assessment

Although this chapter only considers risk of violence, the principles may be applied to the risk of any other behaviour. Assessing risk among sex offenders is considered further in Chapter 13, and among adolescents in Chapter 12.

The World Health Organization (1996) defines violence as:

... the intentional use of physical force or power, threatened or actual, against oneself, another person, or against a group or community, that either results in or has a high likelihood of resulting in injury, death, psychological harm, maldevelopment, or deprivation

It may be subdivided into:

- self-directed violence
- interpersonal violence
- collective violence (perpetrated by groups of people).

This chapter is concerned with interpersonal violence. Many typologies have been proposed, which usually distinguish between violence that is, variously:

- premeditated, planned, instrumental or predatory, and
- impulsive, affective or reactive.

While this dichotomous classification has some heuristic value, it is often too simple to do justice to clinical assessments.

● Approaches to Risk of Violence Assessment in Clinical Practice

Maden (2007) describes three approaches to risk (of violence) assessment:

- unstructured clinical assessment (UCA)
- actuarial risk assessment (ARA)
- structured clinical assessment (SCA), sometimes known as structured professional judgement (SPJ).

SCA is described as providing the right balance between UCA and ARA. This is a somewhat false trichotomy because:

- UCA really exists only as the antithesis of ARA in the minds of those ideologically wedded to the latter:
  - no one ever maintained that a deliberate lack of structure was the best approach to risk assessment.

- The distinction between ARA and SCA is not absolute:
  - actuarial risk assessment instruments (ARAIs) require clinical judgements about the presence of some factors
  - SCA instruments may be used to produce statistical probabilities (the HCR-20, for example).
- Both SCA and ARA depend on the identification of factors that are associated with, or which predict, violence. The factors are the same for both.

Box 6.1 gives examples of violence risk assessment instruments.

Box 6.1 Examples of violence risk assessment instruments

HCR-20 (Webster *et al.*, 1997)

This is the most commonly used risk assessment instrument in the UK. It provides a framework for a SCA approach, based on 20 evidence-based risk factors. The risk factors are separated into 10 historical factors:

- previous violence
- young age at first violence
- relationship instability
- employment problems
- substance misuse
- major mental illness
- psychopathy
- early maladjustment
- personality disorder (PD)
- prior supervision failure

five clinical factors (relating to current functioning):

- lack of insight
- negative attitudes
- active symptoms of major mental illness
- impulsivity
- unresponsive to treatment

and five risk management items (relating to predictions about the future):

- plans lack feasibility
- exposure to destabilizers
- lack of personal support
- non-compliance with remediation attempts
- stress.

PCL-R (Hare, 2003)

The most widely researched instrument, originally developed in order to provide a reliable method of ascertaining the presence of psychopathy to enable brain research. The PCL-R assesses the degree to which an individual matches an archetypal construct based on the cases described by Cleckley (1976):

- glibness or superficial charm
- grandiose sense of self-worth
- proneness to boredom
- pathological lying
- conning or manipulative
- lack of remorse or guilt
- shallow affect
- callous/lack of empathy
- parasitic lifestyle

- poor behavioural controls
- promiscuous sexual behaviour
- early behavioural problems
- lack of realistic long-term goals
- impulsivity
- irresponsibility
- failure to accept responsibility
- many short-term relationships
- juvenile delinquency
- revocation of conditional release
- criminal responsibility.

Psychopathy, the PCL-R and the PCL-SV screening tool are discussed in more detail in Chapter 9.

VRAG (Quinsey *et al.*, 1998)

This was validated on 600 male offenders discharged from a Canadian high security hospital. So, only patients who had been judged fit for discharge were included. Twelve items are scored positively or negatively, to assign individual into one of nine risk categories with an associated risk of violent reoffending over 7 years.

In simple statistical terms, it is perhaps the most accurate instrument, and has been researched in various populations, including UK psychiatric patients.

Positive association with violence:

- elementary school maladjustment
- history of alcohol abuse problems
- never married
- non-violent offence history
- failure on prior conditional release
- severity of victim injury
- personality disorder
- PCL-R score.

Negative association with violence:

- lived with parents to age 16
- older age at index offence
- female victim
- schizophrenia.

OASys

Developed by the National Offender Management Service (NOMS) in the UK, and routinely used by probation and prisons, both to inform sentencing and for sentence planning. It is discussed in more detail in Chapter 17:

- offending history
- current offence
- accommodation
- education, training and employability
- financial management and income
- lifestyle and associates
- relationships
- drug and alcohol misuse
- thinking and behavior
- attitude towards offending
- emotional factors.

OGRS-3 (Howard, 2009)

A strictly actuarial tool developed from the Offender Assessment System which uses a minimum number of factors to produce a likelihood of reoffending for that group of offenders with a similar score. It requires only:

- age
- gender
- current offence
- number of previous cautions/convictions
- time since first caution/conviction.

More recently adjunctive risk assessment tools that look at protective factors have been developed, to be used as part of a SCA approach. These tools may offer more balance in risk assessment, which may better promote collaborative risk assessment with the patient. Examples include:

- Short-Term Assessment of Risk and Treatability (START):
  - a 20-item dynamic risk assessment tool designed to evaluate 7 clinical risk domains: violence to others; suicide; self-harm; self-neglect; unauthorized absence; substance use; victimization.
- Structured Assessment of Protective Factors for violence risk (SAPROF):
  - designed to be used in conjunction with, for example, the HCR-20.

● Actuarial Risk Assessment

The actuarial approach has been appropriated from the insurance industry, where it is used to pool risk, in other words to replace the inevitable uncertainty of individual outcomes with a relative certainty of group outcomes:

- In the group, individually unpredictable bad outcomes are balanced by individually unpredictable good outcomes.
- At first sight this offers little benefit to a clinician seeking to manage individual patients.

In the psychiatric and psychological literature, actuarial has come to be used more loosely (Buchanan, 1999), as a term for assigning a numerical risk:

- either to an individual patient (using correlation data based on regression analyses)
- or to a group to which an individual is assigned.

Actuarial risk assessment is deliberately atheoretical, being solely based on observed associations with no attempt to understand cause:

- Proponents would argue that this is its strength, causal hypotheses of uncertain validity necessarily sometimes leading to error.
- In contrast the idea of cause is key to clinical risk assessment.

Describing predictive accuracy of actuarial risk assessment

The predictive accuracy of ARA instruments (ARAIs) may be assessed using a variety of statistics, all with their advantages and disadvantages. Singh and Fazel (2010) discuss these further in a metareview.

Receiver operator characteristics (ROC) and the statistic of the area under the ROC curve (AUC) are used most often because the AUC is relatively independent of the base rate of the observed outcome:

- The AUC ranges from 0.5 (prediction at the level of chance) to 1.0 (perfect prediction) (Table 6.1):
  - AUC > 0.63 represents a moderate effect size
  - AUC > 0.71 represents a large effect size (Rice and Harris, 2005).

Table 6.1 AUCs of common actuarial risk assessment instruments (ARAIs)

		ARAI	AUC
Douglas *et al.* (2005)	188 non-mentally disordered male offenders released from Canadian prison to community supervision Mean follow-up 7.7 years	HCR-20 VRAG VORAS PCL-R PCL-SV	0.82 0.79 0.61 0.76 0.73
Monahan *et al.* (2005)	157 US acutely hospitalized patients, followed up for 20 weeks after discharge	ICT	0.63
Doyle and Dolan (2006)	112 UK forensic and non-forensic discharges, followed up for 24 weeks	PCL-SV VRAG HCR-20	0.69 0.66 0.79
Snowden *et al.* (2007)	996 discharges from four UK medium secure units (MSUs) Follow-up 6–60 months	VRAG OGRS	0.75–0.86 0.72–0.78
Gray *et al.* (2008)	887 male discharges from UK MSUs 2-year follow-up	HCR-20 H10 C5 R5	0.70–0.76 0.68–0.77 0.54–0.61 0.63–0.69
Coid *et al.* (2011)	1353 male UK prisoners Mean follow-up 2 years	PCL-SV VRAG HCR-20 H10 C5 R5	0.69 0.66 0.79 0.66 0.64 0.59
Where a range of areas under the curve (AUCs) is given, this is dependent on length of follow-up and whether the outcome was violent or general reoffending See Abbreviations for ARAI's name in full			

It is interesting that AUCs seem to be within a similar range for all the commonly used instruments, wherever they are studied and among those with and without mental disorder, men or women and forensic or general psychiatric patients (Buchanan, 2008; Coid *et al.*, 2009):

- Kroner *et al.* (2005) randomly combined items from four established ARAIs including the PCL-R and VRAG, and found that the 'new instruments' predicted as well as the originals.
- It may be that instruments like this cannot achieve a higher predictive accuracy and that they measure a general construct of criminality rather than a specific risk of violence (Coid *et al.*, 2011).

Buchanan (2008) sought to translate the AUC into a clinically meaningful number – the number needed to detain in order to prevent an act of violence. He demonstrates that this number increases as the base rate of the action to be prevented reduces:

- So for the CATIE trial outcome of assault with a weapon or causing serious injury, reported in Swanson *et al.* (2006), use of the VRAG would require 15 people to be detained for 6 months to prevent one incident in that period.

In a systematic review Singh *et al.* (2011) concluded that those instruments designed for use in a highly defined population performed better than those with more general applicability:

- Thus the SAVRY (for adolescents) performed best, while the PCL-R (of general applicability) performed poorly.
- This emphasizes the importance of ensuring that the tool used is appropriate for the case at hand.

ARAIs in clinical practice

ARAIs outperform clinical judgement in research studies (Aegisdottir et al., 2006). For some, this means that they should supplant clinical assessments (Hilton et al., 2006), but:

- This holds only where the relevant question is that which is answered by the ARAI. It must be in the following form:
  - In a group of individuals who share some characteristics with this individual, what is the risk of one of them carrying out a violent act in the next unit time?
- You must be sure that the reference group used in developing the ARAI is applicable to the patient whom you are assessing.
- You must be on the look-out for rare or idiosyncratic risk factors, which are not accounted for by the ARAI.
- Be wary of the pitfalls associated with applying group data to individuals. These may be:
  - statistical pitfalls; see Hart *et al.* (2007), Mossman and Sellke (2007), Harris *et al.* (2008); debate available at http://bjp.rcpsych.org/cgi/eletters/190/49/s60
  - moral/ethical pitfalls relating to prejudice and stereotyping (see Maden, 2007, p75).

For the forensic psychiatrist carrying out risk assessments on patients with a history of violence, or patients whom a colleague has deemed sufficiently dangerous to warrant a forensic opinion, there are other problems that seriously limit the value of a purely statistical approach:

- All these patients are, by definition, relatively high risk. This may limit the ability of an ARAI to distinguish between them.
- ARAIs tend to be dominated by static rather than dynamic factors. This makes them of little use when the need is to moderate and manage risk rather than to state what it is.
- ARAIs do not address the questions that clinical risk assessment must address:
  - when, where, why, how, how bad, to whom, and what to do about it.
- ARAIs do not help where there is cause for concern despite an actuarial categorization of low risk:
  - understanding cause allows sensible predictions to be made even without group data and historical information (Buchanan, 1999).

Maden (2007) suggests that ARA:

- is useful in providing a context or grounding for subsequent clinical assessment, and
- is more useful for those with PD than those with mental illness, because psychosis is too variable and idiosyncratic for ARAIs to cope with.

● Clinical Risk Assessment

A clinical approach to risk assessment may be less reliable than ARA but is likely to be more valid because:

- its flexibility allows account to be taken of idiosyncratic risk factors and risk factors external to the individual
- the assessor may define the target behaviours, the questions to be answered and the associated parameters:
  - for example, different types of violence may be distinguished
- understanding cause allows risk reduction interventions, even where the likelihood is low
- it enables a dynamic assessment, identifying high- and low-risk situations in the future.

Box 6.2 Some risk aphorisms

The best predictor of future violence is past violence:

- the more often it has happened in the past the more likely it is to happen in the future.

Some patients under-report their risk and others over-report it. Very few report it accurately:

- Under-reporting may be motivated by a desire to avoid restrictive interventions.
- Over-reporting tends to serve an internal need, perhaps to be seen as important or powerful, or to attract help and support.
- Always consider whether the patient you are seeing is over-reporting or under-reporting their risk and why.

People who are at low risk of doing something will sometimes do it. The lower the base rate, the more false positives you will get:

- While this is often seen as a problem for ARA, Maden (2007, p99) makes the point that it is just as true for SCA.

Predicting that someone will do something is a safer bet than predicting that they will not:

- The latter cannot be proved wrong until the subject dies. That does not make the former a better prediction.

Risk is always relative. Why and when is more important than whether.

False positives and false negatives are inevitable and qualitatively different:

- Defining the right balance between them is neither a mathematical nor a clinical decision.

Effective clinical practice involves taking risks:

- Deciding what risk to take and how to do it is never a statistical decision.

Sources of error

It is generally held that clinicians overestimate risk, as in the famous Baxstrom patients (Steadman and Cocozza, 1974). For forensic psychiatrists, potential reasons include the following:

- Risk of violence is, in part, what forensic psychiatrists are for, so they may tend to see it more than others.
- Deciding that an individual is high risk is often a low anxiety judgement (Oakley *et al.*, 2009), because it justifies intervention and avoids an assessment of low risk being followed by a serious violent episode.
- A risk-averse, blaming society is likely to promote a risk-averse approach to clinical management.

Otherwise, sources of error in risk assessment mostly result from:

- lack of information, or
- bias.

Information gaps are inevitable and risk assessments must be timely and pragmatic. So you must:

- take reasonable steps to minimize them:
  - collect as much information as reasonably possible in advance of the clinical assessment; consider remaining gaps again afterwards
  - ratify important information from more than one source where possible
  - conduct multidisciplinary assessments, thereby adopting more than a single, potentially narrow perspective
- account for any known gaps in drawing your conclusions, and:
  - bear in mind the possibility of 'unknown unknowns'
  - consider whether any known gap is likely to lead to bias.

Be aware of the common biases in risk assessment:

- Halo effect:
  - Forensic psychiatrists are asked to provide risk assessments on high-risk patients who often have many features in common with the forensic psychiatrist's own patients, all of whom have probably committed serious violence.
  - This will lead to a tendency to overestimate risk.
- Attributional bias:
  - Particularly a tendency to attribute behaviour of others to internal or dispositional factors, and one's own behaviour to external factors.
  - Where the assessor identifies to some degree with the assessed person (same gender, same background, same culture, etc.), they may be more likely to attribute behaviour to external factors, which is likely to lead to a judgement of lower risk.
- Confirmation bias:
  - Weighing up qualitative information related to risk requires judgements about relative importance of information.
  - A prematurely formed opinion may affect these judgements.
- Observer-expectancy effect:
  - A forensic psychiatrist deals with high-risk patients. If they expect their patients to be high risk, they will probably see them as so.
- Illusory correlations:
  - Particularly likely where events are unusual and memorable, violence in one's patients being a good example.
  - Remember that correlation is not the same as causality.

See Moore (1996) for further discussion of error in clinical risk assessment.

Factors important in considering risk of violence

A full psychiatric history and examination is required. The focus of this will depend on the case, but the factors shown in Table 6.2, loosely grouped into four categories, are especially important areas to bear in mind:

- Using a structured risk assessment tool, such as the HCR-20, to guide your consideration of risk factors, may be helpful.
- Most of the areas of enquiry are bipolar, constituting risk factors at one end and protective factors at the other.

Considering previous violence

Previous episodes of violence provide the best indicators of the circumstances in which risk of violence is likely to increase in the future:

- Future risk will increase the more future circumstances resemble those in which violence has occurred before.
- It may be that there are a number of different circumstances in which violence, perhaps of different types, is likely to occur.

Consider:

- The nature of the violence:
  - The frequency of violence, and note any patterns (increasing, decreasing, gaps or spates).
  - The severity of injuries.
  - Have weapons been used?

Table 6.2 Factors in considering the risk of violence

Individual historical and dispositional factors	
• Previous violence • Age • Educational attainment • Psychopathic traits or other PD • Childhood conduct disorder • Childhood abusive experiences • Parental criminality • Impulsiveness	Previous violence is the most important factor to consider in detail (see text) Parenting style, consistency, involvement, loss/separation Sibling relationships, familial attitudes and patterns of conflict and resolution Presence of early maladjustment by way of age at onset of violence and conduct problems. Was conduct disorder socialized or unsocialized? Peer relationships, teacher relationships, sociability, teenage hobbies. Compare school with home
Individual clinical factors	
• Substance misuse • Anger or irritability • Justification of violence • Violent thoughts and fantasies • Insight and understanding • Collaboration with clinical team	Substance misuse is important but the relationship with violence may be complex (see text) Are there reasons why they might be violent – grudges, feelings of resentment or humiliation – and do they justify violence? Collaboration in treatment is an important dynamic determinant of risk (see text)
Explanatory or motivational factors	
• Persecutory delusions • Auditory hallucinations • Threat control over-ride (TCO) symptoms • Morbid jealousy • Delusional misidentification • Negative attitudes	Important symptoms of psychosis are discussed in Chapter 7 Relate episodes of violence to episodes of illness; spend as much time understanding periods of mental health stability as episodes of illness and hospitalization Negative attitudes may be understood in terms of childhood experience or current subcultural influences
Situational or environmental factors	
• Recent victimization • Social network and support • Availability/use of weapons • Availability of victims	The social network, including family and carers, may be absent or present, and it may be violence-promoting or violence-inhibiting Who else should be involved in monitoring and care planning? It is always important to ask about a history of weapon carrying, but answers may be particularly unreliable

- Was the violence more extreme than was necessary to achieve the desired ends?
  - Is there evidence of planning, strong emotion or impulsiveness?
- Situational triggers/precipitants and internal motivations:
  - Think about emotions, places and people.
  - Consider victim types and victim influences on the violence.
  - Where the violence is apparently 'unprovoked' or overt triggers seem trivial, look for an earlier less specific trigger leading to an intervening altered mental state which in turn led on to violence.
  - Identify factors that are necessary for violence (i.e. violence does not occur in their absence), and factors that are sufficient for violence (i.e. if the factor is present, violence will follow).
  - How homogeneous are the circumstances in which violence has occurred?
  - How likely is it that they will encounter similar situations in the future?
- Retrospective attitudes:
  - To the violence.
  - To actual victim(s), or to victim types.

Substance misuse

Where relevant, you need to take a full drug and alcohol history, considering the relationship to episodes of violence.

Box 6.3 *Tarasoff* v *Regents of the University of California* (1976)551 P.2d 334

This famous Californian case placed a duty on health-care professionals to issue warnings in relation to potentially dangerous patients:

- Prosenjit Prodder became obsessed with Tatiana Tarasoff and became a vengeful stalker. He disclosed his violent feelings to his psychotherapist, who notified the relevant police force. But Prodder was not detained and Ms Tarasoff was not informed. Prodder went on to kill her by stabbing, and her parents brought a civil action.
- The majority judgment of the California Supreme Court established that a psychiatrist could be subject to a duty to protect a third party (i.e. someone who was not their patient), Justice Tobriner stating that 'the protective privilege [of confidentiality] ends where the public peril begins'.

Breaching confidentiality in such cases has always been permitted in the UK, but there has not been a similar duty to do so:

- The duty of confidentiality within the doctor–patient relationship is not absolute, being subject to various statutory exceptions and a common law 'public interest' exception.
- But in the latter case the doctor has a discretion, rather than a duty, to breach confidentiality.

See Gavaghan (2007) and Thomas (2009) for further discussion.

Substance use should not be seen as a unidimensional or dichotomous characteristic. There are four possible relationships between substance use and risk of violence in those with mental disorders, which vary according to the substance used:

- Intoxication with drugs leads directly to an increased risk of violence:
  - Stimulant, particularly crack cocaine, and alcohol intoxication are associated with an increased risk of violence.
  - Among non-mentally disordered offenders, cannabis and opiate use are not associated with an increased risk of violent offending.
- Substance use leads to more symptoms of mental illness, which leads to an increased risk of violence:
  - Cannabis and stimulants are clearly associated with greater illness severity on a range of indices, including level of reported symptoms (Kuepper *et al.*, 2011).
  - Opiates and alcohol are less likely to cause deterioration in psychosis directly, but may do so indirectly and over a longer timeframe through socio-economic or other stressful mediators.
- Drug use and violence are associated through other individual characteristics which are associated with both:
  - This may apply to any substance, particularly where the use is heavy and problematic.
  - It is less likely for non-problematic use of those substances that are legally/culturally acceptable (particularly alcohol and cannabis, depending on the culture to which the patient belongs).
- Use of drugs leads to involvement in a social environment where violence is relatively common:
  - This may apply to any substance, particularly where the patient's life is dominated by substance use within a violent/criminal social milieu.

The role of drugs or alcohol in specific episodes of violence should be investigated. Consider (after Moore, 1996):

- Has this violent behaviour occurred only when intoxicated?
- Does it occur every time the patient is intoxicated?
- If not, what are the other necessary conditions?
- Are drugs/alcohol used in order to be violent, or recklessly as to whether he'll be violent?
- Are drugs/alcohol used as a reaction to being violent?

Insight and collaboration

Ongoing engagement in treatment is an especially important risk factor because it is dynamic, modifiable and can generally be readily monitored.

Insight into mental illness should be distinguished from insight into risk of violence. Both are important and they may or may not co-vary:

- Swartz *et al.* (2001) followed up 331 patients after discharge from detention in psychiatric hospital, randomly assigning them to involuntary outpatient commitment or standard follow-up. Those patients who regularly used services and adhered to medication had the lowest rates of violence.
- In the MacArthur study there was a service use effect for patients with PD, rates of violence being lower among those who attended more appointments (Skeem *et al.*, 2002)

Adherence to medication is established as an important factor in a variety of outcomes in schizophrenia, including risk of violence (Ascher-Svanum *et al.*, 2006). Crucial issues include:

- What is the patient's appraisal of the likelihood of future violence or future relapse of mental disorder?
- How motivated are they to reduce these risks?
- What measures do they think are required?
- What is their attitude to ongoing pharmacological and other treatment, including support and monitoring?
- How much commonality of understanding and purpose is there between the patient and the clinical team?
- What is the quality of their relationship with the clinicians involved in their care?

Violent thoughts and fantasies

It is common for disclosure of violent thoughts or fantasies to precipitate a forensic referral. But the relationship between fantasies and violence is not well researched. Violent fantasies are sufficiently common in the normal population that it is difficult to conclude that they predict violence in themselves:

- Up to two-thirds of undergraduates endorsed having had recent homicidal fantasies (Gellerman and Suddath, 2005).

The fantasy must be considered in the context of a broad risk assessment:

- Consider the intensity, persistence and pervasiveness of the fantasy.
- Consider the attitude of the patient to the fantasy.
- Explore any preparatory actions.
- Think about the function that the fantasy is serving for the patient.
- Distinguish between fantasy and intention:
  - Fantasy may include detailed and extreme plans but serves a function in itself – usually leading to some sense of satisfaction.
  - Intentions are more clearly aimed towards guiding action, and are more likely to be associated with a subjective need or urge to act.

Box 6.4 Assessing a patient in a general psychiatric setting to provide advice on risk and risk management

Before the assessment, make sure that you understand the task:

- to provide an independent second opinion on risk, or
- to provide peer support/back-covering for another psychiatric team.

Remember that it is easy to describe a patient as high risk and suggest accordingly restrictive interventions (see discussion in Oakley *et al.*, 2009). It is far better to:

- contextualize your opinion within the referring team's own opinion
- comment on the plans already formulated by the referring team.

It is very common for these not to be detailed within the referral letter:

- a telephone conversation with the referrer is always helpful.

Consider who will carry out the assessment – is a single clinician sufficient? Consider what additional obtainable information you require in advance of your assessment and access this. Then consider what gaps remain and plan your interview, so you know what areas you want to concentrate on with the patient:

- While a full history is always required, there is little need to duplicate information that you already have.
- The time with the patient is precious, and should be used efficiently to gain information that cannot be gleaned from existing sources.

Writing up a risk assessment

Most clinicians develop their own structure with experience, adapting those of others. The following is suggested in that spirit.

Define the target behavior:

- In many cases it is not necessary to subcategorize the violence. Sometimes different types of violence may need to be specified in terms of, for example, victim type, planning and precursors, impulsiveness or method.
- You must consider the likely cost of the behaviour, because management will depend on both likelihood and cost.
- The cost should be considered both to the victim and to the perpetrator.

Acknowledge the limitations of the assessment, in terms of lack of information and possible biases.

Describe previous episodes of violence:

- The frequency and characteristics of the episodes.
- In particular, are they only violent in specific situations that share many characteristics, or are they violent in all sorts of different situations?
- What factors are necessary for violence to occur?
- Are there factors that in themselves are sufficient to cause violence?

Consider other relevant risk and protective factors from Table 6.2 (page 76) and any others that are relevant to the case:

- Think about how they relate to past, and therefore future, violence.
- You should aim to outline an understanding of the causes of violence in terms of these risk factors.

Which factors are modifiable?

- Which ones are potentially susceptible to treatment/intervention?
- What interventions would you recommend? These must be pragmatic and realistic.

What is the residual risk and can it be tolerated in the proposed setting?

- If the modifiable factors are addressed what risk would remain?
- Are there reliably and readily detectable warning signs that would herald an increased risk?
- Could they be detected sufficiently early to allow intervention?
- Who might be involved in monitoring for these?
- What interventions should be considered if an increased risk were detected?
- Consider whether there is any need to disclose information to potential victims or to criminal justice system agencies.

References

Aegisdottir S, White MJ, Spengler PM, Maughermen AS, Anderson LA, Cooke RS, *et al.* (2006) The meta-analysis of clinical judgement project: fifty-six years of accumulated research on clinical versus statistical prediction. *The Counseling Psychologist* **34**(3), 341–82

Ascher-Svanum H, Faries DE, Zhu B, Ernst FR, Swartz MS, Swanson JW. (2006) Medication adherence and long-term functional outcomes in the treatment of schizophrenia in usual care. *Journal of Clinical Psychiatry* **67**(3), 453–60

*Buchanan A. (1999) Risk and dangerousness. *Psychological Medicine* **29**, 465–73

*Buchanan A. (2008) Risk of violence by psychiatric patients: beyond the 'actuarial versus clinical assessment' debate. *Psychiatric Services* **59**(2), 184–90

Cleckley H. (1976) *The Mask of Sanity*, 5th edn. St Louis: Mosby

Coid J, Yang M, Ullrich S, Zhang T, Sizmur S, Roberts C, *et al.* (2009) Gender differences in structured risk assessment: comparing the accuracy of five instruments. *Journal of Consulting and Clinical Psychology* **7**, 337–48

Coid J, Yang M, Ullrich S, Zhang T, Sizmur S, Farrington D, Rogers R. (2011) Most items in structured risk assessment instruments do not predict violence. *Journal of Forensic Psychiatry and Psychology* **22**(1), 3–21

Douglas K, Yeomans M, Boer D. (2005) Comparative validity analysis of multiple measure of violence risk in a sample of criminal offenders. *Criminal Justice and Behavior* **32**(5), 479–510

Doyle M, Dolan M. (2006) Predicting community violence from patients discharged from mental health services. *British Journal of Psychiatry* **189**, 520–6

Gavaghan C. (2007) A Tarasoff for Europe? A European human rights perspective on the duty to protect. *International Journal of Law and Psychiatry* **30**, 255–67

Gellerman DM, Suddath R. (2005) Violent fantasy, dangerousness, and the duty to warn and protect. *The Journal of the American Academy of Psychiatry and the Law* **33**, 484–95

Gray N, Taylor J, Snowden RJ. (2008) Predicting violent reconvictions using the HCR-20. *British Journal of Psychiatry* **192**, 384–7

Hare RD. (2003) *Manual for the Revised Psychopathy Checklist*, 2nd edition. Toronto: Multi-Health Systems

Harris G, Rice M, Quinsey V. (2008) Shall evidence-based risk assessment be abandoned? *British Journal of Psychiatry* **192**(8), 154

Hart S, Michie C, Cooke D. (2007) Precision of actuarial risk assessment instruments. *British Journal of Psychiatry* **190**(suppl), s60–5

Hilton NZ, Harris GT, Rice ME. (2006) Sixty-six years of research on the clinical versus actuarial prediction of violence. *The Counseling Psychologist* **34**(3), 400–9

Howard P. (2009) *Improving the Prediction of Re-offending using the Offender Assessment System. Research Summary 2/09*. London: Ministry of Justice

Kroner DG, Mills JF, Reddon JR. (2005) A coffee can, factor analysis, and prediction of antisocial behaviour: the structure of criminal risk. *International Journal of Law and Psychiatry* **28**, 360–74

Kuepper R, Van Os J, Lieb R, Wittchen H-U, Hofler M, Henquet C. (2011) Continued cannabis use and risk of incidence and persistence of psychotic symptoms: 10 year follow-up cohort study. *British Medical Journal* **342**, d738. doi:10.1136/bmj.d738

*Maden A. (2007) *Treating Violence: A guide to risk management in mental health*. Oxford: Oxford University Press

Monahan J, Steadman HJ, Robbins PC, Appelbaum P, Banks S, Grisso T, *et al.* (2005) An actuarial model of violence risk assessment for persons with mental disorders. *Psychiatric Services* **56**, 810–15

*Moore B. (1996) *Risk Assessment: A practitioner's guide to predicting harmful behavior*. London: Whiting & Birch Ltd

Mossman D, Sellke TM. (2007) Avoiding errors about 'margins of error'. *British Journal of Psychiatry* **191**(6), 561

Oakley C, Hynes F, Clark T. (2009) Mood disorders and violence: a new focus. *Advances in Psychiatric Treatment* **15**, 263–70

Quinsey V, Harris G, Rice M, Cormier C. (1998) *Violent Offenders: Appraising and managing risk*. Washington: American Psychological Association

Rice ME, Harris GT. (2005) Comparing effect sizes in follow up studies: ROC area, Cohen's *d* and *r*. *Law and Human Behavior* **29**, 615–20

Singh JP, Fazel S. (2010) Forensic risk assessment: a metareview. *Criminal Justice and Behavior* **37**(9), 965–88

*Singh JP, Grann M, Fazel S. (2011) A comparative study of risk assessment tools: a systematic review and metaregression analysis of 68 studies involving 25,980 participants. *Clinical Psychology Review* **31**(3), 499–513

Skeem J, Monahan J, Mulvey E. (2002) Psychopathy, treatment involvement, and subsequent violence among civil psychiatric patients. *Law and Human Behavior* **26**, 577–603

Snowden RJ, Gray NS, Taylor J, MacCulloch MJ. (2007) Actuarial prediction of violent recidivism in mentally disordered offenders. *Psychological Medicine* **37**, 1539–49

Steadman HJ, Cocozza JJ. (1974) *Careers of the Criminally Insane*. Lexington: Lexington Books

Swanson JW, Swartz MS, Van Dorn RA, Elbogen EB, Wagner HR, Rosenheck RA, *et al.* (2006) A national study of violent behavior in persons with schizophrenia. *Archives of General Psychiatry* **63**, 490–9

Swartz M, Swanson J, Hiday V, Wagner H, Burns B, Borum R. (2001) A randomized control trial of outpatient commitment in North Carolina. *Psychiatric Services* **52**, 325–9

Thomas M. (2009) Expanded liability for psychiatrists: Tarasoff gone crazy? *Journal of Mental Health Law* **Spring**, 45–56

Webster CD, Douglas K, Eaves D, Hart SD. (1997) *HCR-20 Assessing risk for violence*. Vancouver: Simon Fraser University

World Health Organization (1996) *Violence: A public health priority*. Geneva: WHO

7

Psychosis and Offending

This chapter is concerned primarily with the association between psychosis and violence. Arson and sex offending are considered in Chapter 13.

It is generally held that men with schizophrenia are convicted of criminal offences more often than those without, though the evidence is inconsistent and the increased rate small:

- Lindqvist and Allebeck (1990) compared the inpatient register of a Swedish county with the central criminal records database. Among 644 people with schizophrenia, they found no general increased rate of offending among men with schizophrenia, but violent crime was about four times more likely.
- Wessely *et al.* (1994), using a psychiatric case register in south London, concluded that those with schizophrenia had no increased risk of criminal behaviour as a whole, but only a minor increased risk of violent offending.
- Hodgins *et al.* (1996), using data from a large Danish birth cohort, found an increased rate of criminal convictions among those who had been admitted to psychiatric hospital.
- Mullen *et al.* (2000) compared criminal records of Australian patients with schizophrenia with age-, sex- and residence-matched controls, demonstrating a higher rate of conviction for all offence types except sexual offending.

Much of any general association with offending may be explained by the secondary socio-economic disability that accompanies severe mental illness, and perhaps by an increased risk of being apprehended.

An individual formulation of an offence may draw either direct or indirect links between psychosis and offending. For example:

- There may be a direct link when an individual:
  - takes another's property, delusionally believing it to be their own
  - assaults someone who they delusionally believe has wronged them in some way
  - sets a fire in response to persistent command auditory hallucinations.
- There may be an indirect link when as a result of psychosis:
  - their economic circumstances have broken down and they steal in order to gain money
  - they cannot cope with their poor social circumstances and, while drunk, they set a fire in their flat as a cry for help
  - they are using alcohol and drugs to improve their sense of well-being and become involved in a fight while intoxicated.

Such individual formulations based on causal hypotheses are the basis of effective clinical practice. This should be distinguished from the observational group data showing associations between offending and psychosis.

The research evidence relating to the association between psychosis and violence can be difficult to interpret because of methodological heterogeneity, particularly in terms of:

- various diagnostic categories, such as:
  - schizophrenia
  - (probable) psychosis
  - severe mental illness (which generally includes any affective or non-affective psychosis and mania)
- various definitions of violence:
  - often with no distinction between minor and more severe violence
- various ascertainment strategies for both of the above:
  - self-report and/or criminal records for violence
  - case registers, psychiatric interviews or lay interviews using screening tools for diagnosis.

● Are People with Schizophrenia More Likely to be Violent than Those Without?

This question, at the heart of forensic psychiatry, has preoccupied opinion and research for decades. Three phases can be seen:

- 1970–80s – a dearth of evidence led to a pre-eminence of expert opinion and a broad cross-discipline consensus that the mentally ill were not intrinsically more likely to be violent, and any apparent association was due to confounding co-factors.
  - This consensus may have been maintained by a desire to reduce the stigma of mental illness during deinstitutionalization and the development of community care.
- 1990–2000s – a wealth of research activity using various methodologies, in various settings, produced a similarly broad consensus:
  - That those with severe mental illness, or schizophrenia, had a moderately elevated level of risk of violence compared with the general population (around four to six times greater for men).
  - That this made a relatively small contribution to all the violence in society.
  - That co-morbidities, notably substance use disorders and certain personality disorders, substantially increased this otherwise small increased risk.
  - See Arsenault *et al.* (2000), Brennan *et al.* (2000), Fazel and Grann (2006), Hodgins *et al.* (1996), Stueve and Link (1997), Swanson *et al.* (1990), Tiihonen *et al.* (1997) and Wallace *et al.* (2004).
- Late 2000s – uncertainty over the generality of this consensus, with increasing emphasis on the importance of other risk factors among the mentally disordered:
  - In particular suggesting that schizophrenia may confer no increased risk in the absence of co-morbid substance use.
  - See Elbogen and Johnson (2009) and Fazel *et al.* (2009a,b).
  - This has led to further thought about the heterogeneity of the relationships between severe mental illness and violence, different subgroupings of violent mentally ill patients, and mechanisms by which mental illness might be associated with violence.

Cross-sectional community prevalence surveys

Swanson *et al.* (1990) reanalysed data from the Epidemiological Catchment Area survey (*n* = 10 059; DSM-III diagnoses):

- Violence was ascertained post hoc, from self-report diagnostic questions; no distinction between serious and trivial violence.
- 368 respondents reported violence in preceding year – 55.5 % had a psychiatric disorder, compared with 19.6 % of non-violent respondents.

- There was an increased risk of violence across all diagnostic categories, and co-morbidity was common, making attribution difficult, but:
  - among those with only a single diagnosis, the rate of violence for those with schizophrenia was 8%, compared with 2% for those with no diagnosis
  - those with more than one diagnosis were more likely to have been violent.

Stueve and Link (1997) investigated a community sample in Israel, ascertaining violence by self-reported fighting and weapon use over the previous 5 years:

- Using 'psychosis or bipolar disorders' as a diagnostic category, they gave adjusted odds ratios of 3.3 for fighting and 6.6 for weapon use.
- They found no increased risk of violence for non-psychotic depression, or anxiety disorders.

Elbogen and Johnson (2009) used data from a US national survey about alcohol use, in which 34653 subjects were interviewed twice, 2–3 years apart, relating data on severe mental illness from the first interview to self-reported violence between the interviews. Their multivariate analysis concluded that:

- severe mental illness (psychosis, major depression, bipolar disorder) alone did not predict violence
- various historical, clinical, dispositional and contextual factors were associated with violence, and these were reported more frequently by those with severe mental illness.

Cohort studies based on case registers

These studies (Table 7.1) mostly use established registers of psychiatric diagnosis and criminality to investigate the relationships between the two:

- The advantage is that large numbers of subjects can be included, but
- There is likely to be selection bias related to likelihood of prosecution and need for hospitalization.

Table 7.1 Case register studies of severe mental illness and offending

Author and location	No. of subjects	Diagnostic grouping	Outcome measures	Odds ratio (OR)
Tiihonen et al. (1997) Finland	12058	Schizophrenia	Any conviction	3.0
			Violent conviction	7.2
		Mood psychosis	Any conviction	6.8
			Violent conviction	10.4
Brennan et al. (2000) Denmark	358180	Schizophrenia	Violent arrest/conviction	4.6
Arsenault et al. (2000) New Zealand	961	Psychosis	Conviction or self-reported violence	4.6
Wallace et al. (2004) Australia	2861 patients 2861 controls	Schizophrenia	Any conviction	3.2
			Violent conviction	4.8
Fazel and Grann (2006) Sweden	98082	Psychosis	Violent conviction	3.8
Fazel et al. (2009a) Sweden	8003 patients 80025 controls	Schizophrenia: with substance use* without substance use	Violent conviction	2.0 4.4 1.2

* Among those with co-morbid schizophrenia and substance use, the risk increase was less when non-mentally ill siblings were used as controls, implying that familial factors also contributed to these ORs.

In a meta-analysis of 20 surveys and cohort studies comparing risk of violence among those with schizophrenia or other psychoses with the general population, Fazel et al. (2009b) reported:

- Pooled ORs of
  - 4.7 (range 1–7) (3.8 when adjusted for socio-economic factors) for men, and
  - 8.2 (range 4–29) for women.
- Co-morbid substance use disorders considerably increased this risk.
- The risk among those with schizophrenia and substance use disorders was not different from the risk among those with substance use disorders alone.
- The risk estimates did not vary according to method of ascertainment of violence, the specific diagnosis used or the location of the study.

Discharge follow-up studies

Using data from the MacArthur study, Steadman *et al.* (1998) followed up 1136 people discharged from psychiatric hospital in the USA for 1 year, and compared the rate of violence (ascertained by self-report, collateral informants and police records) with that for 519 controls matched for neighbourhood of residence:

- This study used a very broad diagnostic grouping of 'major mental disorder' which included psychoses, but also depression, dysthymia, mania and cyclothymia.
- There was no significant difference between the prevalence of violence among patients without substance use and the community controls.
- Substance use increased the rate of violence among all groups, and the rate of substance use was greater among patients than controls.
- Among the patients, the overall rate of violence was 27.5 %. The highest rate was in those with 'other mental disorders' (personality disorder/adjustment disorders/suicidality) and substance use:

	Rate of violence (%)
Major mental disorder/no substance use	17.9
Major mental disorder/substance use	31.1
Other mental disorders/substance use	43.0

The grouping of 'Other/no substance use' was too small to be included in the analysis

● What is the Contribution of Schizophrenia to Societal Violence?

The population attributable risk (PAR) is the percentage of violence in the population that can be ascribed to schizophrenia:

- Walsh *et al.* (2002) calculated PARs of between 2 and 10 % from a number of the primary studies referred to above, while noting that co-morbidity with substance use may lead to the contribution of schizophrenia being overestimated.
- Fazel and Grann (2006) gave a PAR of 5.2 % for schizophrenia, noting that it would be higher for women and would increase with increasing age.
- In the UK, Coid *et al.* (2006) found a lower PAR of 1.2 % for 'screening positive for psychosis' in a UK national household survey.

● Homicide, Schizophrenia and the Effect of Deinstitutionalization

The rate of homicide by the severely mentally ill:

- Coid (1983) estimated that the incidence of homicide by the severely mentally ill was about 0.13 per 100 000 per year.
- Wallace *et al.* (1998) estimated that the annual rate of homicide was 1 in 3000 for men with schizophrenia.
- Based on review of psychiatric reports in homicide cases in Finland, Eronen *et al.* (1996) gave ORs for homicide in schizophrenia of 10.0 for men and 8.7 for women.
- Nielssen and Large (2010) conducted a meta-analysis to consider the relationship between homicide and treatment of mental illness. They reported that:
  - nearly 40% of the homicides committed by the severely mentally ill are committed before any treatment is received
  - about 1 in 629 people with psychosis commits a homicide before receiving treatment
  - about 1 in 9090 psychotic patients who have received treatment will commit a homicide each year.

Shaw *et al.* (2006) reported from a UK national survey of 1594 homicides over 3 years:

- 34% had a lifetime mental disorder based on diagnoses given in psychiatric court reports or by current psychiatrist:
  - 5–7% schizophrenia
  - 7–10% affective disorder
  - 9–11% had a personality disorder
  - 7–10% had alcohol dependence
  - 6–8% had drug dependence
- 5–6% were psychotic, and 6–9% were depressed at the time of the offence.

Of people with schizophrenia who committed homicide (Department of Health, 2001):

- 72% were known to services, 51% having been in contact with services within the past year
- mean age 31 years
- 78% not currently married
- 68% unemployed/long-term sick
- 25% living alone
- 37% history of alcohol misuse
- 51% history of drug misuse
- 32% history of violent convictions.

Among 3930 UK homicides, perpetrators with mental illness were more likely to use a sharp instrument or strangulation than those without mental illness (Table 7.2; Rodway *et al.*, 2009).

Table 7.2 Comparison of homicide perpetrators with schizophrenia and affective disorder

	Perpetrators with schizophrenia	Perpetrators with affective disorder
Method	More likely to use a sharp instrument	More likely to use strangulation or suffocation/asphyxiation/drowning
Symptomatic at the time of offence	81%	75%
Relationship of victim	22% spouse/ex-spouse 23% family member 23% acquaintance 9% stranger	52% spouse/ex-spouse 16% son/daughter

Deinstitutionalization and serious violence

In some quarters it has been held that the process of deinstitutionalization of psychiatric care which has taken place throughout much of the developed world has led to an increase in the risk of serious violence committed by those with severe mental illness.

The evidence does not support this assertion:

- Wallace *et al.* (2004) demonstrated that in Australia there was no difference in the proportionate increase in rate of offending during the relevant period, between those with and without mental illness.

With regard to homicide, perhaps the most reliably determined violent crime:

- Shaw *et al.* (2004) reported an increase in the rate of stranger homicides between 1967 and 1997, but found no increase in the numbers subsequently made subject to a hospital order. In comparison with others, perpetrators of stranger homicides were less likely to:
  - have a history of mental disorder or contact with psychiatric services
  - have psychiatric symptoms at the time of the offence.
- Large *et al.* (2008) collated homicide data for England and Wales to illustrate that the UK homicide rate has steadily increased since 1960, but the rate of mentally disordered homicides peaked in the mid-1970s and has since declined:
  - Mentally disordered homicides comprised infanticide, not guilty by reason of insanity (NGBROI) or unfit to plead, and diminished responsibility.

● Psychotic Symptoms and Violence

The search for a relationship between particular psychotic symptoms and risk of violence is driven by anecdotal clinical experience of individual patients who report that an act of violence was caused/precipitated/motivated by a particular psychotic symptom.

This research is problematic because of:

- diagnostic heterogeneity, and the likely variety of confounding factors
- the difficulty of distinguishing psychopathology with sufficient accuracy in groups of patients (delusions as opposed to overvalued ideas, for example)
- the transient nature of individual symptoms, such that demonstrating a causal link with an episode of violence is difficult.

Evidence that risk of violence is associated with changes in mental state

If individual psychotic symptoms lead to violence, then risk should vary according to presence or severity of symptoms.

Humphreys *et al.* (1992) analysed data from the Northwick Park study. Twenty per cent of people presenting with first episode schizophrenia had acted violently and in about half of these cases there was evidence that the violence was motivated by psychotic symptoms.

Link *et al.* (1992) carried out an analysis of data, previously collected for another purpose, from a sample of psychiatric patients and a community sample:

- They found an increased rate of violence among those with a history of psychiatric treatment and concluded that much of this association was attributable to the severity of psychotic symptoms reported.

Mojtabi (2006) examined the association of 'psychotic-like symptoms' (in the absence of psychotic mental disorder) with violence, using data from the US National Household Survey on Drug Abuse:

- 5.1% of adults reported such symptoms and the OR for various forms of self-reported violence was around 5.
- Tentatively, paranoid ideas and perceptual symptoms seemed to be associated most strongly.

Swanson *et al.* (2006) used data from the US CATIE project to examine violence among people with schizophrenia living in the community:

- Both minor (simple assault with no injury or weapon use) and more severe violence were significantly associated with PANSS +ve score, and severe violence was negatively associated with PANSS –ve score:
  - The PANSS symptoms that were associated with serious violence were hostility, suspiciousness and persecutory symptoms, hallucinatory behaviour, grandiosity and excitement.
  - Delusions in general and conceptual disorganization were not in themselves associated with violence.
- Minor violence (simple assault with no injury or weapon use) was significantly associated with younger age, female gender, more years in treatment, reduced vocational activity or functional leisure impairment, housing problems, and not feeling listened to by family members.
- Serious violence was associated with younger age, childhood conduct problems, arrest history.

Delusions

It is common in clinical practice for a patient to report having acted violently as a result of some delusional belief.

Taylor (1985) interviewed UK remand prisoners with psychosis and reported that more than 90% had been psychotic at the time of their alleged offence and about half of them attributed their offence to delusions.

As a whole, the MacArthur study did not find an association between delusions and risk of violence (Appelbaum *et al.*, 2000):

- However, the association was tested across all diagnostic groups and violence was more likely among those with non-psychotic diagnoses.
- Therefore this is of little help to a clinician considering the risk of violence of an individual with a psychotic mental illness.
- Among the 328 deluded subjects (Appelbaum *et al.*, 1999), persecutory delusions were more likely than other delusions to be accompanied by negative affect and acted upon.

A retrospective study of around 80 deluded admissions to a UK general psychiatric ward reported that:

- 60% reported at least one 'delusional action' and this was particularly likely where the patient reported persecutory delusions (Wessely *et al.*, 1993).
- Acting on delusions was associated with (Buchanan *et al.*, 1993):
  - being aware of evidence that supported the delusional belief
  - having actively sought out such evidence
  - a tendency to reduce the conviction with which the belief was held when it was challenged
  - unpleasant mood states consequent to the delusion.

Freeman *et al.* (2007) found that 96 of 100 deluded patients had used 'safety behaviours', that is behaviours intended to avoid a perceived threat, in the previous month. A history of violence and suicidal behavior was associated with greater use of such behaviours.

Box 7.1 Assessing the risk of acting on delusions

Within the context of a general risk assessment, in relation to the delusions themselves you should consider the following:

- The content of the delusion and its significance for the individual, particularly whether it represents a significant threat, either physically or psychologically.
- Is the patient aware of evidence that supports their belief?
- Have they actively sought out such evidence?
- Is there evidence of acting on delusions in a non-dangerous way, or of using safety behaviours?
- What is their response when their belief is challenged? Is there evidence of any uncertainty or ambivalence, and is this expressed with emotion?
- Do they describe a sense of shame, of being wronged or of being denied an entitlement, or is there other evidence of unpleasant mood states?

Hallucinations

There is little evidence that auditory verbal hallucinations in general are associated with an increased risk of violence. In a review article, Rudnick (1999) concluded that:

- there was no convincing evidence for a general association between command hallucinations and dangerous behaviour
- there was evidence for an association between the familiarity and perceived benevolence of the voices and compliance with the commands.

Junginger (1995) reported from a follow-up study of 93 psychiatric inpatients that being able to assign an identity to the voice was associated with compliance with commands. A more recent review (Barrowcliff and Haddock, 2006) reiterated that beliefs about the voices are more important than content in determining compliance.

Junginger and McGuire (2004) suggest that violence is more likely where there are a range of psychotic symptoms consistent with each other, providing a 'a more consistent distortion of reality in which compliance with command hallucinations is more likely to fit'.

Box 7.2 Assessing the risk of acting on auditory hallucinations

Within the context of a general risk assessment, you should consider (adapted from Barrowcliff and Haddock, 2006) the following:

- A detailed account of the content of the hallucinations.
- Does the patient believe the voices to be powerful or of higher social status than the patient?
- Does the patient believe that the commands are justified or reasonable?
- Does the patient seek engagement with the voices, or want to please the voices?
- Do they report any subjective compulsion, urge or drive to comply?
- Can they identify the voices or do they identify with them? Are the voices perceived as benevolent or malevolent?
- What does the patient believe will be the consequences of complying or not complying?
- Have they ever complied with the voices before, either in a dangerous or non-dangerous way?

Threat/control over-ride symptoms

The hypothesis is that psychotic symptoms are especially likely to lead to violence if they lead an individual to think that other people pose a threat, or if they intrude so as to over-ride internal violence-inhibiting controls:

- Link *et al.* (1998) used data from an epidemiological survey in Israel to demonstrate an association between self-reported threat/control over-ride (TCO) symptoms and violence.
- Swanson *et al.* (1996) replicated this work, demonstrating that Epidemiological Catchment Area (ECA) survey respondents who reported TCO symptoms were twice as likely to report violence as those with other psychotic symptoms.

TCO symptoms are usually envisaged as a psychotic construct. But the questions from the Psychiatric Epidemiology Interview Schedule used for ascertainment may not be sufficiently specific for psychosis. Overvalued ideas and other non-psychotic beliefs may have a similar content to psychotic TCO symptoms, and may have a similar relationship to risk of violence:

- The MacArthur study found no association between violence and TCO symptoms (Appelbaum *et al.*, 2000) across all the diagnostic categories.
- Skeem *et al.* (2006) similarly found no evidence for an association in a diagnostically heterogeneous cohort (*n* = 132) of patients from an emergency room.

Stompe *et al.* (2004) compared the prevalence of psychotic TCO symptoms among violent and non-violent patients with schizophrenia. They reported no increased rate of TCO symptoms in the offending patients, but did find an association between the rather non-specific threat component of TCO and more severe violence.

Specific delusional content

There is a wealth of anecdotal evidence from case reports and small series of cases, though little robust epidemiological evidence, that certain specific delusional content is associated with violence:

- Group data is likely to be unreliable when it pertains to the relationship between psychopathology that is uncommon and idiosyncratic (compared with the broad diagnostic grouping of schizophrenia, for example), and behaviour (violence) that is also uncommon.
- The content usually cited would be expected sometimes to lead to extreme behaviour, because of its profound emotional importance. This is irrespective of whether or not it is a pathological delusional belief. For example:
  – delusional jealousy is always said to be associated with a high risk of violence
  – it is very common among non-mentally disordered men who have killed their spouse for the offence to be precipitated by suspected infidelity.

Table 7.3 gives details of delusional content and violence; see Buchanan (1993) for further discussion.

● Developmental Pathways to Violence in Schizophrenia

Most of the studies referred to above take a deliberately broad overview, allowing broad conclusions to be drawn:

- There is an increased rate of violence associated with mental disorder, and with schizophrenia in particular.
- The size of this increase is modest and the contribution of schizophrenia to societal violence is small.
- A very large part of the increased risk is accounted for by substance use, which is more common among people with schizophrenia.

Table 7.3 Delusional content and violence

Delusional jealousy	The association with a risk of violence to the spouse, and less often to her perceived partner, is frequently described. Distinguishing between delusions and overvalued ideas is often difficult in this group, unless the ideas are clearly in the context of a broader psychosis
Erotomania or De Clerambault's syndrome	Commonly leads to nuisance behaviours and stalking behaviours In a series of 29 cases, violence to the object was predicted by a history of general antisocial behaviour and having multiple delusional objects (Menzies *et al.*, 1995)
Delusional misidentification syndromes	Capgras' syndrome is the most common such syndrome and the one most commonly reported in association with violence. Among those who killed, the victim was usually a close family member (Silva *et al.*, 1996)
Delusions of passivity	This is a difficult area of psychopathology to assess retrospectively following violence It is common for patients to report that they were not themselves or not in control; this is also common in non-mentally disordered violent offenders, when it is often best seen as a way of minimizing responsibility

Box 7.3 Morbid jealousy (aka Othello syndrome)

This is a heterogeneous category that includes both psychotic individuals with delusional beliefs and non-psychotic individuals with overvalued ideas, about a spouse's fidelity:

- In the latter group dissocial or paranoid personality disorder and alcoholism are particularly common.
- 'Shakespearean diagnoses' have no place in contemporary psychiatry or courts – clinical cases are complex and generally share few of the features of Shakespeare's tragedy.
- Therefore morbid jealousy/Othello syndrome is an unhelpful clinical construct, because it does not correspond to consistency of psychopathology, treatment, prognosis or indeed risk.
- It is better to give a contemporary diagnosis of a mental illness or personality disorder, and then consider the importance of the particular content of ideation in the case.

Particular aspects to be considered when assessing a patient with morbid jealousy include:

- the form of the jealous psychopathology
- previous episodes of (morbid) jealousy/longevity of this episode, number of previous jealous relationships, and associated threats or risk behaviours
- general antisocial behaviour and criminal/violent history
- personal, familial or subcultural attitudes to infidelity and violence, particularly intramarital violence
- acting on the ideation by way of searching for evidence. This may include following the partner, searching mobile phone, email or social networking sites, setting traps to catch her out, examining clothing and underwear.

The therapeutically nihilistic maxim that separation be recommended is also unhelpful given the heterogeneity of cases:

- In general the treatment depends on the underlying diagnosis; the prognosis may be relatively good in schizophrenia, in contrast to personality disorder.
- It is clearly important to consider confidentiality and sharing of information. Discussing issues of treatment, diagnosis, prognosis and risk carefully with the spouse, and possibly any perceived love-rival, enables them to make informed decisions.
- Supporting the spouse may be an important aspect of a comprehensive treatment plan.

- Those factors that are associated with increased risk of violence, among the non-mentally disordered, are also pertinent to those with mental disorders.

There is relatively little research looking at the relationship in more detail:

- Subgroups of patients with psychosis and violence.

- Longitudinal studies investigating pathways to offending in schizophrenia.
- The temporal relationship between psychotic symptoms and violence.
- The interdependence between particular psychotic symptoms and situational factors

In a records-based review of patients in high security, Taylor *et al.* (1998) perceived two types of psychotic violent patient:

- Those with little previous criminal history whose index offence seemed to have been driven by positive psychotic symptoms.
- Those with established conduct problems in adolescence, whose offence was less likely apparently to be driven by their psychotic symptoms.

Among a cohort of men with schizophrenia and violence, Tengstrom *et al.* (2001) similarly distinguished between early- and late-start offenders:

- The early starters showed:
  − greater and more varied criminality
  − earlier onset of substance use
  − better psychosocial functioning.

Among patients with schizophrenia in the CATIE study, Swanson *et al.* (2008) reported more evidence for this binary typology:

- Among those with childhood conduct problems, violence was associated with substance use at levels that did not reach criteria for substance use disorders.
- Positive psychotic symptoms were associated with violence only in those without childhood conduct problems.

Volavka and Citrome (2008) outline three types of violent behaviour in schizophrenia:

- Violence directly related to positive psychotic symptoms:
  − accounts for about 20% of assaults committed by psychotic inpatients (Nolan *et al.*, 2003).
- Impulsive aggression due to impaired response inhibition:
  − often with a lack of planning and unclear motive
  − may be associated with impaired frontal lobe function and psychotic disorganization symptoms.
- Aggression due to co-morbid psychopathic traits:
  − traits that do not reach diagnostic criteria for disorder may increase the risk in patients who also have schizophrenia.

They note that other subtypes are likely to exist, and emphasize the importance of substance use and non-adherence to medication as contributing factors.

References

Appelbaum PS, Robbin PC, Roth LH. (1999) Dimensional approach to delusions: comparison across types and diagnoses. *American Journal of Psychiatry* **156**, 1938–43

Appelbaum PS, Robbins PC, Monahan J. (2000) Violence and delusions: data from the MacArthur violence risk assessment study. *American Journal of Psychiatry* **157**(4), 566–72

Arsenault L, Moffit T, Caspi A, Taylor PJ, Silva PA. (2000) Mental disorders and violence: results from the Dunedin study. *Archives of General Psychiatry* **57**, 979–86

Barrowcliff AL, Haddock G. (2006) The relationship between command hallucinations and factors of compliance: a critical review of the literature. *Journal of Forensic Psychiatry and Psychology* **17**(2), 266–98

Brennan PA, Mednick SA, Hodgins S. (2000) Major mental disorders and criminal violence in a Danish birth cohort. *Archives of General Psychiatry* **57**, 494–500

Buchanan A. (1993) Acting on delusion: a review. *Psychological Medicine* **23**, 123–34

Buchanan A, Reed A, Wessley S, Garety P, Taylor P, Grubin D, Dunn G. (1993) Acting on delusions II: the phenomenological correlates of acting on delusions. *British Journal of Psychiatry* **163**, 77–81

Coid J. (1983) The epidemiology of abnormal homicide and murder followed by suicide. *Psychological Medicine* **13**, 855–60

*Coid J, Yang M, Roberts A, Ullrich S, Moran P, Bebbington P, *et al*. (2006) Violence and psychiatric morbidity in the national household population of Britain: public health implications. *British Journal of Psychiatry* **189**, 12–19

Department of Health. (2001) *Safety First: Five year report of the National Confidential Inquiry into Suicide and homicide by people with mental illness*. London: DH

Elbogen EB, Johnson SC. (2009) The intricate link between violence and mental disorder: results from the national epidemiological survey on alcohol and related conditions. *Archives of General Psychiatry* **66**(2), 152–61

Eronen M, Tiihonen J, Hakola P. (1996) Schizophrenia and homicidal behavior. *Schizophrenia Bulletin* **22**(1), 83–9

Fazel S, Grann M. (2006) The population impact of severe mental illness on violent crime. *American Journal of Psychiatry* **163**(8), 1397–403

Fazel S, Langstrom N, Hjern A, Grann M, Lichtenstein P. (2009a) Schizophrenia, substance abuse, and violent crime. *Journal of the American Medical Association* **301**(19), 2016–23

Fazel S, Gulati G, Linsell L, Geddes JR, Grann M. (2009b) Schizophrenia and violence: systematic review and meta-analysis. *PLoS Medicine* **6**(8): e1000120doi:10.1371/journal.pmed.1000120

Freeman D, Garety PA, Kuipers E, Fowler D, Bebbington PE, Dunn G. (2007) Acting on persecutory delusions: the importance of safety seeking. *Behaviour Research and Therapy* **45**, 89–99

Hodgins S, Mednick SA, Brennan PA, Schulsinger F, Engberg M. (1996) Mental disorder and crime: evidence from a Danish birth cohort. *Archives of General Psychiatry* **53**, 489–96

Humphreys M, Johnstone EC, MacMillan JF, Taylor PJ. (1992) Dangerous behaviour preceding first admission for schizophrenia. *British Journal of Psychiatry* **161**, 501–5

Junginger J. (1995) Command hallucinations and the prediction of dangerousness. *Psychiatric Services* **46**, 911–14

Junginger J, McGuire L. (2004) Psychotic motivation and the paradox of current research on serious mental illness and rates of violence. *Schizophrenia Bulletin* **30**(1), 21–30

*Large M, Smith G, Swinson N, Shaw J, Nielssen O. (2008) Homicide due to mental disorder in England and Wales over 50 years. *British Journal of Psychiatry* **193**, 13–3

Lindqvist P, Allebeck P. (1990) Schizophrenia and crime: a longitudinal follow-up of 644 schizophrenics in Stockholm. *British Journal of Psychiatry* **157**, 345–50

Link B, Andrews H, Cullen FT. (1992) The violent and illegal behavior of mental patients reconsidered. *American Sociological Review* **57**, 275–92

Link B, Stueve A, Phelan J. (1998) Psychotic symptoms and violent behaviours: probing the components of 'threat/control-override' symptoms. *Social Psychiatry and Psychiatric Epiemiology* **33**, S55–S60

Menzies R, Fedoroff JP, Green CM, Isaacson K. (1995) Prediction of dangerous behaviour in male erotomania. *British Journal of Psychiatry* **166**, 529–36

Mojtabi R. (2006) Psychotic-like experiences and interpersonal violence in the general population. *Social Psychiatry and Psychiatric Epidemiology* **41**, 183–90

Mullen P, Burgess P, Wallace C, Palmer S, Ruschena D. (2000) Community care and criminal offending in schizophrenia. *Lancet* **355**, 614–17

Nielsen O, Large M. (2010) Rates of homicide during the first episode of psychosis and after treatment: a systematic review and meta-analysis. *Schizophrenia Bulletin* **36**(4), 702–12

Nolan KA, Czobor P, Roy BB, Platt MM, Shope CB, Citrome LL, Volavka J. (2003) Characteristics of assaultive behaviour among psychiatric inpatients. *Psychiatric Services* **54**, 1012–16

Rodway C, Flynn S, Swinson N, Roscoe A, Hunt IM, Windfuhr K, *et al.* (2009) Methods of homicide in England and Wales: a comparison by diagnostic group. *Journal of Forensic Psychiatry and Psychology* **20**(2), 286–305

Rudnick A. (1999) Relation between command hallucinations and dangerous behavior. *Journal of the American Academy of Psychiatry and the Law* **27**(2), 253–7

Shaw J, Amos T, Hunt IM, Flynn S, Turnbull P, Kapur N, Appleby L. (2004) Mental illness in people who kill strangers: longitudinal study and national clinical survey. *British Medical Journal* **328**, 734–7

Shaw J, Amos T, Hunt IM, Flynn S, Meehan J, Robinson J, Bickley H, Parsons R, *et al.* (2006) Rates of mental disorder in people convicted of homicide. *British Journal of Psychiatry* **188**, 143–7

Silva JA, Harry BE, Leong GB, Weinstock R. (1996) Dangerous delusional misidentification and homicide. *Journal of Forensic Sciences* **41**(4), 641–4

Skeem JL, Schubert C, Odgers C, Mulvey EP, Gardner W, Lidz C. (2006) Psychiatric symptoms and community violence among high-risk patients: a test of the relationship at the weekly level. *Journal of Consulting and Clinical Psychology* **74**, 967–79

Steadman HJ, Mulvey EP, Monahan J, Robbins PC, Appelbaum PS, Grisso T, *et al.* (1998) Violence by people discharged from acute psychiatric inpatient facilities and by others in the same neighbourhoods. *Archives of General Psychiatry* **55**, 393–401

Stompe T, Ortwein-Swoboda G, Schanda H. (2004) Schizophrenia, delusional symptoms and violence: the threat/control over-ride concept re-examined. *Schizophrenia Bulletin* **30**(1), 31–44

Stueve A, Link B. (1997) Violence and psychiatric disorders: results from a epidemiological study of young adults in Israel. *Psychiatric Quarterly* **67**(4), 327–42

Swanson JW, Holzer CE, Ganju VK, Jono R. (1990) Violence and psychiatric disorder in the community: evidence from the epidemiological catchment area survey. *Hospital and Community Psychiatry* **41**, 761–70

Swanson JW, Borum R, Swartz MS, Monahan J. (1996) Psychotic symptoms and disorders and the risk of violent behaviour in the community. *Criminal Behaviour and Mental Health* **6**, 309–29

Swanson JW, Swartz MS, Van Dorn RA, Elbogen EB, Wagner HR, Rosenheck RA, *et al.* (2006) A national study of violent behavior in persons with schizophrenia. *Archives of General Psychiatry* **63**, 490–9

Swanson JW, Van Dorn RA, Swartz MS, Smith A, Elbogen EB, Monahan J. (2008) Alternative pathways to violence in persons with schizophrenia: the role of childhood antisocial behavior problems. *Law and Human Behavior* **32**, 228–40

Taylor PJ. (1985) Motives for offending among violent and psychotic men. *British Journal of Psychiatry* **147**, 491–498

Taylor P, Leese M, Williams D, Butwell M, Daly R, Larkin E. (1998) Mental disorder and violence: a special (high security) hospital study. *British Journal of Psychiatry* **172**, 218–26

Tengstrom A, Hodgins S, Kullgren G. (2001) Men with schizophrenia who behave violently: the usefulness of an early- versus late-start offender typology. *Schizophrenia Bulletin* **27**(2), 205–18

Tiihonen J, Isohanni M, Rasanen P, Koiranen M, Moring J. (1997) Specific major mental disorders and criminality: a 26-year prospective study of the 1966 Northern Finland birth cohort. *American Journal of Psychiatry* **154**(6), 840–5

Volavka J, Citrome L. (2008) Heterogeneity of violence in schizophrenia and implications for long-term treatment. *International Journal of Clinical Practice* **62**(8), 1237–45

Wallace C, Mullen P, Burgess P, Palmer S, Ruschena D, Browne C. (1998) Serious criminal offending and mental disorder: case linkage study. *British Journal of Psychiatry* **172**, 477–84

Wallace C, Mullen P, Burgess P. (2004) Criminal offending in schizophrenia over a 25-year period marked by deinstitutionalisation and increasing prevalence of comorbid substance use disorders. *American Journal of Psychiatry* **161**(4), 716–27

*Walsh E, Buchanan A, Fahy T. (2002) Violence and schizophrenia: examining the evidence. *British Journal of Psychiatry* **180**, 490–5

Wessely S, Buchanan A, Reed A, Cutting J, Everitt B, Garety P, Taylor P. (1993) Acting on delusions I: prevalence. *British Journal of Psychiatry* **163**, 69–79

Wessely S, Castle D, Douglas A, Taylor P. (1994) The criminal careers of incident cases of schizophrenia. *Psychological Medicine* **24**, 483–502

Mood Disorders, Neuroses and Offending

Non-psychotic mental disorders have an uncertain place in forensic psychiatry. The research effort and clinical service development, at least from the mid-1980s, concentrated on psychosis (see Oakley *et al.*, 2009 for further discussion). Perhaps psychosis is more easily reconciled with the categorical legal approach (see Chapter 21, p268), with an apparently clearer demarcation of the proper boundaries of expert psychiatric evidence, and an unequivocal role for psychiatry in management.

The return of clinical interest in personality disorder since the turn of the century, stimulated by the political driver of the dangerous and severe personality disorder (DSPD) programme (see Chapter 9, p112), has given a new prominence to dispositional neurosis, though not particularly to neurotic mental illness. Nevertheless, much violent offending is driven by affect and emotion, and some non-psychotic mental disorders are partly defined by offending behaviours.

● Mood Disorders and Violence

Mood disorders among violent populations

The prevalence of mood disorders among prisoners is higher than in the general population:

- Major depression is found in 10% of male prisoners and 12% of female prisoners (Fazel and Danesh, 2002).
- Major depression is the most common mental illness among female prisoners.
- 1.2% of male remand prisoners had affective psychosis and all of these were convicted of violent offences (Taylor and Gunn, 1984).
- Older prisoners have higher rates of depressive illness than either younger prisoners or older adults in the community (Hunt *et al.*, 2010).

Among patients of forensic psychiatric services:

- Rates of mood disorder vary considerably between studies (Table 8.1). These studies are all naturalistic surveys relying on clinical diagnoses, and practice may vary between different services.

Table 8.1 Prevalence of mood disorder among forensic psychiatric patients

Coid *et al.* (2001)	Survey of medium secure units (MSUs) in seven English regions	25–42%
Thompson *et al.* (1997)	State Hospital, Carstairs	3.3%
Gow *et al.* (2010)	Scottish MSU	16.5%

Violence among those with mood disorders

Although the association between schizophrenia and violence has received greater attention, mood disorders may also be associated with violence:

- Swanson *et al.*'s (1990) re-analysis of the Epidemiological Catchment Area (ECA) survey data found an equally strong association between schizophrenia, bipolar disorder and depression and self-reported violence.
- Table 8.2 gives the rates of violence in 1 year post-discharge from the MacArthur study (*n* = 1136; multiple sources to ascertain violence; broad criteria for violence) (Monahan *et al.*, 2001).
- In contrast, in the Dunedin birth cohort (Arsenault *et al.*, 2000) the demonstrated associations at age 21, between both mania and violence, and depression and violence, did not persist after controlling for substance use. The numbers of manic patients were low.
- A study of former inpatients using a crime register found that 5.6 % of those with manic disorder and 1 % of those with major depression committed violent crimes in the 7–12 years after their discharge (Graz *et al.*, 2009).
- Tiihonen *et al.* (1997) reported on a Finnish birth cohort unselected for offending or mental illness. Among those who developed an affective psychosis, the odds ratios (OR) for any conviction (6.8) and a violent conviction (10.4) were higher than the respective rates for those with schizophrenia (3.0, 7.2).

Table 8.2 Rate of violence in 1 year post-discharge

Depression	28.5 %
Bipolar affective disorder	22 %
Schizophrenia	14.8 %

In particular, manic patients are likely to show aggression and violence associated with admission:

- Binder and McNeil (1988) reported similar rates of violence pre-admission among patients with mania and those with schizophrenia. Aggression and violence may be determined by irritability, dysphoria and poor impulse control. Manic patients were most likely to be assaultative during the acute phase of an admission.
- The AESOP (Aetiology and Ethnicity of Schizophrenia and Other Psychoses) first episode psychosis study found that nearly two-thirds of patients with mania were aggressive at first contact with services (Dean *et al.*, 2007). They were almost three times more likely to be aggressive at this time than those with schizophrenia. In addition, manic symptoms in schizophrenia were associated with aggression.

Mood disorder and homicide

Analyses of data from the National Confidential Inquiry into Suicide and Homicide by People with Mental Illness (Hunt *et al.*, 2010; Shaw *et al.*, 2006) shows:

- 7 % of perpetrators of homicide have a lifetime diagnosis of mood disorder (5 % have schizophrenia).
- Unlike those with psychotic symptoms at the time of the offence, those with depressive symptoms were unlikely ever to have been in contact with mental health services.
- The proportion of homicide perpetrators with symptoms of mental illness at the time of the offence increased with increasing age:
  - In those over 65 years of age, half were depressed at the time of the offence and nearly half had a past history of a mood disorder.
  - The older homicide perpetrators were much less likely to have previous violent convictions than the younger perpetrators.

- The authors concluded that:
  - there is a need for greater awareness of the potential risk to others posed by elderly patients with mood disorders
  - preventative strategies could include improved training of GPs in the early recognition and management of late-life depression.

Homicide–suicide

Homicide–suicide is rare. It has been commonly associated with depression, one case series finding that 75% of perpetrators were depressed at the time (Rosenbaum, 1990). National Confidential Inquiry data show (Flynn et al., 2009):

- approximately 30 incidents of homicide followed by suicide occur in England and Wales a year
- most perpetrators are male
- men more often killed a partner, while women more commonly killed their children
- 10% had previous contact with mental health services
- the most common diagnoses were mood disorders and personality disorders.

Elderly homicide perpetrators are more likely than younger perpetrators to kill a female partner as opposed to a stranger, and are also more likely to die by suicide after the offence (Hunt *et al.*, 2010). They are sometimes 'mercy killings' to end an ailing partner's suffering.

Infanticide

Depressed mood is common in infanticide:

- Social factors also tend to be important and, overall, the degree of mental illness is perhaps less than is required generally for a defence of diminished responsibility, particularly where the infant was very young:
  - See Chapter 11 (p132) for more details.

Identification of postnatal depression has been improved by midwives and health visitors using tools such as the Edinburgh Postnatal Depression Scale or specific screening questions.

● Neurosis and Offending

Forensic psychiatry tends to be concerned, in particular, with schizophrenia and psychosis, on the one hand, and personality disorder, on the other, neurotic mental illness falling between these two stools. But for many authors, neurosis is a generic category defined by the exclusion of psychotic and organic pathology. Traditionally neurosis is not well demarcated from personality disorder, Schneider (1923), for example, seeing them as indistinguishable. It is unsurprising that, in forensic psychiatry particularly, the dividing line between neurotic mental illness and dispositional neurosis is faint.

Issues for forensic psychiatry in relation to neurosis

Does neurosis constitute mental illness?

Some may argue that while neurotic mental illnesses are clearly defined as mental disorders, in practice they do not mitigate and do not require treatment by virtue of an association with offending in the individual:

- The Butler Committee defined severe mental illness (for medico-legal purposes) in terms aligned closely to the ICD-9 description of psychosis. This was in the context of the future RSU programme being designed primarily to treat those with psychosis:

- Similarly criminal legal concepts related to mental disorder, while adopting a broad approach, also tend to equate mental disorder with psychosis. For example:
  - 'The major mental diseases, which doctors call psychosis such as schizophrenia are clearly diseases of the mind' (*Bratty* v *Attorney General for Northern Ireland* [1963] AC 386).

Psychiatric determinism versus legal free will

- While criminal courts explicitly regard defendants as having free will, a psychiatric formulation is to some degree deterministic, seeing behaviour as the product of inborn characteristics, environmental influences and emotional conflict.
- In neurosis, this may be seen as a more finely balanced, nuanced explanation than when a patient is frankly psychotic at the time of committing an offence.

Psychodynamic formulations of offending behaviour

The benefits of a psychodynamic approach are not limited to those with neurotic, as opposed to psychotic, illness. The fundamental premise of a psychoanalytic approach is that the offence itself has meaning, in the same way that symptoms have meaning for psychoanalysts in other settings. The offending behaviour 'represents an extension of the mind, so that what is not consciously remembered is repeated in action ...' (Blumenthal, 2010).

Psychological defence mechanisms act as psychic buffers, helping to maintain self-esteem, regulate affect and minimize conflict, thus compensating for poor practical coping strategies. As a result of some stressor, these psychological buffers may become stretched to breaking point, and in the absence of practical coping strategies, an individual may shift from their habitual neurotic position to what may be termed a delinquent position, in which offending occurs (Gallwey, 1990).

Bateman (1996) emphasizes, with respect to forensic patients:

- immature defence mechanisms of splitting, projection and projective identification
- reaction formation
- identification with the aggressor.

Early disruption of attachment processes is seen as especially important in offenders with cluster B personality disorders (McGauley and Rubitel, 2006).

Themes of shame and humiliation, in early life and then in adulthood, are often important in psychodynamic formulations:

- Unstable self-esteem, as opposed to high or low self-esteem, leads to vulnerability to feeling threatened in the face of criticism, which in turn leads to shame and humiliation (Baumeister *et al.*, 2000).

Some have sought to explain aggression and violence as a unitary concept:

- Freud – aggression as acting out of an instinctual externalization of the death instinct.
- Object relations theorists – aggression as a reaction to threatened loss of an object.
- Gilligan (1996) – shame as a universal determinant of violence.

Others prefer to acknowledge the polythetic nature of aggression and violence and offer categorizations such as:

- self-preservative violence and sadomasochistic violence (Glasser, 1998)
- affective violence and predatory violence (Meloy, 1992).

Rage-type murder

Assessment of individuals who have killed in the context of explosive rage or anger, but who have little history of criminality or violence, is fertile ground for psychodynamic understanding rooted in neurotic functioning. Some have suggested that explosive violence is cathartic, or that it represents the re-enactment of previous conflicts.

Cartwright (2002) offers a more dynamic model, rooted in a previously rigid defensive structure which denies bad experience, thus maintaining a positive external world as a reflection of an idealized self. Violence represents a psychologically defensive action, aimed at preserving this idealized self; at the moment of violence, destruction of the victim is less important than preservation of the self.

In assessment of risk of violence, Cartwright (2002, pp175–6) emphasizes the importance of, among other factors:

- denial or minimization of an escalating conflict related to loss of an object
- an 'entrapping dyadic situation', excluding any third object
- poor representational capacity – an inability to form coherent internal representations of external objects
- hypersensitivity to a sense of shame
- a lack of alternative sources of self-esteem
- limited flexibility in altering interpersonal functioning.

● Sex Offending in Association with Mood Disorders

While there is no evidence from group data for an association between mood disorders and sex offending, in an individual a mood disorder may lead to sex offending:

- Mania may be associated with sexual disinhibition, an increase in libido, and an enhanced sense of confidence, entitlement and belief in personal attractiveness.
- Depression may present with sex offending, classically in middle-aged men. Often such cases may be understood in terms of a breakdown of established psychological defences under the stressor of an episode of depression.
- Clinically it is common to find indirect sex offending, such as downloading child pornography, to be associated with changes in mood, often in the setting of an inadequate personality style. Depression and alcohol may be seen as weakening internal controls. The behaviour may also be seen as acting out a self-destructive depressive fantasy.

● Shoplifting and Kleptomania

Traditionally, it was held that shoplifting was associated with depression and neurosis:

- Shoplifting in middle-aged women is associated with depression and a range of anxiety symptoms, particularly if it is their only conviction (Gibbens *et al.*, 1971).
- GIbbens and Price (1962) described a typology of depressed shoplifter:
  - isolated young adults under stress
  - older people with chronic depression
  - depression associated with acute loss
  - personality disorder experiencing an aggressive swing.

More recently, shoplifting tends to be seen simply as criminal behaviour, which is strongly associated with problematic drug use. In a US population survey (*n* = 43 093), the lifetime

> **Box 8.1** An illustrative example of depression presenting with late-onset sex offending
>
> A 47-year-old man is charged with sexual assault of his daughter's friend, a 15-year-old girl. She had been staying over one night, when she woke to find the man touching her intimately.
>
> He has no previous convictions. He has no formal psychiatric history, although on close questioning he had a difficult time for a couple of years after leaving university before establishing himself in employment; he may have been depressed then. His subsequent life has been rather staid and uneventful. He has been in the same middle management job for many years. His marriage is longstanding and stable up to now, though on detailed questioning it has been almost sexless for some years. Recent cuts at work have led to an increase in the pressure under which he has been working, he has started drinking more than he used to and has been feeling increasingly sad, de-motivated and profoundly dissatisfied with himself and his life.
>
> Important factors:
>
> - The neurosis in early adult life followed by re-establishment of stable, albeit neurotic, psychological defences and associated lifestyle.
> - Underlying dissatisfaction with his home life.
> - A breaking down of this neurotic defence in response to a stressor in the context of the development of a depressive episode.
> - No evidence of sex offending or other problems with impulse control when well.

prevalence for shoplifting was 11% (Blanco *et al.*, 2008). The odds ratio (OR) for every psychiatric disorder was increased, 89% of shoplifters having a lifetime psychiatric diagnosis:

	Lifetime prevalence (%)	OR (95% CI)
Antisocial personality disorder	21.97	11.98 (10.07–14.25)
Any substance use disorder	76.71	4.33 (3.93–4.77)
Any mood disorder	34.92	2.06 (1.89–2.25)
Any anxiety disorder	30.32	1.80 (1.50–2.16)
Psychotic disorder	0.83	2.93 (1.76–4.89)

Some reported examples of neurotic disorders leading to shoplifting or theft

- Anxiety disorders may lead to distraction or a need to leave a shop quickly (without paying).
- Stealing of food has been reported in anorexia.
- Kleptomania and compulsive states.
- A manic patient may agree to purchase items that they cannot afford, or believe they already own items they do not, or are entitled to take things that they are not.

Pathological stealing or kleptomania

ICD-10 describes this as 'repeated failure to resist impulses to steal objects that are not acquired for personal use or monetary gain', with:

- anticipatory tension and subsequent relief/gratification
- theft usually committed alone
- the stolen items not desired in themselves. They may be discarded, given away or hoarded.

Kleptomania should be distinguished, in particular, from theft due to memory impairment and depression, ICD-10 stating that 'some depressed individuals steal, and may do so repeatedly as long as the depressive disorder persists'.

No robust epidemiology, but of 20 consecutive admissions to psychiatric hospital with kleptomania (McElroy *et al.*, 1991):

- 15 were women
- all had lifetime diagnoses of major mood disorders; 16 of anxiety disorders; 12 of eating disorders
- kleptomanic behaviour abated with resolution of mood disorder.

Clearly the distinction between kleptomania and stealing as a function of depressed mood is not straightforward:

- Clinical descriptions tend to report that chronic neuroticism is common, often with longstanding dispositional dysphoria, unhappy relationships and problems with sexual activity or intimacy.
- This is a good example of the complexity of assessing offending and neurotic disorder, regardless of whether the neurosis is conceptualized as dispositional or an acute mental illnesses.

● Other Habit and Impulse Disorders

The phenomenology overlaps with that of obsessive–compulsive disorder (OCD), tic disorders and the dependence syndrome. The urges in habit and impulse disorder are said to be ego-syntonic, in contrast to OCD. Clinically this distinction is not always so straightforward.

A survey of 204 consecutive admissions to US psychiatric hospitals gave the following rates of lifetime diagnoses, with no associations with any particular primary psychiatric diagnoses (Grant *et al.*, 2005):

	Lifetime prevalence (%)	95% confidence interval (%)
Pathological stealing	9.3	5.3–13.3
Pathological gambling	6.9	3.4–10.4
Pathological fire setting	5.9	2.6–9.1
Intermittent explosive disorder	6.8	3.4–10.4
Compulsive sexual behaviour	4.9	1.9–7.9
Trichotillomania	4.4	1.6–7.3

Pathological fire setting and disorders of sexual preference are dealt with in Chapter 13 (p163 for fire and p158 for sex).

Pathological gambling

The prevalence of problem gambling according to DSM-IV criteria in the UK is around 0.6% (Wardle *et al.*, 2007). ICD-10 defines this in terms that are reminiscent of the dependence syndrome. There should be:

- frequent gambling which dominates the individual's life, and negatively affects their personal and social functioning in various domains
- urge to gamble that is difficult to control
- preoccupation with gambling
- continued gambling despite adverse social consequences.

ICD-10 recognizes that such individuals may sometimes commit offences in order to obtain money or evade debts.

Treatment approaches tend to borrow from the addiction research base, often using the transtheoretical model of stages of behaviour change, motivational interviewing and cognitive–behavioural therapy (CBT), or the 12-step programme as with Gamblers Anonymous.

The natural history of the disorder is very variable. As one might expect, future chronicity is predicted by duration and persistence of past symptoms. Generally, as with addictions, courts are unlikely to consider a diagnosis of pathological gambling to provide significant mitigation for acquisitive offending.

Intermittent explosive (behaviour) disorder

This is mentioned, but not defined, in ICD-10 under the heading 'other habit and impulse disorders'. There is no evidence base on which to support claims of nosological validity. The reports of developmentally immature (increased slow wave activity) EEGs are non-specific.

References

*Arsenault L, Moffit T, Caspi A, Taylor PJ, Silva PA. (2000) Mental disorders and violence in a total birth cohort. Results from the Dunedin Study. *Archives of General Psychiatry* **57**, 979–86

Bateman A. (1996) Defence mechansims: general and forensic aspects. In: Cordess C, Cox M (eds), *Forensic Psychotherapy: Crime, psychodynamics and the offender patient*. London: Jessica Kingsley

*Baumeister RF, Bushman BJ, Campbell WK. (2000) Self-esteem, narcissism and aggression: does violence result from low self-esteem or from threatened egotism? *Current Directions in Psychological Science* **9**, 26–29

Binder R, McNeil D. (1988) Effects of diagnosis and context on dangerousness. *American Journal of Psychiatry* **145**, 728–33

Blanco C, Grant J, Petry NM, Simpson HB, Alegria A, Liu S, Hasin D. (2008) Prevalence and correlates of shoplifting in the United States: results from the National Epidemiologic Survey on Alcohol and Related Conditions (NESARC). *American Journal of Psychiatry* **165**, 905–13

Blumenthal S. (2010) A psychodynamic approach to working with offenders: an alternative to moral orthopaedics. In: Bartlett A, McGauley G (eds), *Forensic Mental Health: Concepts systems and practice*. Oxford: Oxford University Press

*Cartwright D. (2002) *Psychoanalysis, Violence and Rage-type Murder*. Hove: Brunner-Routledge

Coid J, Kahtan N, Gault S, Cook A, Jarman B. (2001) Medium secure forensic psychiatry services: comparison of seven English health regions. *British Journal of Psychiatry* **178**, 55–61

Dean K, Walsh E, Morgan C, Demjaha A, Dazzan P, Morgan K, *et al*. (2007) Aggressive behaviour at first contact with services: findings from the AESOP First Episode Psychosis Study. *Psychological Medicine* **37**, 547–57.

Fazel S, Danesh J. (2002) Serious mental disorder in 23000 prisoners. A systematic review of 62 surveys. *Lancet* **359**, 545–50.

Flynn S, Swinson N, White D, Hunt IM, Roscoe A, Rodway C, *et al*. (2009) Homicide followed by suicide: a cross-sectional study. *Journal of Forensic Psychiatry & Psychology* **20**, 306–21.

Gallwey P. (1990) The psychopathology of neurosis and offending. In: Bluglass R, Bowden P (eds), *Principles and Practice of Forensic Psychiatry*. Edinburgh: Livingston Churchill

Gibbens TCN, Price J. (1962) *Shoplifting*. London: The Institute for the Study and Treatment of Delinquency.

Gibbens TCN, Palmer C, Prince J. (1971) Mental health aspects of shoplifting. *British Medical Journal* **3**, 612–15.

Gilligan J. (1996) Exploring shame in special settings: a psychotherapeutic study. In: Cordess C, Cox M (eds), *Forensic Psychotherapy: Crime, psychodynamics and the offender patient*. London: Jessica Kingsley

Glasser M. (1998) On violence: a preliminary communication. *International Journal of Psycho-analysis* **79**, 887–902

Gow RL, Choo M, Darjee R, Gould S, Steele J. (2010) A demographic study of the Orchard Clinic: Scotland's first medium secure unit. *Journal of Forensic Psychiatry & Psychology* **21**, 139–55

Grant JE, Levine L, Kim D, Potenza MN. (2005) Impulse control disorders in adult psychiatric inpatients. *American Journal of Psychiatry* **162**, 2184–88

Graz C, Etschel E, Schoech H, Soyka M. (2009) Criminal behaviour and violent crimes in former inpatients with affective disorder. *Journal of Affective Disorders* **117**, 98–103

Hunt IM, Ashim B, Swinson N, Flynn S, Hayes AJ, Roscoe A, *et al.* (2010) Homicide convictions in different age groups: a national clinical survey. *Journal of Forensic Psychiatry and Psychology* **21**, 321–35

McElroy SL, Pope HG, Hudson JI, Keck PE, White KL. (1991) Kleptomania: a report of 20 cases. *The American Journal of Psychiatry* **148**(5), 652–7

McGauly G, Rubitel A. (2006) Attachment theory and personality disordered patients. In: Newrith C, Meux C, Taylor P (eds), *Personality Disorder and Serious Offending*. London: Hodder Arnold

Meloy JR. (1992) *Violent Attachments*. London: Jason Aronson

*Monahan J, Steadman HJ, Silver E, Applebaum PS, Robbins PC, Mulvery EP, *et al.* (2001) *Rethinking Risk Assessment. The MacArthur Study of Mental Disorder and Violence*. Oxford: Oxford University Press

*Oakley C, Hynes F, Clark T. (2009) Mood disorders and violence: a new focus. *Advances in Psychiatric Treatment* **15**, 263–70

Rosenbaum M. (1990) The role of depression in couples involved in murder-suicide and homicide. *American Journal of Psychiatry* **147**, 1036–9.

Schneider K. (1923) *Psychopathic Personalities* (translated by M W Hamilton). London: Cassel

*Shaw J, Hunt IM, Meehan J, Robinson J, Bickley H, Parsons R, *et al.* (2006) Rates of mental disorder in people convicted of homicide. National clinical survey. *British Journal of Psychiatry* **188**, 143–7.

Swanson JW, Holzer CE, Ganju VK, Jono R. (1990) Violence and psychiatric disorder in the community: evidence from the epidemiological catchment area survey. *Hospital and Community Psychiatry* **41**, 761–70

Taylor P, Gunn J. (1984) Violence and psychosis I. Risk of violence among psychotic men. *British Medical Journal* **288**, 1945–9.

Thompson L, Bogue J, Humphreys M, Owens D, Johnstone E. (1997) The State Hospital survey: a description of psychiatric patients in special security in Scotland. *Journal of Forensic Psychiatry* **8**(2), 263–84

Tiihonen J, Isohanni M, Rasanen P, Koiranen M, Moring J. (1997) Specific major mental disorders and criminality: a 26-year prospective study of the 1966 northern Finland birth cohort. *American Journal of Psychiatry* **154**, 840–5

Wardle H, Sproston K, Orford J, Erens B, Griffiths M, Constantine R, Pigott S. (2007) *British Gambling Prevalence Survey 2007*. London: National Centre for Social Research

Personality Disorders and Offending

● Diagnostic Issues

The *International Classification of Diseases* 10th revision (ICD-10) and the *Diagnostic and Statistical Manual* 4th edn (DSM-IV) define personality disorders with different phraseology while maintaining similar core concepts:

A severe disturbance in the characterological condition and behavioural tendencies of the individual, usually involving several areas of personality, and nearly always associated with considerable personal and social disruption – ICD 10.

An enduring pattern of inner experience and behaviour that deviates markedly from the expectations of the individual's culture – DSM-IV.

Diagnosis of personality disorder (PD) is in two stages:

- First, the person should fulfil the general criteria for a PD.
- Second, the PD may be categorized into a specific diagnosis.

Reliability and validity of diagnosis

There is no 'gold standard' test for diagnosing PD:

- Structured clinical interviews have good inter-rater reliability.
- The level of agreement is better for diagnosing the presence of PD generally than for categorizing the PD.
- Interview-based and self-report measures suffer with poor validity (convergent and/or discriminant).

Some have called for the conceptualization of PD to be re-examined along with improvements in operationalization and instrumentation (Clark and Harrison, 2001).

Temporal stability

Several studies have indicated that PDs are not necessarily stable over time:

- Tyrer *et al.* (1993) distinguished mature PDs (anankastic, paranoid, schizoid, anxious) from immature PDs (mainly antisocial and emotionally unstable), the latter tending to improve with increasing age.
- Treatment seekers show steady improvement over time, but most patients with PDs in the community are treatment resisters (Tyrer *et al.*, 2007).
- Shea *et al.* (2002) found that fewer than 50% of subjects with borderline, avoidant, obsessive–compulsive or schizotypal PDs persistently satisfied criteria over 1–2 years.

The evidence suggests that, for cluster B PDs, the core symptoms tend to be relatively stable, but secondary characteristics show more attenuation:

- For antisocial personality disorder (ASPD), callousness and lack of empathy are stable, but impulsivity and behavioural controls improve.
- For borderline PD, emotional fluctuations persist, but the intensity and behavioural concomitants, deliberate self-harm (DSH) for example, reduce.

The link with violence

Although it is tempting to assume that certain PDs cause violence, the relationship is complex. Demonstrating causality is difficult because of:

- the variety of PDs involved
- the high co-morbidity
- the difficulty in establishing causative mechanisms (Duggan and Howard 2009).

Categories and dimensions

Diagnosing a disorder necessarily requires a categorical judgement of caseness. However the categorical classifications described in ICD-10 and DSM-IV may be criticized for having:

- inadequate coverage – some people with a general PD not fitting into any specific PD
- excessive overlap between categories
- heterogeneity within diagnoses
- arbitrary and unstable diagnostic boundaries.

Dimensional classifications of personality provide a richer description of an individual's personality structure. Many investigators have sought to bridge this gap between the categorical and dimensional (Livesley, 2007) and it seems likely that DSM-V will adopt a pseudo-dimensional classification (see Widiger *et al.*, 2006, for discussion).

Tyrer (2007) argues for a diathesis model of PD.

Prevalence of personality disorder

Community samples

Huang *et al.* (2009) reported on a cross-sectional community survey (*n* = 21 162) across 13 countries using the International Personality Disorder Examination (IPDE) screening instrument:

- More than half of those with PD also had an axis 1 disorder.

Coid *et al.* (2006) reported data from the British National Survey of Psychiatric Morbidity (*n* = 626; SCID-II diagnoses), giving prevalence rates weighted to control for selection bias:

- Of those with PDs, 53.5% had one PD only, 21.6% had two, 11.4% had three and 14.0% had between four and eight.
- All PDs, except schizotypal, were more common among men than women:

	Huang *et al.* (2009)	Coid *et al.* (2006)
Prevalence of any personality disorder	6.1%	4.4%
Cluster A	3.6%	1.6%
Cluster B	1.5%	1.2%
Cluster C	2.7%	2.6%
Unspecified personality disorder	–	5.7%

Prison samples

The Office for National Statistics (ONS) prison survey (Singleton et al., 1998) suggested that up to 78% of prisoners have a PD:

- ASPD most commonly, followed by paranoid (in men) and borderline (in women).
- See Chapter 18 (p232) for further details.

● Specific Personality Disorders Associated with Offending

Although ICD-10 is widely used for classification of psychiatric disorders in the UK, it is common for DSM-IV to be used for personality disorders and the literature refers to research using DSM-IV diagnostic criteria. Therefore this chapter mostly refers to DSM-IV terminology and criteria.

Antisocial personality disorder

Key characteristics in DSM-IV:

- Failure to conform to social norms with respect to lawful behaviour
- Impulsivity or inability to plan ahead
- Irritability and aggressiveness
- Deceitfulness
- Reckless disregard for safety of self or others
- Consistent irresponsibility
- Lack of remorse.

DSM-IV diagnosis requires that the individual had conduct disorder with onset before the age of 15.

Conduct disorder

Conduct disorder can be classified as either childhood onset (before the age of 10) or adolescence onset.

Key characteristics in DSM-IV:

- Aggression towards people or animals
- Destruction of property
- Deceitfulness or theft
- Serious violations of rules.

Callous–unemotional traits (Frick and Petitclerc, 2009):

- There is mounting evidence that an important distinction can be made within the childhood-onset conduct disorder group, based on the presence of a callous and unemotional affective style.
- This is similar to the distinction made within samples of antisocial adults using psychopathy.
- These callous–unemotional traits can be reliably assessed in children as young as 3 and are relatively stable across extended periods of development.
- Children with these traits show more severe aggression and it is more likely to be pre-meditated and for instrumental gain.
- It is argued that these features have a strong genetic basis and are primarily neurobiological in origin.
- They are associated with persistent antisocial behaviour into adulthood although there is some evidence that the features are amenable to intervention.

The NICE guideline on ASPD (National Collaborating Centre for Mental Health, 2010) emphasizes the importance of conduct disorder:

- The conversion rate from conduct disorder to ASPD is estimated to be between 40% and 70%.
- Recommendations for interventions for children and adolescents with conduct disorder to potentially reduce the risk of later ASPD include:
  - cognitive problem-solving skills on an individual basis for those aged 8 years and older
  - if residual problems after cognitive problem-solving skills, consider anger control groups or social problem-solving groups
  - group-based parent-training/education programmes for the parents
  - functional family therapy should be offered to families of older adolescents at risk of offending behaviour.

Substance misuse

According to the National Collaborating Centre for Mental Health (2010):

- 90% of those with ASPD have a co-morbid disorder and the most common of these co-morbidities is substance misuse.
- Men with ASPD are three to five times more likely to misuse alcohol and drugs.
- Although women have a significantly lower prevalence of ASPD than men, the women with ASPD have an even higher prevalence of substance misuse when compared with men.
- Alcohol misuse is associated with increased violence in people with ASPD.

Relationship to offending

As those with ASPD are generally 'treatment rejecting' rather than 'treatment seeking' they often only come into contact with mental health services in the context of offending behaviour:

- 47% of those with ASPD in the community have significant arrest records (National Collaborating Centre for Mental Health, 2010).
- 50–60% of male prisoners have ASPD (Singleton *et al.*, 1998).
- A relatively small number of life course persistent offenders commit 50–70% of all violent crimes (Odgers, 2009). The life-course persistent pathway is characterized by social, familial and neurodevelopmental deficits, with their onset in early childhood.
- Prisoners with ASPD (Roberts and Coid, 2010):
  - exhibit more criminal versatility
  - are 10–20 times more likely to commit homicide than the general population
  - are significantly more likely to commit violent offences
  - are also more likely to commit robbery, theft, burglary, blackmail, fraud and firearms offences.

Neurobiological basis of antisocial behaviour

- A rapidly growing body of research has considered genetic polymorphisms, neuroimaging and various types of antisocial behaviour.
- There is evidence linking the following genes with violence (Ferguson and Beaver, 2009):
  - dopamine transporter gene
  - serotonin transporter gene
  - monoamine oxidase A (MAO-A) gene
  - catechol-*O*-methyltransferase (COMT) gene.
- Antisocial individuals have:
  - significantly reduced prefrontal structures (Yang and Raine, 2009)
  - larger volumes in posterior brain areas (Tiihonen *et al.*, 2008).

- Psychopathic individuals have:
  - white matter abnormalities in the uncinate fasciculus, which links the amygdala and the orbitofrontal cortex (Craig *et al.*, 2009)
  - significantly reduced volume in the amygdala and the reduced volume correlates with increased affective and interpersonal facets of psychopathy (Yang *et al.*, 2009).

Treatment of ASPD

There is very little evidence for efficacy of psychiatric treatment in ASPD. The NICE guidelines (National Collaborating Centre for Mental Health, 2010) suggest the following:

- For those with a history of offending behaviour consider offering group-based cognitive and behavioural interventions (i.e. accredited offending behaviour programmes, OBPs), in order to address problems such as impulsivity, interpersonal difficulties and antisocial behaviour.
- It is appropriate to consider offering similar groups to non-offenders with ASPD.
- Assess the level of risk and adjust the duration and intensity of the treatment programme accordingly.
- Medication should not be used routinely.
- Co-morbidity should be treated in line with the relevant guidance.
- Psychological interventions should be offered for alcohol and drug misuse.
- Those who meet criteria for psychopathy or dangerous and severe personality disorder (DSPD) should have interventions adapted, for example by lengthening them, with continued follow-up and close monitoring.

Psychopathy

A construct defined by the PCL-R:

- The PCL-R was developed from the clinical descriptions of cases by Hervey Cleckley in his 1941 book *The Mask of Sanity.*
- Intended to provide reliability of diagnosis to allow biological research.

Psychopathy is:

- not the same as the term psychopathic disorder used in the Mental Health Act (MHA) 1983 before the 2007 amendments
- not used in current classificatory systems.

The core characteristics of psychopathy are usually considered in three categories (Feeney, 2003):

- Interpersonal (superficially charming, grandiose, egocentric, manipulative)
- Affective (shallow labile emotions, lack of empathy, lack of guilt, little subjective distress)
- Behavioural (impulsive, irresponsible, prone to boredom, lack of long-term goals, prone to breaking rules).

Relationship to antisocial personality disorder:

- Most, but not all, psychopaths have ASPD.
- Approximately 10% of patients with ASPD are psychopaths (National Collaborating Centre for Mental Health, 2010).

The PCL-R is the standardized method for diagnosing psychopathy (Hare, 1991):

- 20 items (Table 9.1) are scored from interviewing the patient and reviewing their medical and criminal records.

Table 9.1 The 20 items scored on the PCL-R

Glibness and superficial charm	Promiscuous sexual behaviour
Grandiose sense of self-worth	Early behaviour problems
Need for stimulation/proneness to boredom	Lack of realistic long-term goals
Pathological lying	Impulsivity
Conning and manipulative	Irresponsibility
Lack of remorse or guilt	Failure to accept responsibility for own actions
Shallow affect	Many short-term marital relationships
Callous/lack of empathy	Juvenile delinquency
Parasitic lifestyle	Revocation of conditional release
Poor behavioural controls	Criminal versatility

- The frequency, severity and duration of the behaviour over the lifetime should be considered.
- Each item is scored 0 (no), 1 (maybe/in some respects) or 2 (yes).
- A score of 30 or above is considered diagnostic of psychopathy in the USA, whereas a cut-off of 25 is generally used in the UK.
- There is also a shorter screening version (PCL-SV) with good validity as a screening tool.

Relationship to offending

- Approximately 5 % of prisoners in England and Wales are psychopaths:
  - compared with 1 % of the general population.
- Many facets of psychopathy may lead to crime:
  - A lack of guilt and empathy implies an absence of inhibitors to antisocial behaviour.
  - The lack of remorse means that there is no emotional cost to violent behaviour.
  - There is an over-focus on rewards and an under-focus on costs.
  - There may be a desire to control, demean and humiliate.
  - They are likely to engage in impulsive and risky behaviour.
  - Conning others leads to fraud offences.
- Although psychopaths are at high risk of engaging in criminal behaviour not all succumb to that risk. So not all psychopaths are criminals:
  - It has been argued that those psychopaths who have a preponderance of the interpersonal and affective traits, but few of the behavioural traits, may function well in corporate life (Babiak and Hare, 2007).
- However, psychopathy is one of the most researched and most reliable risk factors for violent recidivism among those with a violent history.

Borderline personality disorder

Key characteristics in DSM-IV:

- Efforts to avoid real or imagined abandonment
- Pattern of unstable and intense personal relationships
- Identity disturbance
- Impulsivity
- Inappropriate, intense anger or difficulty controlling anger
- Affective instability
- Chronic feelings of emptiness
- Recurrent suicidal attempts, gestures or threats, or self-mutilating behaviour.

Co-morbidity is particularly common (Leichsenring *et al.*, 2011):

- 84.5 % had a co-morbid axis 1 disorder (especially PTSD [39.2 %] and other mood/anxiety disorders) and 74 % another axis 2 disorder.

Much less is known about the prevalence and characteristics of violence among those with borderline PD than those with ASPD:

- This may be due to borderline PD being seen as a disorder of women, and violence being underestimated among women.
- In clinical practice it is not uncommon for 'difficult' PD patients to be diagnosed as antisocial if they are men and borderline if they are women, but a closer examination of the symptomatology and diagnostic requirements may reveal traits of both disorders.
- Some estimates of the coexistence of borderline PD and ASPD are as high as 60 % (Newhill *et al.*, 2009).

The literature that does exist concerning the relationship between offending and borderline PD primarily considers women:

- Women who have been imprisoned for a major violent offence are four times more likely to have a diagnosis of borderline PD than women whose index offence is one of more minor violence (Logan and Blackburn, 2009).

Newhill *et al.* (2009) reported on a subanalysis of MacArthur study data ($n = 220$, male and female, with borderline PD):

- 73 % were violent during the 1-year period.
- Reported violence was mostly characterized by disputes with acquaintances or significant others.
- The majority of the incidents were relatively minor, not resulting in bodily injury.
- Those with borderline PD were found to be significantly more likely to commit seriously violent and aggressive acts than those without borderline PD:
  - This finding remained significant even after controlling for risk markers such as substance abuse.
  - Increased risk no longer statistically significant when co-morbid ASPD and psychopathy were considered, but there was substantial shared variance among the constructs, suggesting that borderline PD has significant overlap with ASPD and psychopathy.
  - Those with co-morbid ASPD were 3.5 times more likely to be violent.

Treatment of borderline PD is primarily psychological, sometimes with adjunctive psychotropic medication. This is discussed further in Chapter 11 (p139).

Paranoid personality disorder

Key characteristics in DSM-IV:

- Extreme distrust of others
- Bear persistent grudges
- Reluctant to confide in others for fear of malicious use of information given
- Perceive neutral incidents or comments as threatening
- Preoccupied with suspicions that others want to harm or deceive them
- Believe that sexual partners are unfaithful.

Note that jealous overvalued ideas are a diagnostic criterion of paranoid PD, so it is not surprising that paranoid PD commonly underlies morbid jealousy. This nosologically imprecise syndrome is considered further in Chapter 7 (p91).

From Carroll (2009):

- The prevalence in psychiatric outpatient samples is 10% and would be higher in forensic samples.
- In more than half of cases there is a co-morbid PD, commonly ASPD in forensic populations.
- Paranoid thinking is self-perpetuating, self-defeating and very resistant to change.
- Paranoid PD is associated with an increased risk of violence:
  - This risk is increased by co-morbid disorders such as psychosis and ASPD.
- Paranoid PD has also been associated with stalking, making threats, and excessive complaints and litigation.
- Cognitive therapy is a useful management strategy.
- Antipsychotics can sometimes be helpful.

● Dangerous and Severe Personality Disorder

DSPD is a 'diagnosis' invented by politicians and civil servants in 1999 (Maden, 2007). In the following 10 years in excess of £200 million was spent on developing a new programme of treatment for those deemed to have DSPD in England (Tyrer *et al.*, 2010).

In 2010, the DSPD programme consisted of:

- 300 high secure places for men (Broadmoor and Rampton high secure hospitals and HMP Frankland and HMP Whitemoor)
- 75 medium secure and community places
- 12 places for women at HMP Low Newton.

The cost of DSPD treatment in high-security hospitals is over £200 000 per patient per year (Maden, 2007):

- Psychopathy is the key construct of the DSPD initiative.
- The underpinning philosophy of the DSPD programme is that public protection will be best served by addressing the mental health needs of a previously neglected group.
- Treatment is based on a cognitive–behavioural model.

An individual can be admitted to the DSPD programme if they fulfil all three of the following criteria (Department of Health, Ministry of Justice, HM Prison Service, 2008):

- They are more likely than not to commit an offence that might be expected to lead to serious physical or psychological harm from which the victim would find it difficult or impossible to recover.
- They present with a severe disorder of personality (assessed by PCL-R and IPDE):
  - They score 30 or above on the PCL-R, or
  - They score 25–29 on the PCL-R with at least one DSM-IV PD apart from ASPD, or
  - They have two or more DSM-IV PD diagnoses
- There is a link between the personality disorder and the offending.

Challenges in the implementation of the DSPD programme include (Howells *et al.*, 2007):

- the reluctant patient
- maintaining staff morale and a positive therapeutic environment
- meaningful evaluation to demonstrate any effectiveness
- managing expectations of referring agencies and the broader community.

The end of DSPD?

By the end of 2010, the DSPD project was coming to an end. It was seen as not cost-effective (Tyrer *et al.*, 2010) and the Bradley Report (Department of Health, 2009) recommended a re-evaluation. The consequent review led to proposals for a new offender PD strategy, which adopted a broader, more inclusive perspective, encompassing all those offenders with PD, rather than the very small group with DSPD. It emphasized that:

- in the vast majority of cases, offenders with PD should be managed within the CJS rather than in hospital
- management should include:
  - accredited OBPs, delivered within psychologically informed planned environments (PIPEs)
  - psychological treatment in prison for some, and in hospital for a very few.

Other important principles included:

- sharing of responsibility between National Offender Management Service (NOMS) and health care
- training and development of the workforce
- a coherent whole systems pathway.

● Selecting Offenders with PD for Treatment

Treatment for PD is available in prison, in hospital and in the community:

- Availability of treatment in each setting varies considerably geographically.
- There is little evidence of consistency of practice.

Prison therapeutic communities are described further in Chapter 18 (p236) and inpatient management of borderline PD is considered further in Chapter 11 (p139).
  Hospital-based PD units are available in high, medium and low security:

- There is little guidance available to assist with deciding on whether a hospital or prison setting is most appropriate.

The prevalence of PD in prison and the limited available resources mean that only a small proportion can be transferred out for treatment. Clinical decision-making is difficult, and a transfer out is not necessarily a benign option:

- Non-completion of a treatment programme may be associated with an increased risk of recidivism compared with offering no treatment at all (McMurran and Theodosi, 2007).
- Returning a patient to prison after unsuccessful treatment may be experienced as rejecting and lead to considerable iatrogenic harm, especially increased deliberate self-harm (DSH).

High psychopathy scores predict a poor response to all aspects of treatment (Maden, 2007). Of those admitted to a medium secure PD unit (McCarthy and Duggan, 2010):

- one-third completed the treatment programme
- one-third disengaged from treatment
- one-third were expelled from the treatment programme for rule breaking
- 60% reoffended in the 5 years following discharge, with no statistically significant difference observed in those who had completed the treatment programme
- offenders who were less impulsive and had lower levels of psychopathy were more likely to complete treatment programmes.

Box 9.1 Assessing a personality-disordered prisoner for transfer to a hospital setting

The process of assessment:

- It is helpful to undertake a multidisciplinary assessment.
- You may need to assess the person on more than one occasion.
- It will be essential to obtain medical, prison and police records to undertake a thorough risk assessment.
- Discuss with prison health-care staff and with discipline officers – ideally their personal officer.
- Review assessment, care in custody and teamwork (ACCT) documents, noting timing, duration and precipitants of periods on ACCT.
- Establish the length of sentence, and future supervision on licence. How long until they would become a notional s37 patient?

Making a diagnosis of the personality disorder (PD):

- Remember that co-morbidity is very common. The best approach is often to establish that they have a PD and then consider the dominant extreme traits, rather than squeeze the patient into a single ill-fitting taxon.
- This process may be helped by the use of a semi-structured interview schedule such as the IPDE.
- Consider the PCL-R or PCL-SV where there is evidence of psychopathic traits.
- In general the best evidence is for the treatment of borderline PD, so emotional instability may be a good target for treatment.
- Conversely there is little evidence to support the efficacy of treatment for paranoid or antisocial PD, so, where these traits dominate, hospital treatment is less likely to be effective.
- In particular, high levels of psychopathy and high impulsivity are associated with poorer outcome.

Using multiple sources of information, establish the extent in prison of problematic behaviours, which may transfer to a hospital setting and obstruct treatment:

- Incidents of violence to others.
- Incidents of deliberate self-harm or suicidal behaviour.
- Use of drugs within prison.
- Other subversive behaviour, or inciting peers to act out.
- Evidence of manipulative behaviour. This may be evident from health-care interactions and demands for certain treatments, or may be observed by staff in their interactions with other prisoners. They may bargain, make demands or make threats contingent upon some need or wish not being met.
- Consider the motivations for violent and self-harm behaviours. Are they associated with distress, intended to relieve tension, impulsive or planned, or deliberately manipulative?

Is there evidence that they are psychologically minded?

- Are they very focused on medication as the answer to their problems?
- Are they able to frame their problems in psychological terms? Can they draw links between past experiences and current functioning?
- Do they have any capacity for introspection, to consider the way in which they tend to think, or the way in which they relate to other people?
- Do they reflect on why they have certain problems?

Are they able to form effective therapeutic relationships?

- Look for evidence of mature relationships with a variety of staff.
- Sometimes a prisoner with PD will form an intense dependent relationship with one member of staff to the exclusion of others. This may be associated with a tendency to split therapeutic teams in hospital.

What are their motivations for treatment?

- Evidence that they are distressed by their psychological symptoms provides evidence of an internal motivation.
- External motivations might come from family or children.

- What are their longer-term aims and goals in life? Are they realistic? Can they articulate how their PD obstructs realization of these?
- Have they engaged in OBPs or other activities in prison, to back up their claims that they will engage in hospital?

References

Babiak P, Hare R. (2007) *Snakes in Suits: When psychopaths go to work*. New York: Harper Collins

*Carroll A. (2009) Are you looking at me? Understanding and managing paranoid personality disorder. *Advances in Psychiatric Treatment* **15**, 40–8.

Clark L, Harrison J. (2001) Assessment instruments. In: Livesley WJ (ed.), *Handbook of Personality Disorders – Theory, research and treatment*. New York: Guilford Press

Coid J, Yang M, Tyrer P, Roberts A, Ullrich S. (2006) Prevalence and correlates of personality disorders in Great Britain. *British Journal of Psychiatry* **188**, 423–31

Craig MC, Catani M, Deeley Q, Latham R, Daly E, Kanaan R, *et al*. (2009) Altered connections on the road to psychopathy. *Molecular Psychiatry* **14**, 946–53.

*Department of Health. (2009) *The Bradley Report: Lord Bradley's review of people with mental health problems or learning disabilities in the criminal justice system*. Available at: http://www.dh.gov.uk/en/Publicationsandstatistics/Publications/PublicationsPolicyAndGuidance/DH_098694

Department of Health, Ministry of Justice, HM Prison Service. (2008) *Dangerous and Severe Personality Disorder (DSPD) High Secure Services for Men: Planning and delivery guide*. Available at: http://www.dspdprogramme.gov.uk/publications.html

Duggan C, Howard R. (2009). The functional link between personality disorder and violence: a critical appraisal. In: McMurran M, Howard R (eds), *Personality, Personality Disorder and Violence*. London: John Wiley & Sons

Feeney A. (2003) Dangerous severe personality disorders. *Advances in Psychiatric Treatment* **9**, 349–58

Ferguson CJ, Beaver KM. (2009) Natural born killers: the genetic origins of extreme violence. *Aggression and Violent Behaviour* **14**, 286–94

Frick PJ, Petitclerc A. (2009) The use of callous-unemotional traits to define important subtypes of antisocial and violent youth. In: Hodgins S, Viding E, Plodowski A (eds), *The Neurobiological Basis of Violence: Science and rehabilitation*. Oxford: Oxford University Press

Hare RD. (1991) *The Hare Psychopathy Checklist – Revised*. Toronto: Multi-Health Systems

Howells K, Krishnan G, Daffern M. (2007) Challenges in the treatment of dangerous and severe personality disorder. *Advances in Psychiatric Treatment* **13**, 325–32.

Huang Y, Kotov R, de Girolamo G, Preti, A, Angermeyer M, Benjet C, *et al*. (2009). DSM-IV personality disorders in the WHO World Mental Health Surveys. *British Journal of Psychiatry* **195**, 46–53

Leichsenring F, Leibing E, Kruse J, New AS, Leweke F. (2011) Borderline personality disorder. *Lancet* **377**, 74–84

Livesley WJ. (2007) A framework for integrating dimensional and categorical classifications of personality disorder. *Journal of Personality Disorders* **21**, 199–224

Logan C, Blackburn R. (2009) Mental disorder in violent women in secure settings: potential relevance to risk for future violence. *International Journal of Law and Psychiatry* **32**, 31–8.

Maden A. (2007) Dangerous and severe personality disorder: antecedents and origins. *British Journal of Psychiatry* **190**(suppl 49), s8–s11

McCarthy L, Duggan C. (2010) Engagement in a medium secure personality disorder service: a comparative study of psychological functioning and offending outcomes. *Criminal Behaviour and Mental Health* **20**, 112–28

McMurran M, Theodosi E. (2007) Is treatment non-completion associated with increased reconviction over no treatment? *Psychology, Crime and Law* **13**, 333–43

*National Collaborating Centre for Mental Health. (2010) *Antisocial Personality Disorder: The NICE guideline on treatment, management and prevention*. London: NICE

Newhill CE, Eack SM, Mulvey EP. (2009) Violent behaviour in borderline personality disorder. *Journal of Personality Disorders* **23**, 541–54

Odgers CL. (2009) The life-course persistent pathway of antisocial behaviour: risks for violence and poor physical health. In: Hodgins S, Viding E, Plodowski A (eds), *The Neurobiological Basis of Violence: Science and rehabilitation*. Oxford: Oxford University Press

Roberts ADL, Coid JW. (2010) Personality disorder and offending behaviour: findings from the national survey of male prisoners in England and Wales. *Journal of Forensic Psychiatry and Psychology* **21**, 221–37

Shea MT, Stout, R, Gunderson J, Morey LC, Grilo CM, McGlashan T, *et al.* (2002) Short-term diagnostic stability of schizotypal, borderline, avoidant and obsessive-compulsive personality disorders *American Journal of Psychiatry* **159**, 2036–41

Singleton N, Meltzer H, Gatward R, Coid J, Deasy D. (1998) *Psychiatric morbidity among prisoners. Summary report*. London: Office for National Statistics.

Tiihonen J, Rossi R, Laakso MP, Hodgins S, Testa C, Perez J, *et al.* (2008) Brain anatomy of persistent violent offenders: more rather than less. *Psychiatry Research: Neuroimaging* **163**, 201–12

Tyrer P (2007) Personality diatheses: a superior explanation than disorder. *Psychological Medicine* **37**, 1521–5

Tyrer P, Casey P, Ferguson B. (1993) Personality disorder in perspective. In: Tyrer P, Stein G (eds), *Personality Disorder Reviewed*. London: Gaskell

Tyrer P, Coombes N, Ibrahimi F, Mathilakath M, Bajaj P, Ranger M, *et al.* (2007) Critical developments in the assessment of personality disorders. *British Journal of Psychiatry* **190**, s51–s59

Tyrer P, Duggan C, Cooper S, Crawford M, Seivewright H, Rutter D, *et al.* (2010) The successes and failures of the DSPD experiment: the assessment and management of severe personality disorder. *Medicine, Science, and the Law* **50**, 95–9.

Widiger TA, Simonsen E, Sirovatk PJ, Regier DA. (2006) *Dimensional Models of Personality Disorders: Refining the research agenda for DSM*. Washington DC: American Psychiatric Association

Yang Y, Raine A. (2009) Prefrontal structural and functional brain imaging findings in antisocial, violent, and psychopathic individuals: a meta-analysis. *Psychiatry Research: Neuroimaging* **174**, 81–8.

Yang Y, Raine A, Narr KL, Colletti P, Toga AW. (2009) Localization of deformations within the amygdala in individuals with psychopathy. *Archives of General Psychiatry* **66**(9), 986–94.

10

Learning Disability, Autistic Spectrum Disorders and Offending

● Learning Disability

Emerson *et al.* (2010) reported that in England in 2010, there were:

- 1 198 000 people with learning disability (LD), 900 000 of whom were adults.
- Of the adults:
  - 58 % were male
  - 21 % were known to LD services.
- There were 1246 NHS residential care beds for people with LD, down from 3703 in 2000–1.
- There were 3501 people in LD provider services, a drop of 21 % from 4435 people identified in 2006.

Various terms are used relatively synonymously, which is particularly important when reviewing the literature:

- learning disability
- intellectual disability
- mental retardation
- developmental disability.

'Learning difficulty' tends to be used to describe a broader group.

Identifying rates of LD among offender populations is problematic because ascertainment of cases is difficult:

- The diagnosis of LD requires:
  - significant intellectual impairment, and
  - significant impairment in social functioning
  - both being present from childhood.
- The validity and reliability of the WAIS (and other IQ assessment tools) may be affected by level of education, culture, language barrier, co-morbid mental health problems and psychotropic medication.
- There is no definitive tool for assessing the presence of impairment of social functioning. LD services often use their own 'eligibility assessment' tools, with uncertain reliability.
- Official rates of offending generally underestimate the true rate of offending, and this may be particularly true among the learning-disabled population.

Holland *et al.* (2002) have reviewed prevalence studies of offending in learning-disabled populations:

- Up to 5% of those attending day services or living in group homes had contact with the criminal justice system (CJS).
- Of those awaiting interview in police stations:
  - 9% had IQ ≤ 70
  - 34% had IQ ≤ 75.
- There are no relevant studies of defendants in Crown or magistrates' courts.
- A small survey of a probation sample found 6% with IQ < 70 and 11% <75.

Rates in prisons have varied greatly, depending on varying methodology. In a survey across a local male prison, a women's prison and a young offenders' institution (YOI), Mottram (2007) found a mean IQ of 86:

- 6.5% had IQ < 70
- 25% 70–79
- 29% 80–89
- 35% 90–109
- 4% ≥ 110.

According to the Prison Reform Trust (Talbot, 2008):

- 20–30% of offenders have learning disabilities or difficulties that interfere with their ability to cope within the criminal justice system.
- 23% of prisoners under 18 years of age have an IQ of less than 70.
- 20% of the prison population has a 'hidden disability' that 'will affect and undermine their performance in both education and work settings'.
- dyslexia is three to four times more common among prisoners than among the general population.

Characteristics of learning-disabled offenders

In their review Holland et al. (2002) found the following factors to be common among learning-disabled offenders (as they are among non-learning-disabled offenders as well):

- mostly young men
- borderline or mild (rather than more severe) LD
- background of psychosocial deprivation
- childhood behavioural problems
- co-morbid psychiatric disorders
- family history of offending
- low socio-economic status
- a history of behavioural problems or previous offending
- homelessness.

Wheeler *et al.* (2009) reviewed 237 referrals to a LD team because of antisocial or offending behaviour in three geographical areas over 2 years:

- Those whose offending had led to contact with the CJS represented an estimated 0.8% of all adults with LD in the relevant areas.
- 62% had mild, borderline or no LD.
- 44% had a co-morbid psychiatric condition.
- The range of behaviours included:
  - physical (52%) and verbal (40%) aggression
  - damage to property (24%)
  - inappropriate sexual behaviour (18%)

Box 10.1 Assessment of individuals with LD

Before the assessment:

- An appointment letter should be in a larger font, written in simple English and include a pictorial list of contraband items.
- A family member, carer or solicitor (for court reports) should also be informed so that they can remind the person of the appointment.
- Always request the attendance of an informant who knows the person well, preferably from childhood.
- Check if the patient suffers from any sensory abnormalities and consider use of an interpreter, such as in cases with hearing difficulties.
- Sometimes it may be more feasible to review the patient in a familiar non-domestic environment such as their community learning disability team (CLDT) base, their GP surgery or their solicitor's offices.

During the assessment

- Consider any sensory abnormality that may impede their participation in the interview process such as hearing loss, speech impediment or poor eyesight.
- Use simple language, short phrases and short sentences. Be aware of the use of technical words or jargon.
- Talk slowly and give the person time to process information. You may have to repeat or rephrase questions.
- Check the understanding of the person as you go along. Certain gestures (e.g. nodding head) and expressions (e.g. saying 'yes' or 'no') may be learnt social responses, and may not reflect the true understanding of the questions being asked.
- It may be helpful to start the interview by asking the individual about innocuous subjects that they like to talk about such as their hobbies or interest.
- Focus particularly on developmental history, early childhood, schooling and adaptive functioning.
- You may need to allow breaks in the interview, or conduct more than one assessment, depending on the ability to concentrate and attend to the interview.

After the assessment collateral information from the family is particularly important:

- Pregnancy-related complications, prematurity, birth, birth weight.
- Postnatal complications and early development. Focus on attainment of developmental milestones.
- Details about play activities and interactions with peers and parents.
- Details about schooling and educational difficulties.
- Risk behaviours even though they may not have resulted in being charged by the police.

If they are available, school records and a copy of the special educational needs assessment are helpful.

– cruelty and neglect relating to children (11 %), mostly involving women
– fire setting (1 %).

Commissioning of secure services and care pathways

The provision of secure inpatient facilities for people with LD varies geographically:

- For services without secure inpatient facilities, out-of-area placements, often in the independent sector, are used:
  – this may lead to more difficult integration with local community learning disability teams (CLDTs), and lack of suitable local step-down facilities
  – potentially this may lead to increased lengths of stay.
- Active gate-keeping of new referrals, both at clinical assessment level and at commissioning level, has the benefit of reducing unnecessary out-of-area placements, and active monitoring of cases can help streamline care pathways, thereby reducing delayed discharges.

25

More recently some community forensic LD teams have been developed and tasked with gate keeping and monitoring of cases requiring secure care.

There is limited data on outcome following admission to secure LD placements. Alexander *et al.* (2006) reported on outcomes following discharge from a LD medium secure service, with 12 years of follow-up:

- 11 % of the sample were reconvicted:
  - Risk factors for reconviction were personality disorder, a history of theft or burglary, and young age.
  - Contact with the police was less likely in those with schizophrenia.
- 58 % showed offending-like behaviour that did not lead to police contact.
- 28 % were currently detained in hospital under the Mental Health Act (MHA):
  - Readmission to hospital was associated with the presence of offending-like behaviours, rather than any specific diagnosis.

● Challenging Behaviour

The Royal College of Psychiatrists (2007) gives the following definition:

Behaviour can be described as challenging when it is of such an intensity, frequency or duration as to threaten the quality of life and/or the physical safety of the individual or others and is likely to lead to responses that are restrictive, aversive or result in exclusion.

Observed prevalence rates of challenging behaviour among learning-disabled populations (Tsiouris, 2010):

- tend to vary, from 10 % to as much as 60 %
- point prevalence rates have been reported at:
  - 9.8 % for aggressive behaviour towards others or objects
  - 4.9 % for self-injurious behaviour.

The Royal College of Psychiatrists emphasizes the following factors in assessing challenging behaviours:

- Factors unique to the individual:
  - degree and nature of learning disability
  - communication difficulties
  - sensory or motor disabilities
  - co-morbid mental health problems
  - physical health problems
  - emotional needs and strength
  - social competency
  - insight
  - strengths and coping strategies.
- Environmental factors:
  - geographical location of the placement and its perceived importance for the patient
  - physical structure of the placement, e.g. room sizes, communal areas, facilities available, open spaces, time-out room or sensory room
  - environmental adaptations to meet the needs of the person including their sensory needs or physical health needs
  - other patients in the placement.
- Staff, support and intervention:
  - training and experience of staff

Box 10.2 Assessment of challenging behaviour

1. Collect information from all possible sources

- Patient
- Carers
- Nursing staff
- Psychiatric or psychological reports
- Speech and language therapy assessments
- OT reports.

2. Record the frequency, intensity and duration of behaviours

- These will serve as a baseline for ongoing evaluation.

The next step is to record the behaviour systematically:

- by breaking it down into antecedents, behaviours and consequences (ABC), or
- setting, triggers, action and response (STAR).

It is important to collect this data over a period of time to be able to identify any emerging patterns.

3. This information is collated into a formulation, which includes a causal hypothesis for the challenging behaviour:

- The hypothesis is tested by modulating the identified problematic contributory factors, the outcome being compared with the baseline data.
- If unsuccessful, review the formulation with the multidisciplinary team, and change other factors.

It is important to have small goals and realistic expectations, with adequate supervision and support for staff.

- constancy of staff group and in particular the key or named worker
- procedural consistency meeting the needs of the individual
- opportunities for planned and regular constructive activities and sessions
- individualized care plans to meet the particular needs of the patients
- functional analysis of the challenging behaviour.

Management strategies

There is a limited evidence base for psychological and environmental strategies, which may include:

- focusing on individual strengths and weaknesses
- CBT and behavioural modification
- environmental modification:
  - creating capable and supportive environments with adequate organizational structures
  - adequate number of well-trained staff members
  - a supportive ethos with clear values
- specialist placements.

According to Tsiouris (2010):

- Antipsychotic medications are not anti-aggressive drugs so they should not be used unless indicated for an underlying mental disorder.
- Patients with autism show improvement in irritability and aggressive behaviour on risperidone.
- Selective serotonin reuptake inhibitors (SSRIs) led to improvement in aggressive behaviours in 50% of cases with LD.

● Offending and LD

There is no convincing evidence that LD is, in itself, a risk factor for offending, though those with borderline ability are over-represented in offender populations. Factors that may mediate this relationship include:

- behaviours may be appropriate to the developmental stage but not the chronological age of the individual
- reduced capacity to delay gratification or resist temptation
- reduced capacity to modify behaviour according to experience
- social naivety
- difficulty coping with socio-economic, interpersonal or other normal life stresses, leading to frustration.

Sexual offending

Sexual offending is covered generally in Chapter 13. Earlier studies (Hayes, 1991) found similar rates of sexual offending in learning-disabled and non-learning-disabled populations. A large meta-analysis (Cantor *et al.*, 2005) of sex offenders, found that:

- overall adult males who commit sexual offences have a lower IQ than non-sexual offenders
- but if offenders against children are excluded, the difference was not statistically significant
- the association between low IQ and sexual offending is particularly strong for paedophilic offences.

Sexual offending is common among those admitted to secure LD care:

- Up to 40% (Day, 1988), compared with perhaps 10% for an adult mental illness secure service (see Chapter 3).

Day (1997) proposed the following typology of learning-disabled sexual offenders:

- Developmental:
  - shy and immature
  - little or no sexual experience
  - offence due to poor adaptation.
- Sociopathic:
  - more serious and persistent sexual offender, perhaps with other offences as well
  - lack of impulse control.
- Sexually deviant:
  - exclusively paraphillic behaviour
  - a small proportion.

The evidence base for interventions for learning-disabled sex offenders is weak:

- There are no randomized controlled trials of interventions for learning-disabled sex offenders (Ashman and Duggan, 2008).
- Many studies were deemed methodologically flawed, with variation in inclusion criteria, no standardized outcomes and small sample sizes (Courtney and Rose, 2004).

Psychological interventions:

- Depending on the need and ability of the patient, they may be offered individual or group CBT-based programmes:
  - These adapted sex offender treatment programmes (SOTPs) are altered from standard programmes for non-learning-disabled offenders (see Chapter 13)

- May be accompanied by other interventions, such as social skills training, enhancing thinking skills and problem solving.

Pharmacological treatment:

- Discussed in Chapter 13.
- Most of the evidence is from non-learning-disabled populations.

Published outcomes are focused heavily on recidivism rates:

- Huge variation is reported, depending on the sample size and the duration of the follow-up (up to 68 % – Gibbens and Robertson, 1983).
- Some have argued that the reoffending rates following organized treatment were not any lower than following a non-therapeutic prison sentence. However, learning-disabled patients may be vulnerable in a prison setting. Learning-disabled sex offenders suffered abuse double the rate of non-learning-disabled sex offenders; and mostly the abuse was sexual.
- At least 2 years in hospital and planned discharge have been associated with better outcomes.

Arson

See Chapter 13 for information on psychiatric diagnoses and arson generally:

- In his series of people charged with arson, Rix (1994) found that 11 % had an LD.

Reasons for setting fires are similar in learning-disabled and non-learning-disabled arsonists. In a small descriptive study, Devapriam *et al.* (2007) gave the following reasons among 15 learning-disabled arsonist patients:

- revenge – nine (60 %)
- mental illness – one (6.6 %)
- suggestibility – three (20 %)
- pyromania – two (13.3 %).

Management is primarily psychological, usually in a cognitive–behavioural therapy (CBT)-based group setting:

- Hall *et al.* (2005) described an example of a treatment programme consisting of three sections of five sessions each, with a final session evaluating patient's perspective, and evaluation and maintenance sessions at 6 weeks and 6 months:
  - Introduction to fires : the expectations of the group, general dangers of fire, good/bad fires, media and fire setting, others' view of fire.
  - Personal fire setting: history and pattern, details of the index offence or the main fire set, focus on ABC, develop personal fire focus.
  - Alternative ways of coping: issue of risk, fire setting as a risky behaviour, identify individual risk patterns, safe ingredients and alternative ways of coping, role plays.

● Legal Issues

Mental Health Act 1983 and LD

A learning disability is defined (s1(4)) as a 'state of arrested or incomplete development of the mind, which includes significant impairment of intelligence and social functioning':

- This is broadly in line with contemporary classification systems.

A learning disability does not constitute a mental disorder for the purposes of the MHA unless it is associated with 'abnormally aggressive or seriously irresponsible conduct':

- The behaviour should be understood within the social and cultural aspect.
- The nature, intensity and frequency of the behaviour should be observed.
- This should take into account the potential impact of the behaviour on the person and/or others.

LD in the police station

- The safeguards relating to mentally disordered people in police stations, particularly the role of the appropriate adult, are covered in Chapter 16.
- LD may lead to greater suggestibility (Gudjonsson and Henry, 2003) and consequent unreliability at interview:
  - However, some suggest that LD tends to affect episodic memory less than semantic memory (White and Willner, 2005), so scales assessing primarily semantic memory may be of limited importance.

Fitness to plead and stand trial (role of the intermediary)

A low IQ does not determine unfitness to plead. In particular the courts can make reasonable adjustments to help a defendant participate effectively in a trial (see Chapter 21 for further details).

The role of an intermediary is particularly important for defendants with LD:

- Section 104 of the Coroners and Justice Act 2009 amends s33 of the Youth Justice and Criminal Evidence Act 1999 to provide that:
  - where the accused 'suffers from a mental disorder … or otherwise has a significant impairment of intelligence and social function and … is for that reason unable to participate effectively in the proceedings as a witness giving oral evidence in court'
  - the court may order that any examination is conducted through an intermediary, whose function is to communicate and explain questions to the accused, and communicate their answers.

Mental Capacity Act 2005 (MCA)

The principles of the MCA (s1) are:

- A person is assumed to have capacity until it is established that they do not.
- All practicable steps to assist a person to make their own decision must be taken.
- Making an unwise decision should not be taken to imply lack of capacity.
- Those acting on behalf of an incapacitated person:
  - must act in their best interests
  - must act in the way that is least restrictive of the person's rights and freedom.

Capacity must be assessed in relation to a particular decision and a particular time:

- a person may have the capacity to make some decisions but not others
- capacity may vary over time.

A two-stage test:

- Is there an impairment of, or disturbance in, the functioning of the person's mind or brain?
- Is the impairment or disturbance sufficient to cause the person to be unable to make that particular decision at the relevant time?

In considering best interests, all relevant circumstances must be taken into account, including:

- if and when the person is likely to regain capacity
- the person's past and present wishes, beliefs and values
- consultation with carers.

The test of capacity (s3) requires the ability to:

- understand the relevant information i.e. information about reasonably foreseeable consequences of the decision
- retain the information related to the decision to be made even if only for a short period
- use or weigh that information as part of the process of making the decision
- communicate that decision by any means, including blinking an eye or squeezing a hand.

Deprivation of liberty safeguards (DOLS)

Introduced into the MCA by the MHA 2007, to provide a legal framework for those who are deprived of their liberty which satisfies Article 5 of the European Convention on Human Rights (ECHR) by providing:

- a procedure prescribed by law and
- access to a speedy review of the lawfulness of the detention by a court.

The safeguards were introduced following the judgement in the 'Bournewood case' (*HL v United Kingdom* [2004] 40 EHRR 761):

- a man with autism and learning difficulties who lacked capacity to agree to informal admission to hospital. His admission was challenged by his carers and was found by the European Court of Human Rights to be in breach of his rights under Article 5 (1) and Article 5 (4) of the ECHR.

The person to be detained must be an adult with a mental disorder who lacks capacity to consent to the arrangements made for their care or treatment:

- Receiving care and treatment in circumstances that amount to a deprivation of liberty must be:
  - necessary to protect them from harm
  - proportionate to the likelihood and seriousness of the harm
  - in their best interests.
- There must be no less restrictive alternative available.

Deprivation of liberty has not been clearly defined. But:

- the difference between deprivation of and restriction of liberty is one of degree
- the deprivation of liberty has an objective element (which includes whether a person is free to leave) as well as a subjective element (which takes into account whether the person has the capacity or not).

● Autistic Spectrum Disorders

As with LD, several terms are in use, including autistic spectrum disorders (ASDs), autistic spectrum conditions, autistic spectrum difference and neuro-diversity:

- The code of practice (CoP) to the MHA 1983 considers that 'the Act's definition of mental disorder includes the full range' of ASDs:
  - but detention in the absence of an additional mental disorder 'is likely to happen only very rarely'.

The National Audit Office (2009) indicated that:

- there are 400 000 adults with ASD, with around half of them having LD
- the male to female ratio (M:F) is around 3–4:1.

Brugha *et al.* (2009) estimated:

- The overall prevalence of ASD, using the threshold of a score of 10 on the Autism Diagnostic Observation Schedule (ADOS) to indicate a positive case, was 1 % of the adult population in England:
  - M – 1.8 % ; F – 0.2 %.

Dein and Woodbury-Smith (2010) describe the very inconsistent prevalence rates reported in various secure mental health and custodial settings, concluding that:

- there probably is an increased rate of ASD in such settings, but
- this does not reflect a raised rate of offending in the community.

The Autism Act 2009 placed a duty on the Secretary of State for Health to introduce a strategy for improving outcomes for adults with autism:

- The resultant strategy (Department of Health, 2010) emphasizes:
  - increasing awareness and understanding of autism
  - developing a clear, consistent pathway for diagnosis of autism
  - improving access for adults with autism to the services and support that they need to live independently within the community
  - helping adults with autism into work
  - enabling local partners to develop relevant services for adults with autism to meet identified needs and priorities.

ASD and offending

Berney (2004) considers the relationship between ASD and offending. He

- suggests that the following offence types might indicate the presence of ASD:
  - obsessive harassment or stalking
  - inexplicable violence
  - computer crime
  - offences arising from misjudged social relationships
- cites the following as characteristics of ASD that are liable to lead to offending:
  - lack of concern for or awareness of the likely outcome of actions
  - lack of empathy
  - apparently impulsive violence resulting from rapidly escalating anxiety
  - social naivety leading to exploitation by others
  - sexual offending may result from misinterpretation of social rules and norms and difficulty judging others' ages
  - obsessive interests may lead to stalking or theft.

Management of ASD

The evidence base for specific therapies for ASD is weak. However, the following aspects are important:

- Setting – mainstream secure units or specialist secure ASD units.

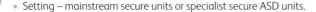

Box 10.3 Assessment of an individual with autistic spectrum disorders (ASD)

As with all psychiatric evaluations the diagnosis is based upon the account given by the person, their presentation during the interview and information from other sources such as:

- an informant who knows the person well (preferably from childhood)
- school records
- past medical and psychiatric notes.

In some cases it may be important to see the individual for several sessions before a diagnosis can be made reliably. The assessment should particularly focus on the autistic triad of symptom clusters.

Reciprocal social interactions:

- Ask about interactions with others at school, college and work. Try to evaluate the quality of their interactions with others including what characteristics of other people they tend to like, dislike, ignore, copy, idolize.
- Ask about friends (how many, how long for, best friend, how easy it was to make friends, reasons for disagreements, etc.) and their understanding of friendship (what is a friend, differences between social friends and boy-/girlfriends, what makes a good friend, etc.).

Communication:

- As part of developmental history focus on any delay in speech (when first words spoken, difficulties in hearing as a child or requiring a speech therapist).
- Check for qualitative difficulties – literal thinking, difficulty in understanding implied meaning, jokes or sarcasm, reciprocity of conversation.
- Ability to pick up how the other person talking to them may be feeling, use of non-verbal gestures, eye contact, understanding of body language or non-verbal cues.

Restrictive and repetitive interests:

- Enquire about hobbies and interests (what, how long for, how much time spent, what others think of it, exclusion of other pastimes, etc.).
- Ask about routines or rituals and response to enforced or unexpected changes.

Consider the use of structured assessment tools such as:

- The Diagnostic Interview for Social and Communication Disorders (DISCO) – for children and adults. The most commonly used instrument for diagnosing broad-spectrum ASD.
- Autism Diagnostic Interview, Revised (ADI-R) – children from > 2 years old, takes 1.5–2.5 hours. Focuses mainly on core autistic features, leading to relatively restrictive diagnosis.
- ADOS (Autism Diagnostic Observation Schedule) – from toddlers to adults, takes 30–45 minutes.
- Adult Asperger's Assessment – tool designed specifically for use in adults.

Howlin (2000) discusses the limitations of these assessment tools in terms of validity, reliability, specificity and sensitivity.

- Psychological treatment:
  - CBT, music or art therapy
  - role playing
  - mind reading
  - social skills training
  - specific interventions for the offending behaviour
  - support for carers and family members.
- Pharmacological treatment:
  - only indicated for treatment of co-morbid mental disorders.
- Environmental factors:
  - reasonable adaptations to avoid sensory overload.
  - sensory room

- predictable and consistent regimens
- structured daily programmes
- specifically trained staff.
- Following an inpatient episode:
    - suitable placement (trained staff, gradual transition, ongoing support)
    - employment
    - adequate support structures for follow-up, monitoring and implementing contingency plans (including re-admission and respite care).

References

Alexander RT, Crouch K, Halstead S, Piachaud J. (2006) Long-term outcome from a medium secure service for people with intellectual disability. *Journal of Intellectual Disability Research* **50**(4), 305–15

Ashman LLM, Duggan L. (2008) Interventions for learning disabled sex offenders. *Cochrane Database of Systematic Reviews* 2008, Issue 1. Art. No.: CD003682. DOI: 10.1002/14651858. CD003682.pub2

*Berney T. (2004) Asperger syndrome from childhood into adulthood. *Advances in Psychiatric Treatment* **10**, 341–51

*Brugha T, McManus S, Meltzer H, Smith J, Scott FJ, Purdon S, et al. (2009). *Autism Spectrum Disorders in Adults living in Households throughout England. Report from the Adult Psychiatric Morbidity Survey 2007*. Available from: http://www.ic.nhs.uk/statistics-and-data-collections/mental-health/mental-health-surveys

Cantor JM, Blanchard R, Robichaud LK, Christensen BK. (2005). Quantitative reanalysis of aggregate data on IQ in sexual offenders. *Psychological Bulletin* **131**, 555–68

Courtney J, Rose J. (2004) The effectiveness of treatment for male sex offenders with learning disabilities: a review of the literature. *Journal of Sexual Aggression* **10**(2), 215–36

Day K. (1988) A hospital based treatment programme for male mentally handicapped offenders *British Journal of Psychiatry* **153**, 635–44.

Day K. (1997). Sex offenders with learning disabilities. In: Read SG (ed.), *Psychiatry in Learning Disability*. London: WB Saunders Company Ltd

*Dein K, Woodbury-Smith M. (2010) Asperger syndrome and criminal behaviour. *Advances in Psychiatric Treatment* **16**, 37–43

Department of Health. (2010) *Fulfilling and Rewarding Lives. The strategy for adults with autism in England*. Available at: http://www.dh.gov.uk/en/Publicationsandstatistics/Publications/PublicationsPolicyAndGuidance/DH_113369

Devapriam J, Raju LB, Singh N, Collacott R, Bhaumik S. (2007) Arson: characteristics and predisposing factors in offenders with intellectual disabilities. *British Journal of Forensic Practice* **9**(4), 23–7

*Emerson E, Hatton C, Robertson J, Roberts H, Baines S, Glover G. (2010) *People with Learning Disabilities in England 2010*. London: DH

Gibbens CN, Robertson G. (1983) A survey of the criminal careers of hospital order patients. *British Journal of Psychiatry* **143**, 362–9

Gudjonsson GH, Henry L. (2003) Child and adult witnesses with intellectual disability: the importance of suggestibility. *Legal and Criminological Psychology* **8**(2), 241–52

Hall I, Clayton P, Johnson P. (2005) Arson and learning disability. In: Riding T, Swann C, Swann B (eds), *The Handbook of Forensic Learning Disability*. Oxford: Radcliffe Publishing

Hayes S. (1991) Sexual offenders. *Australia and New Zealand Journal of Developmental Disabilities* **17**(2), 221–7

*Holland T, Clare CH, Mukhopadhyay T. (2002) Prevalence of criminal offending by men and women with intellectual disability and the characteristics of the offenders: implications for research and service development. *Journal of Intellectual Disability Research* **46**(S1), 6–20

Howlin P. (2000) Assessment instruments for Asperger syndrome. *Child and Adolescent Mental Health* **5**(3), 120–9

Mottram PG. (2007) *HMP Liverpool, Styal and Hindley Study Report.* Liverpool: University of Liverpool

National Audit Office. (2009) *Supporting People with Autism through Adulthood.* London: The Stationery Office

Rix K. (1994) A psychiatric study of adult arsonists. *Medicine Science and the Law* **4**(1), 21–34

Royal College of Psychiatrists. (2007) *Challenging Behaviour: A unified approach CR144.* London: Royal College of Psychiatrists

Talbot J. (2008) *No One Knows: Experiences of the criminal justice system by prisoners with learning disabilities and difficulties.* London: Prison Reform Trust

*Tsiouris JA. (2010) Pharmacotherapy for aggressive behaviours in persons with intellectual disabilities: treatment or mistreatment? *Journal of Intellectual Disability Research* **54**(1), 1–16

Wheeler JR, Holland AJ, Bambrick M, Lindsay WR, Carson D, Steptoe L, *et al.* (2009) Community services and people with intellectual disabilities who engage in anti-social or offending behaviour: referral rates, characteristics, and care pathways. *Journal of Forensic Psychiatry and Psychology* **20**(5), 717–40

White R. Willner P. (2005) Suggestibility and salience in people with intellectual disabilities: an experimental critique of the Gudjonsson Suggestibility Scale. *Journal of Forensic Psychiatry and Psychology* **16**, 638–50

11

Women in Secure Care

● Female Offenders

There are significant differences in patterns of offending between genders:

- Women offend less often than men:
  - in 2004–5 there were 1 120 200 (83%) men arrested for recorded criminal offences compared with 233 600 (17%) women (Home Office, 2007).
- Female offenders are more likely to commit acquisitive offences and are less likely to commit violent offences and sexual offences.
- Home Office (2006) conviction figures show that women commit only 6% of murders, 1.5% of attempted murders, 16% of manslaughters and 7% of woundings.

The female prison population

In August 2010, women constituted 5% of the total prison population (Ministry of Justice, 2010):

- However, there was a disproportionate rise in the prison female population from the early 1990s, reaching a peak in 2005.
- Women are more likely to be remanded in custody and to receive a custodial sentence than male equivalents (Home Office, 2007).
- Women on remand are most likely to be charged with drug offences (26%) or acquisitive offences (24%) (Singleton *et al.*, 1998).
- One-third of female sentenced prisoners are serving a sentence for drug offences, 18% for violent offences and 17% for theft.
- Women in prison are more likely to be from ethnic minorities or be foreign nationals compared with the male prison population (Singleton *et al.*, 1998).

Psychiatric morbidity among female prisoners

Data on the prevalence of mental disorder among female prisoners is given in Chapter 18:

- For all diagnostic groups the rates are higher than in the community.
- Among prisoners, women have higher rates of mental illness and lower rates of personality disorder (PD) than men.
- Women have a lower rate of hazardous alcohol use but the same rate of drug dependence.

The rate of both deliberate self-harm (DSH) and parasuicidal behaviour among women is higher than that of male prisoners:

- Up to half of women within prison have a lifetime history of DSH and 46% have attempted suicide.

- Self-harm and attempted suicide were more common among white women but the highest rate was found in black/mixed race women with a history of substance dependence (Borrill *et al.*, 2003).
- Although representing only 5% of the prison population, women represent half of all incidents of DSH within prisons (Fossey and Black, 2010).
- Fazel and Benning (2009) reported a suicide rate among female prisoners of 163/100 000 between 1978 and 2004. This was just over 20 times the rate in the general population.

Women in prison suffering from severe borderline personality disorder (PD) present particular challenges to the prison service and those working within that setting. They sometimes present with unusually severe DSH and parasuicidal behaviour.

- Fossey and Black (2010) highlight the limited provision within the prison service of treatment compliant with the NICE guidelines.

● Women, Mental Disorder and Violence

The rate of violence among female psychiatric patients

Although the rate of violence in men is much higher within the normal population, these differences are less clear among psychiatric populations, suggesting that the impact of mental disorder on risk is greater among women:

- Lidz *et al.* (1993) in a study of patients discharged from short-term psychiatric facilities found no significant difference in the rates of community violence by male and female patients.

The MacArthur study (Monahan *et al.*, 2001) found, over 1-year follow-up post-discharge:

- Violence (battery leading to injury, sexual assault, threat/assault with weapon in hand) was more common among men (29.7%) than women (24.6%).
- Aggressive acts (battery not resulting in physical injury) were more common among women (37.0%) than men (30.1%).
- Women in the sample were more likely to have a diagnosis of depression and less likely to have a diagnosis of or a co-occurring diagnosis of alcohol/drug dependence.
- In comparison to male violence, women's violence:
  - was more likely to occur in the home, and the victims were more likely to be family members
  - was less likely to have been preceded by alcohol/drug use, or to be followed by arrest. The victims were less likely to seek medical treatment.

Female homicide

Women are less likely to commit homicide than men:

- In 2006 there were 516 male perpetrators of homicide compared with 40 women (National Confidential Inquiry, 2010).

Female perpetrators of homicide are more likely to kill someone with whom they are in a close relationship. Of 55 women who committed homicides in Victoria, Australia between 1997 and 2005 (Bennett *et al.*, 2010):

- 20 (36.4%) killed their partner
- 13 (23.6%) killed another relative (including their children)
- 20 (36.4%) killed an acquaintance or friend
- 2 killed a stranger (3.6%).

Psychiatric factors are more likely to be associated with female homicide:

- Between 1997 and 2006 14% of women convicted of homicide had been in contact with mental health services during the previous year (compared with 10% overall).
- According to d'Orban (1990), between 1980 and 1987 the average annual number of murder convictions for women was 6 (154 for men). Women accounted for:
  - 4% of convicted murderers
  - 12% of manslaughter convictions
  - 20% of convictions for manslaughter on the grounds of diminished responsibility.
- In Bennett's study, 20% had been diagnosed with a psychotic illness of whom:
  - 16.4% had schizophrenia (compared with 7.9% of male perpetrators).
- Studies by Eronen (1995) and Schanda *et al.* (2004) have shown generally higher rates of mental disorder among female perpetrators of homicide.
- In a review of 125 Finnish psychiatric reports in homicides, Putkonen (2001) reported that 27% had a psychotic disorder and 70% a PD.

Box 11.1 Battered woman syndrome (Walker, 1999)

This term is sometimes applied to women in violent relationships who kill their abusive partner. It describes a characteristic pattern of psychological and behavioural responses by a woman to severe abuse inflicted upon her by her partner.

It has two stages:

- the 'cycle of violence' – the tension-building stage → the acute battering incident → kindness and contrite loving behaviour stage
- 'learned helplessness', as an explanation for why the woman is unable to leave the relationship.

The concept has been criticized for stereotyping women and ignoring the other factors which might make it difficult for women to leave a violent relationship.

It is neither a psychiatric diagnosis nor in itself a legal defence to a charge of murder:

- It has been used successfully to support a defence of provocation, to explain why women who kill their abusers may not fit into the usual sudden loss of control of the old provocation defence.
- The new partial defence to murder of loss of control explicitly allows that the loss of control may not be sudden (see Chapter 20), thus maintaining battered woman syndrome potentially within the defence.
- Women who are the victims of repeated violence within relationships experience depression, anxiety and PTSD which may sometimes amount to abnormality of mind, and may allow a defence of manslaughter on the grounds of diminished responsibility.

Filicide, infanticide and neonaticide

Parental child killing is described throughout history and across cultures:

- Filicide is the killing of a child by his or her parent.
- Infanticide means the killing of a child soon after birth. The legal definition is contained in s1(1) Infanticide Act 1938:

> *Where a woman by any wilful act or omission causes the death of her child being a child under the age of twelve months, but at the time of the act or omission the balance of her mind was disturbed by reason of her not having fully recovered from the effect of giving birth to the child or by reason of the effect of lactation consequent upon the birth of the child, then, if the circumstances were such that but for this Act the offence would have amounted to murder or manslaughter, she shall be guilty of felony, to wit of infanticide, and may for such offence be dealt with and punished as if she had been guilty of the offence of manslaughter of the child.*

- Neonaticide is the killing of a child within 24 hours of birth (Resnick, 1970).

On average there are 32 cases of filicide per year in England and Wales, approximately half of all child homicides (National Confidential Inquiry, 2009):

- These figures may be an underestimate due to the difficulties in recording and determining cause of death, for example in cases of sudden infant death syndrome.
- Children under the age of 1 year are at greatest risk (Friedman *et al.*, 2005) representing approximately 55% of all cases of filicides.
- Men are more likely to commit filicide than women, who represent about one-third of all cases.

Parental filicide is associated with suicide:

- Stack (1997) reported that filicide constituted 2% of all homicides, but that they represented 7.6% of homicide followed by suicide.
- Friedman *et al.* (2005) showed between 16% and 29% of maternal filicides died by suicide and between 40% and 60% of fathers took their own life.
- Over an 8-year period, 17% of perpetrators who committed filicide subsequently took their own life (National Confidential Inquiry, 2009).

Women who have killed their children have the following characteristics:

- They are usually between the ages of 20 and 40.
- There are no clear associations with marital status in case series of filicide overall, but women committing neonaticide are more often single.
- There is a strong association with poverty and a fifth of offenders are from a minority ethnic group.
- They often have depressed mood:
  - however, in infanticide, the degree of psychological disturbance is generally less than is required for a defence of diminished responsibility
  - Friedman and Resnick (2009) reported that neonaticide was most often committed by poor, young, single women who lacked prenatal care.

In a sample of 254 filicides (National Confidential Inquiry, 2009):

- affective disorder was the most common diagnosis (38, 23%) followed by
- PD (27, 16%) and schizophrenia (21, 13%).

Over a third were mentally ill at the time of offence (54, 35%), including 19 (13%) who were psychotic.

Attempts to classify filicide according to motive tend to founder in the complexity of relevant factors. Resnick (1969), Scott (1973) and d'Orban (1979) all used a similar typology in their studies:

- Altruistic/mercy killing:
  - to relieve the suffering of a sick child or filicide, or
  - suicide where the motive is not to abandon the child.
- Unwanted children:
  - death may be caused by passive neglect or active aggression
  - neonaticide is common.
- Accidental:
  - impulsive acts leading to the death of the child, e.g. within the context of child abuse.
- Retaliation or spousal revenge:
  - occurring usually within the context of a relationship breakdown where the child becomes the object of retaliation.
- Mental illness.

D'Orban (1979) surveyed 89 consecutive female remands charged with killing or attempted killing of their infants, 44% of whom were less than 12 months old:

- The most common group was a killing resulting from loss of temper and consequent child battering; depression was common among them.
- In the second group a more severe depressive or psychotic illness directly caused the killing.
- A verdict of infanticide was more likely the younger the victim.

Munchhausen syndrome by proxy

A form of child abuse in which parents (usually mothers) fabricate or induce illness in their children. This may take the form of:

- giving false accounts of symptoms
- fabricating symptoms
- inducing symptoms of illness.

It is associated with harm through:

- iatrogenic procedures
- the psychological harm caused to the child.

According to McClure *et al.* (1996) the combined annual incidence of fabricated or induced illness, non-accidental poisoning and non-accidental suffocation in the UK and Ireland in children under 16 years of age was 0.5 per 100 000.

There is no clear relationship with any specific mental disorder, although, as with all forms of child abuse, perpetrators are more likely to have a diagnosis of PD. According to Bools *et al.* (1994) in a study of 47 individuals who had fabricated illness in children:

- 72% had somatoform disorders
- 55% self-harmed
- 21% misused alcohol and/or drugs
- 89% had a PD.

Diagnosis relies on paediatric assessment and investigation rather than psychiatric examination:

- Psychiatrists should resist requests to provide opinions where the diagnosis is merely suspected as there is no established association with maternal mental disorder.

● The Characteristics of Women Detained in Secure Mental Health Services

Women detained in secure mental health services are often described as having complex mental health-care needs. They often have more than one mental disorder, a history of severe prolonged abuse and significant experience of separation and loss, including that of their children. They have disturbed attachments and present with parasuicidal behaviour, pervasive anger, depression, mood instability, dissociation and/or anxiety.

Legal characteristics

Women represent the minority of patients detained under the Mental Health Act (MHA):

- Men and women are detained in roughly equal numbers under Part 2 of the Act, but women tend to be detained for shorter periods.
- Fewer women than men are detained within secure mental health services across the three levels of security. According to the Healthcare Commission (2008), there were:
  - 47 women detained in high security (compared with 686 men)
  - 643 detained in medium security (2611 men)
  - 1007 detained in low security (2787 men).

Correspondingly, women represent the minority of patients detained in hospital under restriction orders (Ministry of Justice, 2007):

- Women represent between 11 and 13% of restricted patients.
- In 2007 there were 458 female restricted patients in hospital (compared with 3448 men).
- Female restricted patients are less likely to be detained on the grounds of mental illness and more likely to be detained on the grounds of PD:
  - 56% detained under the then legal category of mental illness (compared with 69% men)
  - 20% under the then legal category of psychopathic disorder (compared with 12% men).

Clinical characteristics

Women detained in secure mental health services are more likely than men:

- to have been transferred from other NHS facilities
- to have a history of fire setting or criminal damage, but less likely to have committed a violent or sexual offence
- to have a history of abuse and/or self-harm – estimates suggest that at least 70% of women in high secure care may have histories of child sexual abuse and over 90% self-harm
- to have physical ill-health
- to be admitted after behaviours for which they were not charged or convicted and be detained under civil sections of the MHA
- to have a diagnosis of PD, particularly borderline PD.

Coid *et al.* (2000) reported on the characteristics of 471 women admitted to high and medium secure mental health services over a 7-year period. Cluster analysis identified seven subgroups according to primary diagnosis (Table 11.1).

Of 781 patients in low and medium secure care in London (Bartlett *et al.*, 2007):

- 9.6% were women, 25% of whom were not offenders
- women were more likely than men to be admitted with a diagnosis of PD
- one-third of the women had committed serious violence (homicide, attempted murder and grievous bodily harm) but they were less likely to have killed than the men.
- 13% had committed arson.

Long *et al.* (2010) described a series of 65 consecutive admissions to an independent sector women's medium secure service between 2002 and 2008:

- 45% detained under s37, 23% civil sections, 20% sentenced prisoners, 12% pre-sentence prisoners
- 39% were admitted from other medium secure units (MSUs), 26% from prison, 22% from high security, 19% from low or non-secure hospital
- mean age at admission was 31 years
- 92% were white, 2% black, 6% of mixed heritage
- 79% were single, 25% were in some contact with their children
- 85% reported a history of emotional, physical or sexual abuse

Table 11.1 Seven groups of women in secure psychiatric services by primary diagnosis (Coid *et al.*, 2000)

Primary diagnosis	No. in group	Other features
Antisocial personality disorder (ASPD)	51	A substantial number had co-morbid borderline personality and a smaller number co-morbid psychotic disorder Usually young, UK-born, white women, with a history of substance misuse Usually admitted as a result of criminal behaviour; many had an index offence of arson and had more extensive offending histories (including violence) than the other groups
Borderline PD	98	A subgroup of these had a co-morbid psychotic illness Younger than other groups except ASPD Three-quarters admitted due to criminal behaviour, some from less secure inpatient settings due to behavioural disturbance Extensive criminal histories, but less than ASPD group
Manic/hypomanic	48	15% had co-morbid borderline PD Relatively likely to be admitted due to violence within a less secure setting
Schizophrenia/ paranoid psychosis	160	More likely to be non-UK-born or non-white More likely to have been admitted following serious acts of violence Generally older than the other groups with previous admissions under Part 2 of the MHA
Other PDs	37	A subgroup having co-morbid ASPD and a quarter co-morbid psychotic disorders
Depression	53	Approximately half had co-morbid borderline PD and a quarter co-morbid psychosis
Organic brain syndrome	24	Many had co-morbid psychotic illness or PD

- 89% were diagnosed with a PD as either a primary or secondary diagnosis, with borderline PD being most common
- 88% had a history of alcohol or drug misuse, and 15% were diagnosed with dependence or harmful use
- 60% had a violent index offence, 22% arson
- 94% had previous convictions, 60% serious offence against the person, 35% arson
- 97% had histories of DSH.

● Secure Mental Health Services for Women

A number of Department of Health policy documents have focused on the needs of women requiring secure mental health services, notably:

- *Secure Futures For Women: Making a difference* (Department of Health, 1999)
- *Women's Mental Health into the Mainstream* (Department of Health, 2002)

These highlighted that:

- women were unnecessarily detained in high security
- women's treatment needs were different from those of men
- women required more relational security and less physical security.

Consequently, during the past decade there has been a major reconfiguration of women's secure services (Parry-Crooke and Stafford, 2009):

- The closure of the female beds in two of the three high secure hospital sites with Rampton Hospital providing the National High Secure Hospital Service for Women with approximately 50 beds.
- An increase in the number of female medium and low secure beds both within the NHS and the independent sector.
- Secure services are now gender-specific, with women's services either in separate hospitals or in specific units within existing secure services.
- A national pilot project has produced three enhanced medium secure units which provide higher levels of relational and procedural security than standard MSUs. These are at:
  - the Orchard Clinic in London
  - Arnold Lodge in Leicester
  - Edenfield Centre in Manchester

In January 2009 there were

- 29 women-only MSUs comprising 543 beds:
  - 9 provided by the independent sector (261 beds)
  - 17 services within the NHS (282 beds).

Characteristics of women's secure mental health services:

- Have a philosophy and model of care that takes into account the impact of life trauma and abuse on women's mental health.
- Ward sizes should be generally smaller with higher staff to patient ratios.
- The physical environment should be designed in a way that minimizes the risk of parasuicidal behaviour. Some services are designed to enable 'zonal' nursing observation to minimize the use of continuous one-to-one (or greater) observation, which sometimes reinforces patterns of DSH.
- The use of crisis suites or extra care areas as alternatives to the use of seclusion.
- An appropriate gender mix of staff working within services (70:30% female to male).
- Clinical staff should receive gender-specific training.
- Gender-specific therapeutic interventions to reflect the high rate of:
  - parasuicidal behaviour
  - PD diagnosis
  - histories of trauma/abuse
  - differing offending patterns.
- Availability of female-only therapeutic areas.
- Availability of gender-specific occupational and leisure activities.
- Availability of primary care services to meet the specific needs of women.

Assessment processes

As in other secure services, referrals may be to consider a patient's suitability for inpatient treatment or to provide advice to other services on risk management. Patients being considered for admission:

- Are usually assessed by a psychiatrist, a senior nurse and, in those patients identified as having significant axis 2 psychopathology, a clinical psychologist.
- In addition to risk of violence, emphasis is placed on assessment of risk to self, including DSH and suicide.

Deciding to admit a patient is dependent on:

- the individual treatment needs of the patients, and
- the context of the existing patient group in the service, including, for example:
  - the ability of the service to manage high numbers of patients on constant observations

– particular vulnerabilities of the assessed patient or patients already on the ward, in relation to each other.

Generally, decisions about admission are more straightforward for those with mental illness than those with PD:

- A proportion of women with severe borderline PD within prison require diversion to secure mental health services. However, there are considerable challenges in selecting the most appropriate cases from a population where the prevalence of PD is very high.
- Admission for a trial of treatment is often useful in cases of PD, under s38, s47 or perhaps s45A, though the last is rarely used in practice.

> **Box 11.2** Assessing a female patient with borderline personality disorder (PD) for transfer from prison to hospital
>
> There are no standardized assessment criteria. The decision is made following a careful and considered multidisciplinary assessment. See Box 9.1.
>
> Factors of particular importance among women which might favour admission include the following:
> - High risk of suicide or extreme deliberate self-harm, which cannot be managed within a custodial setting.
> - An index offence that can be formulated within the context of the patient's PD, e.g. arson within the context of a suicide attempt in a woman with borderline PD.
> - The patient has characteristics that may suggest a good response to treatment, e.g. evidence of motivation and ability to engage in psychological treatment.
> - Absence of co-morbid disorders which suggests a poor response to treatment, e.g. ASPD.
> - Specific treatment is available within the hospital that is not available within the prison setting.

Risk assessment in women

The principles of risk assessment are the same among women as men. However, there is debate about the use of violence risk assessment tools in women:

- There are no gender-specific risk assessment tools.
- The evidence base for available tools is mostly derived from men.

Nevertheless, the PCL-R and HCR-20 are routinely used in women's secure services.

De Vogel and de Ruiter (2005) compared the predictive validity for violent recidivism post-discharge of the HCR-20 and the PCL-R, in 42 women and a matched sample of men, from a Dutch forensic psychiatric service:

- The base rate for inpatient violence in male (29%) and female (30%) patients was the same, but the rate of violent recidivism was greater among male (43%) than female patients (13%).
- The areas under the curve (AUCs) (see Chapter 6) in relation to predicting a violent outcome were:
  - HCR-20 total score – 0.59 for women and 0.88 for men
  - HCR-20 final risk judgement – 0.86 for women and 0.91 for men
  - PCL-R total score – 0.34 for women and 0.74 for men.

The appropriateness of applying the concept of psychopathy to women is considered in Nicholls *et al.* (2005). They advised cautious use of the PCL-R.

Treatment issues

Seeman (2004) reviewed gender differences relevant to prescribing antipsychotic drugs, highlighting that the pharmacokinetics and pharmacodynamics of antipsychotic drugs differ in women and men:

- Women need lower doses than men.
- Prolactin levels are higher in women and have gender-specific side effects, e.g. abnormalities of menstrual cycle, fertility, lactation and gynaecomastia.
- Obesity is particularly common, leading to greater risk of the metabolic syndrome.
- Women require additional investigations, e.g. mammograms and bone density scans (in addition to cardiovascular and metabolic monitoring).
- Dose needs to be modulated in ageing women.

Medication regimes need to take into account the possibility of pregnancy following discharge. Kohen (2004) has provided a useful review of psychotropic prescribing in pregnancy.

Treatment for women with borderline PD

The high rate of borderline PD within secure women's services necessitates specific therapeutic interventions:

- NICE (2009) recommends considering a comprehensive dialectical behaviour therapy (DBT) programme for women with borderline PD for whom reducing recurrent self-harm is a priority:
  - This is usually a 12-month programme of weekly individual therapy and weekly group skills training.
  - Although much of the original evidence base for DBT is based on non-forensic and outpatient populations' modified inpatient programmes exist in women's forensic settings. Swenson *et al.* (2007) describe the successful adaption of DBT within inpatient settings.

In a recent review, Leichsenring *et al.* (2011) acknowledge the lack of empirical evidence but suggest that three clusters of symptoms may be targeted by adjunctive pharmacotherapy:

- Cognitive–perceptual symptoms by antipsychotics
- Affective symptoms by selective serotonin reuptake inhibitors (SSRIs)
- Impulsive–behavioural dyscontrol by SSRIs or low-dose antipsychotics.

Patients with borderline PD suffer transient psychotic symptoms, which are sometimes described as dissociative psychotic symptoms. The nosology is complicated further because a proportion also goes on to develop schizophrenia:

- There is considerable clinical experience in the use of clozapine within these patient groups in women's forensic services although published data is limited to small case series or single case studies. Frankenburg and Zanarini (1993), Chengappa *et al.* (1999), Swinton (2001) and Parker (2002) all describe the use of clozapine in severe borderline PD.

Outcomes

Mezey *et al.* (2005) compared the experiences of women in single and mixed-sex medium secure units. The women in single sex units:

- did not feel safer from physical violence than women in mixed-sex settings
- did feel less vulnerable, in relation to actual or threatened sexual assault and harassment
- complained of bullying, intimidation and aggressive behaviour by other women patients.

Maden *et al.* (2004) examined reoffending over one year in 959 individuals (116 women) discharged between 1997 and 1998, 116 of whom were women:

- The rate of conviction in women, at 9%, was lower than in men, at 16%.

Coid *et al.* (2007) studied reoffending rates of 1344 patients discharged from 7 of 14 MSUs in England and Wales over a follow-up period of 6.2 years. Outcome data was obtained from the offender's index, hospital case-files and the central register of deaths:

- 1 in 7 women committed a criminal offence (compared with one-third of men).
- 1in 16 women committed a grave offence (compared with 1 in 8 men).
- Women with previous convictions for arson and a history of substance misuse were more likely to be convicted of arson.

References

Bartlett A, Johns A, Fiander M, Jhawar H. (2007) *Report of the London Forensic Unit's Benchmarking Study*. London: NHS

*Bennett D, Ogloff J, Mullen P, Thomas S. (2010). A study of psychotic disorders among female homicide offenders. *Psychology, Crime & Law*. First published on 23rd July 2010 (iFirst)

Bools CN, Neale BA, Meadow SR. (1994) Munchausen syndrome by proxy: a study of psychopathology. *Child Abuse and Neglect G* **18**, 773–88

Borrill J, Burnett R, Atkins R, Miller S, Briggs D, Weaver T, Maden A. (2003). Patterns of self-harm and attempted suicide among white and black/mixed race female prisoners. *Criminal Behaviour and Mental Health* **13**, 229–40

Chengappa KNR, Ebeling T, Kang JS, Levine J, Parepally H. (1999). Clozapine reduces severe self-mutilation and aggression in psychotic patients with borderline personality disorder. *Journal of Clinical Psychiatry* **60**(7), 477–84

Coid J, Kahtan N, Gault S, Jarman B. (2000). Women admitted to secure psychiatric facilities 2: Identification of categories using cluster analysis. *Journal of Forensic Psychiatry and Psychology* **11**(2), 296–315

Coid J, Hickey N, Kahtan N, Zhang T, Yang M. (2007) Patients discharged from medium secure forensic psychiatry services: reconvictions and risk factors. *British Journal of Psychiatry* **190**, 223–9

Department of Health. (1999) *Secure Futures for Women: Making a difference*. Available at: http://www.dh.gov.uk/en/Publicationsandstatistics/Publications/PublicationsPolicyAndGuidance/DH_4077724

*Department of Health. (2002) *Women's Mental Health Into the Mainstream. Strategic development of mental health care for women*. Available at: http://www.dh.gov.uk/prod_consum_dh/groups/dh_digitalassets/@dh/@en/documents/digitalasset/dh_4075487.pdf

d'Orban PT. (1979). Women who kill their children. *British Journal of Psychiatry* **134**, 560–71

d'Orban PT. (1990) Female homicide. *Irish Journal of Psychological Medicine* **7**(1), 64–70

de Vogel V, de Ruiter C. (2005) The HCR-20 in personality disordered female offenders: a comparison with a matched sample of males. *Clinical Psychology and Psychotherapy* **12**, 226–40

Eronen M. (1995) Mental disorders and homicidal behaviour in female subjects. *American Journal of Psychiatry* **152**, 1216–18.

Fazel S, Benning R. (2009) Suicides in female prisoners in England and Wales, 1978–2004. *British Journal of Psychiatry*, **194**, 183–4

*Fossey M, Black G. (2010) *Under the Radar: Women with borderline personality in prison*. London: Centre for Mental Health

Frankenburg F, Zanarini M. (1993) Clozapine treatment of borderline patients: a preliminary study. *Comprehensive Psychiatry* **34**, 402–5.

Friedman SH, Resnick PJ. (2009) Neonaticide: phenomenology and considerations for prevention. *International Journal of Law and Psychiatry* **32**, 43–7

Friedman SH, Hrouda DR, Holden CE, Noffsinger SG, Resnick PJ. (2005) Filicide-suicide: common factors in parents who kill their children and themselves. *Journal of the American Academy of Psychiatry and the Law* **33**, 496–504.

Healthcare Commission. (2008) *Count me in Census 2008*. Available at: http://www.cqc.org.uk/guidanceforprofessionals/mentalhealth/countmeincensus.cfm

Home Office. (2006) *Criminal Statistics 2005*. Available at: http://rds.homeoffice.gov.uk/rds/crimstats05.html

*Home Office. (2007) *The Corston Report*. London: Home Office

Kohen D. (2004) Psychotropic medication in pregnancy. *Advances in Psychiatric Treatment* **10**, 59–66

Leichsenring F, Leibing E, Kruse J, New AS, Leweke F. (2011) Borderline personality disorder. *Lancet* **377**, 74–84

Lidz CW, Mulvey EP, Gardner W. (1993) The accuracy of predictions of violence to others. *Journal of American Medical Association* **269**(8), 1007–11

Long C, Hall L, Craig L, Mochty U, Hollin CR. (2010) Women referred for medium secure inpatient care: a population study over a six-year period. *Journal of Psychiatric Intensive Care* **7**(1), 17–26

Maden A, Scott F, Burnett R, Lewis GH, Skapinakis P. (2004) Offending in psychiatric patients after discharge from medium secure units: prospective national cohort study. *British Medical Journal* **328**, 1534

McClure RJ, Davis PM, Meadow SR, Sibert JR. (1996) Epidemiology of Munchausen syndrome by proxy, non-accidental poisoning, and non-accidental suffocation. *Archives of Disease in Childhood* **75**, 57–61

Mezey G, Hassell Y, Bartlett A. (2005) Safety of women in mixed-sex and single-sex medium secure units: staff and patient perceptions. *British Journal of Psychiatry* **187**, 579–82

Ministry of Justice. (2007) *Statistics of Mentally Disordered Offenders 2007 England and Wales*. Available at: www.justice.gov.uk/publications/mentally-disordered-offenders.htm

Ministry of Justice. (2010) Population in custody monthly tables August 2010 England and Wales. *Ministry of Justice Statistics Bulletin*. Available at: http://www.justice.gov.uk/publications/docs/pop-in-custody-aug2010.pdf

Monahan J, Steadman HJ, Silver E, Appelbaum PS, Robbins PC, Mulvey EP, *et al.* (2001) *Rethinking Risk Assessment: The MacArthur study of risk assessment and violence*. Oxford: Oxford University Press

*National Confidential Inquiry. (2009) *Filicide: A literature review*. National Confidential Inquiry into Suicide and Homicide by People with Mental Illness. Available at: http://www.medicine.manchester.ac.uk/mentalhealth/research/suicide/prevention/nci/inquiry_reports/

National Confidential Inquiry. (2010) *Annual Report: England and Wales 2010*. National Confidential Inquiry into Suicide and Homicide by People with Mental Illness. Available at: http://www.medicine.manchester.ac.uk/psychiatry/research/suicide/prevention/nci/inquiryannualreports/AnnualReportJuly2010.pdf

National Institute for Health and Clinical Excellence. (2009) *Borderline Personality Disorder: Treatment and management*. NICE Clinical Guideline 78. Available at: http://guidance.nice.org.uk/CG78/NICEGuidance/pdf/English

*Nicholls TL, Ogloff JRP, Brink J, Spidel A. (2005) Psychopathy in women: a review of its clinical usefulness for assessing risk for aggression and criminality. *Behavioral Sciences and the Law* **23**, 779–802

Parker GF. (2002) Clozapine and borderline personality disorder. *Psychiatric Services* **53**, 348–9

Parry-Crooke G, Stafford P. (2009) *My Life: In safe hands? Dedicated women's medium secure services in England.* NHS National R&D Programme on Forensic Mental Health. Available at: http://www.londonmet.ac.uk/fms/MRSite/acad/dass/CSER/Report % 20of % 20an % 20evaluation % 20 of % 20women's % 20medium % 20secure % 20services % 202009.pdf

Putkonen H. (2001) Personality disorders and psychoses form two distinct subgroups of homicide among female offenders. *Journal of Forensic Psychiatry* **12**(2), 300–12

Resnick P. (1969) Child murder by parents. *American Journal of Psychiatry* **126**, 325–34.

Resnick P. (1970) Murder of the newborn: a psychiatric review of neonaticide. *American Journal of Psychiatry* **126**, 1414–20

Schanda H, Knecht G, Schreinzer D, Stompe T, Ortwein-Swoboda G, Waldhoer T. (2004) Homicide and major mental disorders: a 25-year study. *Acta Psychiatrica Scandinavica* **110**, 98–107.

Scott PD. (1973) Parents who kill their children. *Medicine, Science and the Law* **13**, 120–6

Seeman MV. (2004) Gender differences in the prescribing of antipsychotic drugs. *American Journal of Psychiatry* **161**, 1324–33

Singleton N, Meltzer H, Gatward R, Coid J, Deasy D. (1998) *Psychiatric Morbidity Among Prisoners. Summary report.* London: Office for National Statistics

Stack S. (1997) Homicide followed by suicide: an analysis of Chicago data. *Criminology* **35**(3), 435–53

Swenson CR, Witterholt S, Bohus M. (2007) Dialectical behaviour therapy on inpatient units. In: Dimeff LA, Koerner K (eds), *Dialectical Behavior Therapy in Clinical Practice.* New York: Guilford Press

*Swinton M. (2001) Clozapine in severe borderline personality disorder. *Journal of Forensic Psychiatry & Psychology* **12**(3), 580–91

Walker LE. (1999) *The Battered Woman Syndrome*, 2nd edn. New York: Springer

12

Children and Adolescents in Secure Care

● Setting the Context

Legal context

The age of criminal responsibility varies considerably among jurisdictions worldwide, generally from 7 years to around 15 years. In England and Wakes it is 10; in Scotland it is 12.

Currently, children and adolescents constitute 25% of the total UK population. The Offending, Crime and Justice Survey investigates offending among 10–25 year olds. The 2006 survey (Roe and Ashe, 2008) showed that:

- the peak age of offending was 14–17 years; males were more likely to have offended than females
- 22% reported committing at least 1 of 20 core offences in previous 12 months
- 10% had committed at least one serious offence (serious offenders)
- 6% had committed an offence six or more times in the past 12 months (frequent offenders)
- 4% were both frequent and serious offenders.

There are three statutory routes through which a young person can be deprived of their liberty:

- criminal justice system (CJS) – remanded or sentenced following criminal charge or conviction
- health – detention under the Mental Health Act (MHA)
- local authority (LA) – placement via Secure Accommodation Order.

Custodial Settings (the Secure Estate) for young people consists of:

- local authority secure units/children's homes (LASUs or LASCHs) – provisions are for 12- to 14-year-old boys and girls up to 16; support is tailored to individual needs
- secure training centres (STCs) – four purpose-built centres for up to 17 year olds; focus is on education and rehabilitation
- young offender institutions (YOIs) – provisions are for 15- to 17-year-old boys and girls over 16; deemed inappropriate for vulnerable or high-risk groups.

In June 2009 there were (Berman, 2009):

- 2102 juveniles (15–17 year olds) in prison:
  - 353 of whom were awaiting trial and 163 awaiting sentence
- 258 12–15 year olds in privately run STCs and 175 in LASCHs.

Mental health context

Office for National Statistics (ONS) surveys of the mental health of children and young people (Green *et al.*, 2005; Meltzer *et al.*, 2000) showed that:

- 10% of 5–16 year olds had a 'clinically diagnosed mental disorder':
  - 4% emotional disorder
  - 6% conduct disorder
  - 2% hyperkinetic disorder
  - 2% had 'more than one type of disorder'.
- Boys had a higher prevalence of mental disorders than girls (10–13% compared with 5–10%)
- Higher rates of mental disorder were found in those:
  - from single parent, reconstituted families and low-income families
  - with parents who were unemployed and had little or no education
  - who lived in 'deprived' areas.

Rates of mental health problems among young offenders are higher:

- According to the Mental Health Foundation (Leon, 2002):
  - prevalence rates for mental health problems in young offenders are significantly higher (at least three times) compared with the general population
  - figures range from 25% to 81%, with highest rates reported for those in custodial settings
  - the most common disorders are emotional disorders, conduct disorders and attentional disorders, although substance misuse is also a significant issue in this group.
- Harrington and Bailey (2005) found that:
  - over 50% of young offenders appeared to have borderline or mild learning difficulties
  - 33% 'had a mental health need' which included depression (20%), self-harm (10%), anxiety and post-traumatic stress symptoms (10%), hyperactivity (7%) and psychotic-like symptoms (5%)
  - female offenders had more mental health needs than male.
- Chitsabesan *et al.* (2006) highlighted the additional unmet needs of young offenders, particularly:
  - education/work (36%)
  - social relationships (48%).

The higher rates of mental health problems in young offenders are thought to be due to:

- pre-existing factors related to parents and parenting, the child (hyperactivity, learning difficulties) and the psychosocial environment
- offending related factors such as negative lifestyle choices and stress
- stressful interactions with the CJS and environments such as custody.

It is argued that, in the absence of appropriate services and help, young offenders are likely to demonstrate:

- continuation or escalation of offending behaviour and mental health problems,
- increased vulnerability to psychosocial stresses
- worsening in social circumstances
- propensity to engage in self-harm/suicidal behaviour and behaviours likely to result in harm to others.

● Youth Justice System

The rules and procedures for dealing with juvenile offenders began to become distinguished from those for adults in the nineteenth century.

The Criminal Justice Act 1998 reviewed the whole youth justice system, creating the Youth Justice Board (YJB) and Youth Offending Teams (YOTs):

- The YJB was an independent body tasked to oversee youth justice in England and Wales and to be responsible for secure facilities.
- The YJB was abolished in 2011, its functions to be subsumed within the Ministry of Justice.

Youth Offending Teams

Each LA in England and Wales has a YOT, which is a multidisciplinary team including representatives from police, probation service, social services, health, education, substance misuse services and housing. YOTs:

- conduct assessments of all young offenders using Asset – a standardized structured tool focusing on criminogenic needs
- provide appropriate adults for police interviews
- provide pre-sentence reports (PSRs) for court
- implement court diversion schemes and community sentences
- provide bail supervision, and supervision after release from custody
- work with local authorities to impose acceptable behaviour contracts and ASBOs for young people engaging in low-level antisocial behaviour.

Young people in the police station

The Police and Criminal Evidence Act 1984 provides guidance on dealing with young people who have been arrested and detained in a police station, including:

- considering whether the matter can be dealt with by police via:
  - a reprimand – a formal verbal warning for first offence, or a
  - final warning – a formal verbal warning for further offence(s)
- considering whether the young person suffers with any mental health problems
- considering alternatives to being held in a cell
- the need to inform parent(s) as soon as possible
- the requirement for an appropriate adult for all those under 17, and for over 17 year olds if they are mentally disordered
- assessment of a young person's fitness to be interviewed.

There are similarities with adults in relation to:

- being issued with a caution on arrest
- the right to silence until a solicitor has been consulted
- adverse inferences (negative inferences drawn from silence or refusal/failure to explain evidence).

Bail or remand into custody or to a secure unit?

The criteria for considering remand into custody or to a secure unit for a young person are (Nacro, 2008):

- Has young person been charged with violent or sexual offence(s) punishable with imprisonment for 14 years or more in adults?
- Does the young person have a recent history of absconding?
- Is such a course of action needed to protect the public from harm and to prevent further offences?

Although a young offenders institution (YOI) may be suitable for the older age group, remand in a secure unit is considered for boys aged 12–14 years, 'vulnerable' boys up to 15 or 16 years and girls up to 16 years.

Youth or Crown court?

The youth court is a section of the magistrates' court:

- that deals with the majority of offenders under the age of 18, unless they have been charged with an adult, or the offence is particularly serious
- where proceedings are less formal and more open, but there is no public access and rules for press reporting are more stringent
- where judges have specialist training on dealing with young people
- that upholds young people's right to legal representation and right to a fair trial but not to a litigation friend (an individual to represent and instruct in a civil case on behalf of someone who is unable to do so).

The Crown court hears:

- cases sent from the youth court due to the seriousness of the offence
- cases sent for sentencing due to insufficient powers of the youth court
- appeals against sentences given in the youth court.

Box 12.1 Crown court proceedings involving juveniles

James Patrick Bulger (born 16 March 1990) was abducted, tortured and murdered in February 1993 by two 10-year-old boys, Jon Venables and Robert Thompson. They were arrested and charged with murder on 20 February, appeared at South Sefton Youth Court on 22 February and subsequently remanded in a secure setting to await trial.

The trial at Preston Crown Court was conducted in the same manner as an adult trial with the accused in the dock away from their parents, and Judge and court officials in legal regalia. Each boy sat in view of the court on raised chairs during the proceedings.

Venables and Thompson were found guilty on 24 November 1993 and sentenced to Detention at Her Majesty's pleasure. At the close of the trial, the judge ruled that their details should be released to the public.

In *T and V* v *UK* (2000) 30 EHRR 121 the European Court of Human Rights held that the trial process had led to a breach of the defendants' right to a fair trial (Article 6.1) because, given their immaturity and the tense public scrutiny of the court, they would have been unable freely to consult with their lawyers.

In response to this judgment a practice direction was issued by the Lord Chief Justice:

- A young defendant should usually be tried separately from their adult co-defendant, unless the court decides that this would not be prejudicial to their welfare.
- The young defendant may visit the courtroom out of hours to familiarize themselves with it.
- The police should protect a high-profile young defendant from 'intimidation, vilification or abuse'.
- If possible all participants in the trial should be at the same level.
- The young defendant should be free to sit with their family so as to allow informal communication with their lawyers.
- The trial should be conducted in language that the young defendant can understand.
- Frequent and regular breaks should be taken to allow for reduced ability to concentrate.
- Gowns and wigs should not be worn and police/custody staff should not be in uniform.
- The court may seek to restrict access by the public and press to the courtroom.

Fitness to plead and stand trial

This is dealt with in the same way and using the same criteria as for adults (see Chapter 20). However, assessments should take into account:

- the young person's age
- the overall emotional and intellectual development
- the previous contact with the CJS.

Disposal options available for juvenile offenders

Fines and absolute and conditional discharges operate in the same way as for adults (see Chapter 15).

Community sentences:

- Reparation order:
  - reparation may be direct to the victim or indirect to the community
  - wide range of potential actions (writing a letter of apology, cleaning up graffiti, clearing litter, etc.)
  - available only where the victim agrees
- Referral order:
  - for most juvenile offenders on their first time in court
  - requires attendance at a youth offender panel, which draws up a contract (3–12 months' long) aiming to repair the damage caused by the offence and address causes of offending
  - conviction is spent once contract successfully completed
- Youth rehabilitation order:
  - the juvenile equivalent of the community order, with a similar list of potential additional requirements, including a mental health treatment requirement
  - maximum duration of 3 years.

Custodial sentences:

- Detention and Training Order (DTO):
  - For 12–17 year olds
  - 4–24 months' duration, with automatic release under supervision at halfway point
- Section 90 (Powers of Criminal Courts Act [PCCA] 2000):
  - Following conviction for murder, a mandatory life sentence applies as for adults
  - For juveniles, this is termed 'detention at Her Majesty's pleasure'
- Section 91 (PCCA):
  - following conviction for an offence which for an adult would carry a maximum sentence of 14 years imprisonment or more
  - may include custody for life (for those aged 18–21), or detention for life (for those under 18)
  - the sentence is imposed and managed in the same way as for adults
- extended sentences and indeterminate sentences are available for 'dangerous offenders' under 18 in much the same way as for adults (see Chapter 20):
  - the sentence of imprisonment for public protection is termed 'detention for public protection' for those under 21 years
  - the qualifying criterion of a previous schedule 15A conviction is not applicable for those under 18.

MHA disposals are available for those under the age of 18 where appropriate.

● Social Care System

The Children Act 1989

The Children Act 1989 provides the basis of the law relating to the care of and provision of services for children:

- It brings together legislation concerning care and upbringing of children in private and public law.
- The main principles are:
  - children's welfare is the paramount consideration
  - children are best brought up within their own families wherever possible
  - unwarranted interference in family life should be avoided.
- It is addressed mainly to local authority social services departments and courts but also has important implications for the NHS.
- It refers to partnership among children, parents and local authorities.
- It stipulates that local authorities (LAs) should provide services for 'Children (and families) in Need' and 'Looked After Children'.
- It serves to protect rights of parents with children who are looked after by an LA.
- It aims to ensure that children looked after by an LA or living away from home are provided with a good standard of care.
- It improves the way in which courts deal with children and families.
- It stipulates that family court proceedings, presided by judges who are specialists in family law, should avoid delays, be more flexible, have a friendlier atmosphere and make an order only if it is best for the child.
- It requires that children are kept informed of the proceedings and are allowed to participate, and that parents have the right to appear in court, access available information, have their views heard, appeal against court decisions and access automatic legal aid.

Parental responsibility:

- is defined at s3(1) as 'all the rights, duties, powers, responsibilities and authority which by law a parent has in relation to a child and his property'
- the mother automatically has parental responsibility, as does the father if they were married at the time of birth:
  - otherwise, the father may acquire it, by being registered as the child's father, by making a formal agreement with the mother, or by court order
- in most cases, someone with parental responsibility does not lose it, even if another individual or body also gains it.

The Children Act expects health authorities and their professionals to:

- have knowledge of the Children Act and its provisions
- be aware of issues relating to the use of the Children Act and the MHA:
  - e.g. stigma, social/family issues or mental disorder, need for compulsory treatment and available safeguards
- collaborate with social services departments in providing services to children and families
- liaise with social services departments in relation to risk (child abuse/protection), and meeting a child's and family's needs
- provide expert opinions on cases in court if deemed suitably qualified and appropriate
- inform if a child has been an inpatient in hospital for over 3 months
- consider applying Children Act 1989/Children Regulations 1991 if liberty of a child or young person is being restricted other than under the MHA.

The 1989 Act has been amended by the Children Act 2004, which established a Children's Commissioner and various new powers and duties on agencies relating to the wellbeing of children.

Private law

This refers to private disputes between parents, usually after separation, about the child's care, particularly where the child should live and how often parents should see the child. The Children Act 1989 provides:

- Section 8 Orders:
  - Residence Orders
  - Contact Orders, requiring the person with whom the child lives to allow contact with another
  - Prohibited Steps Orders, requiring the permission of the court to take specified steps in relation to the child
  - Specific Issue Orders, relating to any aspect of parental responsibility
- Additional Orders:
  - Parental Responsibility Order, to give a father parental responsibility
  - Family Assistance Orders, to provide support to families struggling to reach agreement over arrangements for their children.

Public law

Sometimes, attempts to help children in their own families may not be enough to protect their welfare. Under such circumstances, local authorities can apply to the court for permission for further action. The Orders used are:

- Supervision Orders, including:
  - Education Supervision Orders, to support a child in education
  - Child Assessment Orders, where there is concern that a child may be at risk of significant harm
- Care Orders:
  - the LA is required to receive the child into care for the duration of the order and has parental responsibility
- Emergency Protection Orders
- Secure Accommodation Orders.

Children and young people may be placed in secure accommodation through the CJS, or for welfare reasons:

- Section 25 of the Children Act 1989 allows an LA to apply for an order to keep a 'Looked After Child' in secure accommodation if the child or young person:
  - is aged 13–17 years on admission (if it is being considered for a 10–13 year old, it requires approval from Secretary of State)
  - has a history of absconding and is likely to abscond from any other type of accommodation
  - should they abscond, is likely to suffer significant harm
  - if kept in any other type of accommodation, is likely to injure themselves or others.
- Secure Accommodation Orders initially last for 3 months but can be renewed every 6 months.

● Mental Health System

The causes of mental health problems in young people include:

- genetic and temperamental factors such as impulsivity and intelligence
- adverse childhood experiences such as neglect and abuse
- disrupted and unhappy family relationships due to abandonment, institutional care, loss of caring adults
- negative family and peer influences including substance misuse and offending behaviour
- social and community disadvantages such as poverty and marginalization
- drug and alcohol use
- ongoing stressful situations and interactions.

Box 12.2 Assessment framework for children and young people

It is particularly important to collate information from a variety of sources, including:

- parents and other adults involved with the child
- school records
- records from social services and from the criminal justice system
- medical records from the GP.

Clinical assessment must include:

- developmental assessment taking into account motor, language, emotional, cognitive and intellectual, physical, behavioural and moral aspects
- upbringing and family history
- personal history including education, temperament, peer relationships and interactions, substance misuse, antisocial behaviour
- past behavioural problems, particularly hyperactivity, impulsivity
- index offence and past offending behaviour (level, frequency, variety, triggers/protective factors, cruelty/empathy)
- past medical and psychiatric history
- presenting complaint
- mental state examination.

Also consider the use of structured/standardized assessments:

- Checklists – Child Behaviour Checklist (Achenbach and Edelbrock, 1983) and Strength and Difficulties Questionnaire (Goodman, 1997).
- Rating scales – Conner's parents and teachers versions for hyperactivity.
- Structured interviews – Diagnostic Interview Schedule for Children (DISC; Costello *et al.*, 1985).

Risk assessment in young people

The principles are the same as in adults, but there is a lack of validated actuarial risk assessment instruments (ARAIs) available for young people.

The Structured Assessment of Violence Risk in Youth (SAVRY; Borum *et al.*, 2003) is the most commonly used structured clinical approach. It is:

- useful for male or female adolescents between 12 and 18 years
- composed of 24 risk factors in three risk domains scored as low, moderate or high
  - historical factors
  - social/contextual factors
  - individual/clinical factors
- and six protective factors rated as either present or absent.

Sheldrick (2004) proposes an alternative structure composed of:

- predisposing factors in the form of genetics, problems before, during or after birth or during early development

- 'upbringing', particularly parenting style, experiences of abuse, exposure to deviant behaviour
- past behavioural problems, especially cruelty, violence, fire setting
- details of index offence, particularly use of threats, violence and weapons
- specifics of past offending such as age of onset, number and variety of offences
- clinical factors, including symptoms of mental illness, substance use, 'interests/fantasies' involving violence or sex
- compliance, ability to learn from experience and motivation to change
- availability of treatment
- protective factors such as supportive relationships, achievements, non-deviant peers.

Other tools may be applicable for particular subgroups, for example:

- Estimate of Risk of Adolescent Sexual Offense Recidivism (ERASOR; Worling and Curwen, 2001)
- Psychopathy Checklist – Youth Version (PCL-YV; Forth et al., 1996)

Needs assessment

This is best completed with young person and parent/carer, using an assessment tool such as the Salford Needs Assessment Schedule for Adolescents (SNASA; Kroll *et al.*, 1999):

- It covers 21 areas including physical and mental health, psychological and behavioural aspects, personal, family and social issues, daily living skills and constructive daytime activities.

Mental disorders in adolescence

Particular disorders to consider in young people include:

- specific and pervasive disorders of psychological development:
  – particularly autistic spectrum disorder (ASD) (see Chapter 10)
- behavioural and emotional disorders of childhood:
  – hyperkinetic and conduct disorders
  – emotional disorders
  – disorders of social functioning
  – tic disorders.

Conduct disorder is described in the ICD-10 (World Health Organization, 1992) as a repetitive and persistent (more than 6 months) pattern of dissocial, aggressive or defiant conduct, including the following sorts of behaviours:

- excessive fighting or bullying
- cruelty to animals or people
- fire setting
- stealing
- repeated lying
- truancy and running away from home
- frequent or severe temper tantrums or uncontrolled rages.

Conduct disorder is discussed further in relation to adult antisocial personality disorder in Chapter 9. Hyperkinetic disorder is commonly associated with behavioural problems and may lead to conduct disorder either:

- as a direct manifestation of hyperactivity and attentional problems, or
- as a secondary disability.

Depression and conduct disorder may coexist, the nosological relationship between them being complex and possibly heterogeneous (see Dubicka and Harrington, 2004, for further discussion). In adolescence the depressive syndrome generally resembles the adult syndrome, but:

- the young person may appear irritable rather than sad
- subjective complaint may be of boredom rather than sadness
- academic performance may decline due to poor concentration
- increased misbehaviour at school, fighting or other conduct problems may dominate the presentation.

● Child and Adolescent Forensic Mental Health Services

Child and Adolescent Mental Health Services consist of four 'tiers':

- Tier 1 – any professional with knowledge of and training in children's issues but who is not a specialist CAMHS practitioner (e.g. social worker, GP).
- Tier 2 – a specialist individual practitioner working with children and their families who may be attached to a CAMHS or non-CAMHS team or network (e.g. professional working within a YOT).
- Tier 3 – specialist CAMHS practitioners working in a multidisciplinary team (e.g. any member of a community CAMHS team).
- Tier 4 – specialist CAMHS operating on an outpatient and inpatient basis (e.g. inpatient CAMHS, inpatient or outpatient Child and Adolescent Forensic Services).

Specialist Child and Adolescent Forensic Mental Health Services

Currently provided in England as part of a national framework, services are based in:

- Manchester (Gardener unit)
- Newcastle (Roycroft unit)
- Birmingham (Ardenleigh unit)
- London (Bill Yule and Wells units)
- Southampton (Bluebird unit).

The multidisciplinary teams working within these services are similar to those in adult forensic services, but with the addition of teaching staff and a greater educational and developmental perspective.

Each of these units provides most if not all of the following:

- Consultation/liaison to Tier 3 CAMHS and other agencies such as local YOTs and social care teams.
- Outpatient services largely providing specialist needs and risk assessments.
- In-reach mental health services to LASUs/STCs/YOIs.
- Medium secure inpatient care for young people who are:
  - under 18 years of age
  - detainable under the MHA, excluding detention solely for learning disability
  - present a risk of harm to others through direct violence, including homicide, seriously sexually aggressive behaviour, destructive/life-threatening use of fire.

Recently, a similar nationally commissioned provision for young people in need of Forensic Learning Disability Services was developed, to provide for an estimated need of 36 referrals a year. Beds became available in mid-2007 in Newcastle and Northampton-based units.

Treatment issues and approaches

Pharmacological treatment in young people encompasses most of the medications that are available for treating illness in adults, with a few exceptions such as paroxetine:

- Additional treatments include:
  - stimulants for hyperkinetic disorder
  - clonidine for tic disorders
  - desmopressin for enuresis.
- Baseline height, weight and vital parameters are especially important, together with, when necessary, blood tests and ECG.
- Most drugs are prescribed off-licence and off-label.
- Side effects and reactions may be different in young people.
- Electroconvulsive treatment is rarely used in this age-group.
- Antipsychotic prescribing in children and adolescents is considered in detail by James (2010).

Psychological treatment (Dogra *et al.*, 2002) includes:

- individual treatments:
  - behavioural therapies for anxiety disorders, behaviour and conduct disorders, and behavioural aspects of psychotic disorders
  - cognitive therapies for aggression, anxiety disorders and depression, especially in adolescents
  - solution-focused therapy and motivational interviewing for substance misuse and other problems
  - other talking therapies such as interpersonal and psychodynamic therapy
  - non-talking therapies such as play, music, dance, art and drama therapies (see Aulich, 2004, for discussion of these)
- group interventions:
  - psychoeducation, social skills, anger management, conflict resolution, dealing with voices/ psychosis
- family therapy.

Legislation related to mental health

The MHA 1983 has no lower age limit so it generally applies to children and young people. Note:

- Before making a community treatment order (CTO), the responsible clinician (RC) should involve the patient's parent to ensure that they are ready and able to provide assistance and support.
- A guardianship application may only be made in respect of a person aged 16 or over.

The MCA 2005:

- does not generally apply to people under the age of 16, except:
  - the Court of Protection may make financial or property decisions where the child lacks capacity and is likely still to lack capacity by the age of 18
  - offences of ill-treatment or wilful neglect of a person who lacks capacity do apply to young victims
- does generally apply to those between 16 and 18, except:
  - in relation to making a lasting power of attorney or advance decisions about medical treatment
  - the Court of Protection may not make a statutory will.

Otherwise, capacity and best interest assessments apply to children and young people just as to adults, while bearing in mind developmental issues and parent/carer involvement.

References

Achenbach TM, Edelbrock CS. (1983) *Manual for the Child Behaviour Checklist and Revised Child Behaviour Profile*. Burlington, VT: University of Vermont

Aulich LP. (2004) Arts therapies. In: Bailey S, Dolan M (eds), *Adolescent Forensic Psychiatry*. Arnold: London

Berman, G. (2009) *Prison Population Statistics updated 22nd December 2010*. House of Commons Library. Available at: http://www.parliament.uk/briefingpapers/commons/lib/research/briefings/snsg-04334.pdf

Borum R, Bartel P, Forth A. (2003) *Manual for the Structured Assessment of Violence Risk in Youth (SAVRY)*. Tampa: University of South Florida

Chitsabesan P, Kroll L, Bailey S, Kenning C, Sneider S, MacDonald W, Theodosiou L. (2006) Mental health needs of young offenders in custody and in the community. *The British Journal of Psychiatry* **188**, 534–40

Costello E J, Edelbrook C, Costello AJ. (1985) Validity of the NIMH Diagnostic Interview Schedule for Children: a comparison between psychiatric and paediatric referrals. *Journal of Abnormal Child Psychology* **13**, 579–95

Dogra N, Parkin A, Gale F, Frake C. (2002) *A Multidisciplinary Handbook of Child and Adolescent Mental Health for Front-line Professionals*. London: Jessica Kingsley

*Dubicka B, Harrington R (2004) Affective conduct disorder. In: Bailey S, Dolan M (Eds) *Adolescent Forensic Psychiatry*. London: Arnold

Forth AE, Kossen DS, Hare RD. (1996) *The Hare Psychopathy Checklist – Youth Version (PCL-YV)*. New York: Multi-Health Systems Inc.

Goodman R. (1997) The Strengths and Difficulties Questionnaire: a research note. *Journal of Child Psychology and Psychiatry* **38**, 581–6

Green H, McGinnity A, Meltzer H, Ford T, Goodman R. (2005) *Mental Health of Children and Young People in Great Britain, 2004*. London: HMSO

Harrington R, Bailey S. (2005) *Mental Health Needs and Effectiveness of Provision for Young Offenders in Custody and in the Community*. Youth Justice Board for England and Wales. Available at: http://www.yjb.gov.uk/publications/Resources/Downloads/MentalHealthNeedsfull.pdf

James AC. (2010) Antipsychotic prescribing for children and adolescents. *Advances in Psychiatric Treatment* **16**, 63–75

Kroll L, Woodham A, Rothwell J, Bailey S, Tobias C, Harrington R, Marshall M. (1999) Reliability of the Salford Needs Assessment Schedule for Adolescents. *Psychological Medicine* **29**, 891–902

Leon L. (2002) *The Mental Health Needs of Young Offenders. Updates 3 (18)*. The Mental Health Foundation. Available at: http://www.mentalhealth.org.uk/publications/mental-health-needs-young-offenders/

Meltzer H, Gatward R, Goodman R, Ford T. (2000) *The Mental Health of Children and Adolescents in Great Britain*. London: Office for National Statistics

Nacro (2008) *Remands to Local Authority Accommodation: Secure and non-secure. Youth Crime Briefing*. Available at: http://www.nacro.org.uk/data/files/nacro-2009070904-185.pdf

Roe S, Ashe J. (2008) *Young People and Crime: Findings from the 2006 Offending, Crime and Justice Survey*. London: Home Office

*Sheldrick C. (2004) The assessment and management of risk. In: Bailey S, Dolan M (eds), *Adolescent Forensic Psychiatry*. London: Arnold

World Health Organization (1992) *The ICD-10 Classification of Mental and Behavioural Disorders: Clinical descriptions and diagnostic guidelines.* Geneva: WHO

Worling JR, Curwen T. (2001) Estimate of Risk of Adolescent Sexual Offense Recidivism (ERASOR). In: Calder MC (ed.), *Juveniles and Children who Sexually Abuse: Frameworks for assessment.* London: Russell House Publishing

13

Sex Offenders, Stalkers and Fire Setters

● Sex Offenders

Rules, traditions and norms relating to sexual behaviour vary among cultures, and this impacts on a society's attitude to sexual offences and offenders (Grubin, 1992).

Soothill (2003) described societal changes in England and Wales over the last 60 years:

- 1950s: focused on the visibility of prostitution in society
- 1960s: saw the decriminalization of homosexuality
- 1970s: the feminist movement highlighted issues relating to the rape of women
- 1980s: increasing publicity of the extent of childhood sexual abuse (CSA) within families
- 1990s: public attention focused on the length of sentences given to those convicted of rape
- 2000s: saw public attention shift to the risk posed to children by sex offenders living in the community and the risks posed by 'strangers'.

The 2000s have also seen the advent of Internet-based offending, including downloading of child pornography and grooming, together with consequent changes in legislation and police operation.

There have been several major political turning points:

- Sexual Offenders Act 1997: introduced the Sex Offenders Register, requiring all convicted or cautioned sex offenders to notify police of their address and any changes in it.
- In 2003 the Sexual Offences Act expanded the offences that could be prosecuted. It also changed the Sex Offender Register to the Violent and Sexual Offenders Register (ViSOR) and allows police, prison and probation services access to information on registered offenders.
- In response to public pressure in August 2010 the Government announced that a pilot scheme, allowing parents to request a police check on anyone (such as a new partner) who has unsupervised access to their children, would be rolled out across England and Wales (*The Independent*, 2010).

Classification of sexual offending

A general definition of a sexual offence was given by O'Connell *et al.* (1990):

A criminal offence involving sexual behaviour occurs when one party does not give, or is incapable of giving, fully informed consent or where the difference in power between two parties is such that one is not in a position to make a truly free choice.

The police recording system for sexual offences divides such offences into two categories (Home Office, 2010):

- serious sexual offences: including rapes, sexual assaults and sexual activity with children
- other sexual offences: including soliciting, exploitation of prostitution and other unlawful sexual activity between two consenting adults.

The legal classification of sexual offences is considered in Chapter 15.

Indecent images of children are classified by severity (Sentencing Guidelines Council, 2010):

- Level 1 – images of erotic posing, with no sexual activity.
- Level 2 – non-penetrative sexual activities between children, or solo masturbation by a child.
- Level 3 – non-penetrative sexual activity between adults and children.
- Level 4 – penetrative sexual activity involving a child or children, or both children and adults.
- Level 5 – sadism or penetration of, or by, an animal.

Frequency of sexual offending

Of a random sample of 2019 adults, 12% of females and 8% of males reported having had unwanted sexual contact before the age of 16 (Baker and Duncan, 1985). Perhaps only 11% of all victims of serious sexual assault told the police about the incident (Povey *et al.*, 2009).

The British Crime Survey 2009–10 (Home Office, 2010) reported that 2% of women and less than 1% of men aged 16–59 had experienced a sexual assault within the last 12 months. Recorded offences in the year 2009–10 (Home Office, 2010) showed:

- There were 54 509 sexual offences recorded by the police, a 6% increase on the previous year:
  - 43 579 were serious sexual offences (7% increase on previous year)
  - 10 930 other sexual offences (2% increase on previous year).

These apparent increases in sexual offending may be due to police efforts to improve rates of reporting of sexual offences: national crime statistics underestimate the extent of sexual offending particularly. Under-reporting may be due to:

- shame and fear of the criminal justice system (CJS) process
- the fact that most victims are known to the offender.

Home Office research (Feist *et al.*, 2007) showed that of a sample (*n* = 676) of alleged rapes in 2003–4:

- 8% were shown to be a false allegation
- 70% were not charged, mostly due to either:
  - withdrawal of the complaint, or
  - insufficient evidence
- 13% led to a conviction (not necessarily for rape)
- the figure most commonly quoted is that 6% of rape allegations lead to a conviction for rape.

Types of sex offender

There are no convincing typologies of sex offender. Sexual offenders are a widely heterogeneous group (Lockmuller *et al.*, 2008):

- It is unhelpful to categorize and make judgements about sexual offenders based on offence type.
- It is far more useful to consider individual circumstances and motivations for offending.

Female sexual offenders

- Eldridge (2000) estimated that 3% of convicted sexual offenders are women:

- This is probably an underestimation due to under-reporting and a differential response of the CJS and other professionals to women who offend sexually.
- These factors, compounded by societal attitudes to women as caregivers and views on women as being sexually submissive, have contributed to the paucity of research in this area. See Denov (2004) for further discussion of these issues.

Sexual offending and mental disorder

Risk assessment tools for sexual offending, in contrast to those for violence, tend not to cite mental illness as a risk factor. Personality disorder, learning disability and organic brain disease may be important.

A comparison of rates of hospitalization in Sweden between 1988 and 2000 (Fazel *et al.*, 2007) showed that, compared with matched population controls, sexual offenders had odds ratios (ORs) of:

- 6.3 for psychiatric hospitalization
- 4.8 for schizophrenia
- 5.2 for other psychoses
- 3.4 for bipolar affective disorder.

A typology of sexual offenders with schizophrenia is given by Drake and Pathe (2004):

- Those with a pre-existing paraphilia.
- Those whose deviant sexuality arises in the context of illness and/or its treatment.
- Those whose deviant sexuality is one manifestation of more generalized antisocial behaviour.
- Factors other than the above (including degenerative organic conditions and substance misuse).

Mood disorders occasionally lead to sex offending (see Chapter 8). Depending on the relationship between a mental illness and sex offending in the individual, effective psychiatric treatment may reduce the risk, increase the risk or have little effect on the risk of sexual offending.

Disorders of sexual preference in ICD-10 (paraphilias)

Paraphilias refer to recurrent, intense, sexually arousing fantasies, urges or behaviours (Table 13.1). The subject engages in the paraphilic activity repetitively, either instead of or as well

Table 13.1 Paraphilias

Fetishism	Reliance on an inanimate object for sexual arousal or gratification
Fetishistic transvestism	Wearing of clothes in order to create the appearance of the opposite gender, for the purposes of sexual arousal. In contrast to transsexual transvestism, the clothes are removed with decline of sexual arousal
Exhibitionism	Recurrent tendency to expose genitalia to strangers in public places, without a desire for contact. Sexual excitement at the time is usual, and masturbation commonly follows
Voyeurism	Recurrent tendency to watch unsuspecting people engaging in sexual or intimate activity. Usually associated with masturbation
Paedophilia	A persistent sexual preference for pre-pubertal or early pubertal children. About 20% are gender non-specific, and they tend to be attracted to younger (less physically differentiated) children
Sadomasochism	A preference for sexual activity involving the infliction of pain or humiliation either on the subject (masochism), on the subject's partner (sadism), or both
Other paraphilias	Includes frotteurism, necrophilia, zoophilia, coprophilia, urophilia; many others have been described

as engaging in 'normal' sexual activity. The stimulus is culturally considered to be outside the range of 'normal' sexual practices.

Problems such as hypersexuality, compulsive masturbation, excessive promiscuity and reliance on pornography are not paraphilias, because the arousing stimulus in itself is not abnormal. They may nevertheless lead to relationship problems, distress and, occasionally, offending.

The assessment of sex offenders

Thornton (2002) proposes four domains of psychological problem to consider:

- Sexual interests:
  - deviant sexual interests (e.g. children or violence)
  - a high sexual drive or preoccupation with sexual thoughts.
- Distorted attitudes:
  - cognitive distortions are commonly used to minimize the impact of their offending, and resolve feelings of guilt or shame
  - implicit theories are the beliefs that underlie the cognitive distortions (e.g. children as sexual beings or a sense of entitlement that men should be able to have sex with women when they want).
- Problems with socio-affective management:
  - problems with adult intimacy and difficulty regulating emotions
  - self-esteem.
- Problems with self-management:
  - poor impulse control
  - difficulty coping with stress
  - poor problem solving.

Risk assessment in sex offending follows the same principles as discussed in Chapter 6. Commonly used actuarial risk assessment instruments (ARAIs) (see Craig and Beech, 2009, for a more detailed account) include the following:

- Static-2002 (14 items) adds to and modifies items used in the previous Static-99; predicts risk of sexual, violent and other recidivism.
- Risk Matrix 2000, used by prison, probation and police services nationally. Has separate sections for sexual offending (RM2000-S) and violent offending (RM2000-V), or they can be combined (RM2000-C). Has been shown to have good predictive accuracy.
- The Sex Offender Risk Appraisal Guide (SORAG) using 14 items was developed in Canada, but validated for use in the UK.
- Rapid Risk Assessment for Sex Offender Recidivism (RRASOR) uses four factors with demonstrated predictive accuracy (Hanson and Harris, 1997):
  - sexual offending history
  - age less than 25
  - unrelated to victim
  - gender of victim.

Hanson (2004) categorizes dynamic risk factors as stable or acute:

- Stable risk factors have the potential to change, but typically endure for months or years (e.g. personality disorder).
- Acute risk factors may exist for minutes to days and can signal the timing of offences (e.g. negative mood state, intoxication).

The most commonly used dynamic risk assessment tool is the Risk of Sexual Violence Protocol (RSVP) (Hart *et al.*, 2003):

- An updated version of the Sexual Violence Risk-20 (SVR-20).
- 22-item measure assessing items in five domains: sexual violence history, psychological adjustment, mental disorder, social adjustment and manageability.
- Items are coded as to their presence and relevance to the offender's risk.
- Risk formulation and scenarios allow for hypothesizing about future offending; these inform future management plans.

Box 13.1 The psychiatric assessment of sexual offenders

Common issues for a psychiatrist:

- Is the person suffering from a mental illness and what is the impact of this on their offending?
- What is the risk of reoffending and who is potentially at risk?
- What types of treatment or intervention are available?
- How effective have previous interventions been?

Assessment is often complicated by the level of denial displayed by many offenders. Use a non-judgemental style, while not colluding, and use collateral information (witness statements and police records) when exploring their accounts of past and recent offences.

In addition to the normal history and mental state assessment a comprehensive assessment of a sexual offender should include the following:

- Family background and early developmental experiences. Consider sexual boundaries within the family and behaviour or attitudes learned from parents or others.
- A detailed psychosexual history including sexual experiences and intimate relationships. It is also important to explore sexual fantasies and use of pornography.
- A more general assessment of interpersonal relationships, social skills and self-image.
- Psychiatric history.
- An analysis of patterns of offending behaviour, including precipitants and victim types. Look for evidence of escalation in offending.
- Criminal history, particularly frequency and range of sex offending, as well as current attitudes to past offences and victims.
- An alcohol and drug history. Consider whether offending has occurred as a result of being intoxicated, or whether they get intoxicated in order to offend.

The aim of the assessment is to provide an individualized formulation of the sexual offending, considering:

- early life experiences that may have predisposed to sexual offending
- factors that precipitate offending
- underlying beliefs that may impact on offending
- the relationship between any mental illness and offending
- key cognitive distortions, particularly relating to victim empathy and degree of denial
- other (particularly dynamic) risk factors.

The role of penile plethysmography (PPG) and polygraphy in the assessment and management of sex offenders is not established in mainstream UK practice. See Gordon and Grubin (2004) and Grubin and Madsen (2006) respectively for further discussion.

Psychological treatment

The aim is to reduce risk by identifying and modifying dynamic risk factors. The principles of therapy (after Abel and Osborn, 2003) are as follows:

- The offender should accept personal responsibility for offending. Denial, rationalization or minimization will obstruct treatment.
- The aim is not to cure, but to teach the offender better control of their sex offending behaviour. The time frame is life-long.
- Treatment should be offender-specific.
- Multiple factors may lead to sex offending; it is not just related to sexual gratification.

Most therapy is carried out by psychologists, prison and probation officers within the CJS.

Sex offender treatment programme (SOTP)

- A standardized treatment programme, introduced in the prison service in England and Wales in 1991 (Spencer, 2000), and also delivered in the community by probation.
- All prisoners convicted of a sexual offence and serving a sentence of 1 year or more should be offered SOTP as part of their sentence plan.
- Usually delivered in groups, but the same interventions can be delivered individually.
- Delivered in four stages (diagram developed using information from Spencer, 2000), as shown in Figure 13.1.

The adapted-SOTP is designed for offenders with an IQ of 65–80. It has less emphasis on victim empathy; more emphasis on sexual knowledge, modified belief patterns and avoidance of risk factors (Henson, 2008). The evidence about efficacy is conflicting. Conclusions from the Sex Offender Treatment Evaluation Project (Friendship *et al.*, 2003) are:

- reconviction rates were reduced for SOTP completers, but not significantly
- SOTP seemed more effective for offenders classified as medium risk, than those classified as high risk
- interventions need to be intensive and long term both in prisons and in the community.

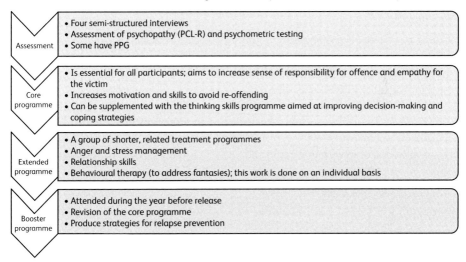

Figure 13.1 Sex offender treatment programmes (SOTP): delivered in four stages (PPG = penile plethysmography, PCL-R = psychopathy checklist – revised) (diagram developed using information from Spencer, 2000)

Pharmacological treatment

Pharmacological treatment should be used only as part of a comprehensive treatment and monitoring package. The aim is to suppress deviant sexual fantasies, urges, drive and behaviour. There are three classes of treatment:

- Selective serotonin reuptake inhibitors (SSRIs) are first line, used to suppress sexual fantasies and urges, particularly those with an obsessional or compulsive quality. The effect on general sexual drive is minor, and normal sexual activity may continue.
- Antiandrogens lead to suppression of fantasies and urges and a greater, dose-dependent reduction in sexual drive. Cyproterone acetate (blocks testosterone receptors) is mostly used in Canada and Europe. Medroxyprogesterone acetate (induces metabolism of testosterone) is used more often in the USA.
- Luteinizing hormone-releasing hormone agonists (e.g. goserelin) are less well established. They may have a place in patients resistant to antiandrogens. Effects on available androgens are very similar to those resulting from surgical castration (Bradford and Harris, 2003).

Reconviction rates

A meta-analysis of 61 follow-up studies of sexual offenders ($n = 28\,972$) (Hanson and Bussiere, 1998) showed that the overall recidivism rate was 13.4% with an average follow-up period of 4–5 years.

Of 192 sex offenders (60% had offended against children) released from determinate prison sentences in the UK, followed up for 4–6 years (Hood *et al.*, 2002):

- 8.5% were convicted of a sexual offence
- 18.1% were imprisoned for any offence type
- reconviction rates were lower for:
  - those who had offended against a child in their own family (0%) rather than outside the family (26.3%)
  - those who had offended against adults (7.5%).

● Stalkers

Stalking may be defined as repeated intrusions involving unwanted contacts and/or communications (Mullen *et al.*, 2001). Epidemiology is subject to poor criterion reliability and sampling bias, but 15% lifetime prevalence of being stalked among women has been suggested in Australia (Mullen *et al.*, 2000).

Stalking (rather like violence) is a behavioural end point that stems from very diverse motivations and underlying issues. An individual formulation is required. Mullen *et al.* (2000) have offered the typology given in Table 13.2 while Mohandie *et al.* (2006) categorize by relationship with the victim, although their rates for each group may be affected

Table 13.2 Mullen *et al.*'s (2000) typology

Rejected	An angry, dependent man pursuing an ex-partner. Unable to accept rejection, stalking maintains a semblance of a relationship
Intimacy seekers	Socially incompetent fantasist seeking a relationship with somebody with whom they are in love, or they believe to be in love with them. Delusional erotomania forms a subgroup
Incompetent suitor	Pursue intimate relationships inappropriately due to poor social skills and/or a sense of entitlement. May occur in learning disability or autistic spectrum disorder (ASD). May be easy to persuade them to stop stalking one victim, but the behaviour may well recur with someone else
Resentful	Motivated by revenge for some slight or insult, so well aware of distress or fear of the victim. Likely to threaten, but relatively less likely to carry out violence. Paranoid personality disorder common
Predatory	Stalking is preparatory to a sexual assault

Table 13.3 Mohandie *et al.*'s (2006) typology

Ex-Intimate	50% of their sample Considered to present the greatest risk. Threats, drug abuse and criminality are common
Acquaintance	13% of the sample; 21% of this group were women
Public figure	27% of the sample. The least likely to threaten violence, but where it occurs violence may be serious
Private stranger	10% of their sample, with a greater prevalence of mental illness than the other groups

by selection bias (Table 13.3). Based on a sample of 211 stalkers referred to a forensic psychiatric service in Australia, McEwan *et al.* (2009) reported that risk factors for violence particularly included previous violence, and threats by ex-intimate stalkers.

● **Fire Setters**

In 2008–9 (Fire Statistics Monitor, 2010):

- Fire and rescue services responded to 722 000 fires or false alarms:
  - a total of 326 000 fires
  - 52 000 were deliberate primary fires (fires in buildings, cars or structures, any involving casualties)
  - 148 000 deliberate secondary fires (fires outdoors and in derelict buildings).
- There were 322 fire fatalities.

Legal aspects of the criminal offence of arson are discussed in Chapter 15. Figure 13.2 shows the frequency of arson offences in England and Wales.

Frequency of arson correlates with (Arson Control Forum, 2009):

- levels of antisocial behaviour in a community
- economic stability
- fire safety interventions.

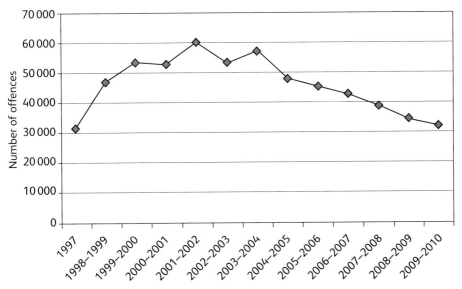

Figure 13.2 Frequency of offences of arson recorded in the Crime in England and Wales Report 2009–10 (Home Office, 2010)

In the year 2009–10 (Home Office, 2010):

- arson offences accounted for 4% of all police recorded criminal damage offences, a fall of 6% on the previous year:
  - life was endangered in 11% of the 32 579 cases
- only 28% of the incidents of arson endangering life and 7% of arson not endangering life were 'cleared up by the police' (including charging or cautioning).

Fire setting and mental disorder

Psychiatric studies tend to find high levels of mental disorder in those convicted of arson. Rix (1994) assessed 153 arsonists referred for pre-trial reports in Yorkshire (Table 13.4).

Table 13.4 Mental disorders in arsonists

Diagnosis (some had more than one)	Percentage
Personality disorder	54
Learning disability	11
Psychosis	8
Alcohol misuse	8
Depressive disorder	5
Substance misuse	3
Conduct disorder	1
Not known	1
No diagnosis	13

- Jayaraman and Frazer (2006) found a similar pattern; Dickens *et al.* (2007) found higher levels of mental disorder in female fire setters.
- Fire setting is considered to be particularly associated with learning disability. Observed prevalence rates vary according to study setting:
  - Hogue *et al.* (2006) found rates of 2.8% in the community and 21.4% in medium/low secure settings.
- The most common diagnosis in children and adolescents is conduct disorder (Kolko and Kazdin, 1991).
- Using Swedish national registers for convictions and hospital discharge diagnoses, Anwar *et al.* (2011) demonstrated odds ratios after correction for socio-demographic factors:

	Men	Women
Schizophrenia	22.6 (14.8–34.4)	38.7 (20.4–73.5)
Other psychosis	17.4 (11.1–27.5)	30.8 (18.8–50.6)

Motivations for fire setting

A curiosity about fires and some fire play is normal during childhood development. Persistence into a more deviant pattern of behaviour is associated with (Glancy *et al.*, 2003):

- male gender
- young age
- dysfunctional family background
- stressful life events
- low socio-economic status
- academic or vocational difficulties.

Motivations for fire setting may be thought of as either criminal or psychopathological (Table 13.5):

Table 13.5 Motivations for fire setting

Criminal motivations	Psychopathological motivations
For financial compensation or to earn money	To commit suicide
To hide or destroy evidence of something	Psychosis
Politically motivated (animal rights, for example)	A way of communicating distress or seeking support
As part of a wider pattern of vandalism or other antisocial behaviour	To boost self-esteem perhaps by saving a pet or property (may coexist with pyromania)
Emotionally driven, through anger or jealousy, or for revenge, whether planned or impulsive	Pyromania

- Rix (1994) found that revenge was the most common motivation.
- Jayaraman and Fraser (2006) found anger compounded by substance misuse to be more common.
- Despite the earlier psychodynamic association of fire with sexual imagery, it is rare for arsonists to show sexual arousal in association with fire setting.

Pyromania or pathological fire setting

Repetitive fire setting without external motivation

- Classified as a habit and impulse disorder in ICD-10 (World Health Organization, 1992; see Chapter 8).
- The interest is in the fire itself and associated things. The subject is likely to watch the fire burn, call the fire brigade and watch the fire service intervention.
- There is a compulsive quality, with anticipatory subjective tension, followed by excitement after setting the fire. Subjects may describe an irresistible impulse or urge to set a fire.
- More common in men, particularly in those with:
  - learning disability
  - inadequate personality, for whom fire setting tends to relieve deep-seated despondency, perhaps leading to compensatory feelings of increased self-importance and potency.

Treatment

There is a dearth of evidence about potentially modifiable dynamic risk factors for adult arsonists. Palmer *et al.* (2007) reviewed available interventions for arsonists and young fire setters, in the community, CJS and forensic mental health units:

- There were two broad approaches used: educational and psychological.
- Most interventions for children and adolescents were provided by fire and rescue services, often in conjunction with youth offending services.
- Some forensic mental health services provided interventions for arsonists, but little available in either prison or probation services.

Educational approaches

Educational approaches are typically used with children, and provide teaching on fire safety skills and information on risks and consequences:

- For example: the FACE UP (Fire Awareness Child Education UP) programme developed in 1991 by the Merseyside Fire and Rescue service for young offenders. Palmer *et al.* (2007) reported that this has been adapted for use in the adult prison population in HMP Liverpool in 1998.

Psychological interventions

Psychiatric units use mostly CBT-based group interventions. They are more common in learning disability services:

Box 13.2 Psychiatric assessment of fire setters

The aim is to:

- diagnose mental disorder
- understand the relationship between mental disorder and the fire setting
- formulate the motivation for fire setting
- set out dynamic risk factors associated with fire setting
- suggest interventions that may impact upon those risk factors.

Unlike violent and sexual offending there are no specifically designed risk assessment tools to assess risk in those who set fires; however, some tools such as the HCR-20 specify that arson can be included within their risk assessment schedules (Gannon, 2010).

Fire setters, particularly those with predominantly psychopathological motivations, often give poor histories, and struggle to recognize or acknowledge their motivations. Adopting a sensitive interviewing style is most likely to be fruitful, but ensure that all available collateral information is used. Seek an informant history to ascertain, in particular:

- childhood fireplay
- previous acts of fire setting (including undetected)
- previous threats or targets
- types of fires set (use of accelerants, single or multiple seats)
- motivations for previous acts.

A careful functional assessment of the index incident should concentrate on:

- recent psychosocial stressors
- affect and circumstances surrounding event
- intoxication or other disinhibiting factors
- acts of planning and preparation
- fascination/preoccupation with fire and associated items
- feelings immediately before and after the act.

Motivations may be complex, such that more than one of the motivational categories may be important. In particular pyromania and a desire to be a hero may coexist.

- Swaffer *et al.* (2001) described an arson intervention group at Rampton High Secure Hospital used with a mixed gender group. It comprises four modules of both group and individual work:
  - danger of fire – assessing and developing insight (12 sessions)
  - skills development – coping without fire setting (social skills, problems solving, conflict resolution) (24 sessions)
  - insight and self-awareness – assessing and developing (12 sessions)
  - relapse prevention – practical strategies to help break offence cycles (14 sessions).
- Taylor *et al.* (2006) described the Fire Setter Treatment Programme (FSTP) designed for those with learning disabilities:
  - preparatory work: establishing the group, group cohesion exercises, family and related issues (9 sessions)
  - review of offence cycle (12 sessions)
  - education, skills acquisition and development including anger management and self-esteem work (15 sessions)
  - relapse prevention: personalized risk assessment and relapse prevention plan (4 sessions).

There is little good evidence to support the efficacy of these programmes, except for face validity and acceptability to participants.

Reoffending

Brett (2004) reviewed the available literature (24 studies) on re-offending among fire setters in various environments:

- Reoffending rates varied from 4% to 60%, depending on the populations studied.
- There is no empirical support for the assumption that arsonists are inherently dangerous.
- There is a clear need for more research in specific groups.

Dickens *et al.* (2007) suggested that the following factors were associated with recidivism:

- youth
- single
- developmental history of family violence or substance misuse
- early onset of criminal convictions
- lengthier prison stays
- relationship problems
- more previous convictions for property offences.

References

Abel GG, Osborn CA. (2003) Treatment of sex offenders. In: Rosner R (ed.), *Principles and Practice of Forensic Psychiatry*, 2nd edn. London: Arnold

Anwar S, Langstrom N, Grann M, Fazel S. (2011) Is arson the crime most strongly associated with psychosis? – A national case-control study of arson risk in schizophrenia and other psychoses. *Schizophrenia Bulletin* **37**(3), 580–6

Arson Control Forum. (2009) *Annual Report to the Fire Minister*. Available at: http://www.arson controlforum.gov.uk/129

Baker A, Duncan S. (1985) Child sexual abuse: a study of prevalence in Great Britain. *Child Abuse and Neglect* **9**, 457–67

Bradford J, Harris VL. (2003) Pharmacologic treatment of sex offenders. In: Rosner R (ed.), *Principles and Practice of Forensic Psychiatry*, 2nd edn. London: Hodder Arnold

Brett A. (2004) 'Kindling Theory' in arson: how dangerous are firesetters? *Australian and New Zealand Journal of Psychiatry* **38**, 419–25

Craig LA, Beech A. (2009) Best practice in conducting actuarial risk assessments with adult sexual offenders. *Journal of Sexual Aggression* **15**(2), 193–211

Denov MS. (2004) *Perspectives on Female Sex Offending: A culture of denial*. Hampshire, UK: Ashgate Publishing Limited

Dickens G, Sugarman P, Ahmad F, Edgar S, Hofberg K, Tewari S. (2007) Gender differences amongst adult arsonists at psychiatric assessment. *Medicine Science & Law* **47**, 233–8.

Drake CR, Pathe M. (2004) Understanding sexual offending in schizophrenia. *Criminal Behaviour and Mental Health* **14**, 108–20

Eldridge HJ. (2000) Patterns of offending and strategies for effective assessment and intervention. In: Itzin C (ed.), *Home Truths about Child Sexual Abuse*. London: Routledge

Fazel S, Sjostedt G, Langstrom N, Grann M. (2007) Severe mental illness and risk of sexual offending in men: a case-control study based on Swedish national registers. *Journal of Clinical Psychiatry* **68**(4), 588–96

Feist A, Ashe J, Lawrence J, McPhee D, Wilson R. (2007) *Investigating and detecting recorded offences of rape. Home Office online Report 18/07*. Available at: http://rds.homeoffice.gov.uk/rds/pdfs07/rdsolr1807.pdf

Fire Statistics Monitor. (2010). *Revised data for 2008–09 and the first data for April to September 2009. Communities and Local Government National Statistics.* Available at: http://www.communities.gov.uk/documents/statistics/pdf/1576231.pdf.

Friendship C, Mann R, Beech A. (2003) *The Prison-base Sex Offender Treatment Programme – an evaluation.* London: Home Office. Available at: http://rds.homeoffice.gov.uk/rds/pdfs2/r205.pdf

Gannon TA. (2010) Female arsonists: key features, psychopathologies, and treatment needs. *Psychiatry* **73**(2), 173–89

Glancy GD, Spiers EM, Pitt SE, Dvoski JA. (2003) Commentary: models and correlates of firesetting behaviour. *Journal of the American Academy of Law and Psychiatry* **31**, 53–7

Gordon H, Grubin D. (2004) Psychiatric aspects of the assessment and treatment of sex offenders. *Advances in Psychiatric Treatment* **10**, 73–80

Grubin D. (1992) Cross-cultural influences on sex offending. *Annual Review of Sex Research* **3**, 201–17.

Grubin D, Madsen L. (2006) Accuracy and utility of post-conviction polygraph testing of sex offenders. *British Journal of Psychiatry* **188**, 479–83.

Hanson RK. (2004) Sex offender risk assessment. In: Hollins CR (ed.), *The Essential Handbook of Offender Assessment and Treatment.* Chichester: John Wiley & Sons

Hanson RK, Bussiere MT. (1998) Predicting relapse: a meta-analysis of sexual offender recidivism studies. *Journal of Consulting and Clinical Psychology* **66**, 348–62

Hanson RK, Harris AJR. (1997) *Dynamic Predictors of Sexual Recidivism.* Ottawa: Department of the Solicitor-General of Canada

Hart S, Kropp P, Laws, D. (2003) *The Risk for Sexual Violence Protocol (RSVP): Structured professional guidelines for assessing risk of sexual violence.* Vancouver: The Institute Against Family Violence

Henson T. (2008) Do sexual offenders with learning disabilities benefit from sex offender treatment programmes? *British Journal of Learning Disabilities* **37**, 98–107

Hogue TE, Steptoe L, Taylor JL, Lindsay WL, Mooney P, Pinkney L, *et al.* (2006) A comparison of offenders with intellectual disability across three levels of security. *Criminal Behaviour and Mental Health* **16**, 13–28

Home Office (2010) *Crime in England and Wales 2009/10.* Available from http://rds.homeoffice.gov.uk/

Hood R, Shute S, Feilzer M, Wilcox A. (2002) *Reconviction rates of serious sex offenders and assessments of their risk.* Home Office. Available at: http://rds.homeoffice.gov.uk/

Independent, The. (2010) 'Sarah's Law' may backfire, say campaigners. 2 August 2010. Available at: http://www.independent.co.uk/news/uk/crime/sarahs-law-may-backfire-say-campaigners-2041217.html

Jayaraman A, Frazer J. (2006) Arson: A growing inferno. *Medicine Science and the Law* **46**(4), 295–300

Kolko DJ, Kazdin AE. (1991) Motives of childhood firesetters: firesetting characteristics and psychological correlates. *Journal of Child Psychology and Psychiatry* **32**, 535–50.

Lockmuller M, Beech A, Fisher D. (2008) Sexual offenders with mental health problems: epidemiology, assessment and treatment. In: Soothill K, Rogers P, Dolan M (eds), *Handbook of Forensic Mental Health.* Deacon: Willan Publishing

McEwan TE, Mullen PE, MacKenzie RD, Ogloff JRP. (2009) Violence in stalking situations. *Psychological Medicine* **39**, 1469–78

Mohandie K, Meloy JR, McGowan MG, Williams J. (2006) The RECON typology of stalking: reliability and validity based on a large sample of North American stalkers. *Journal of Forensic Science* **51**(1), 147–55

Mullen P, Pathe M, Purcell P. (2000) *Stalkers and their Victims.* Cambridge: Cambridge University Press

Mullen P, Pathe M, Purcell P. (2001) The management of stalkers. *Advances in Psychiatric Treatment* **7**, 335–42

O'Connell MA, Leberg E, Donaldson CR. (1990) *Working with Sex Offenders: Guidelines for therapist selection.* Newbury Park: Sage Publications

Palmer EJ, Caulfield LS, Hollin C. (2007) Interventions with arsonists and young fire setters: A survey of the national picture in England and Wales. *Legal and Criminological Psychiatry* **12**, 101–16

Povey D, Coleman K., Kaiza P, Roe S. (2009) *Homicides, Firearm Offences and Intimate Violence 2007/08 (Supplementary Volume 2 to Crime in England and Wales 2007/08.* Home Office Statistical Bulletin 02/09. London: Home Office

Rix K. (1994) A psychiatric study of adult arsonists. *Medicine Science and the Law* **4**(1), 21–34

Sentencing Guidelines Council (2010) *Sexual Offences Act 2003. Definitive Guideline.* Available at: http://www.sentencingcouncil.org.uk/docs/web_SexualOffencesAct_2003.pdf

Soothill K. (2003) Serious sexual assault: using history and statistics. In: Matravers A (ed.), *Sex Offenders in the Community Managing and Reducing Risks.* Deacon: Willan Publishing

Spencer A. (2000) *Working with Sex Offenders in Prisons and through Release to the Community.* London: Jessica Kingsley

Swaffer T, Haggett M, Oxley T. (2001) Mentally disordered firesetters: a structured intervention programme. *Clinical Psychology and Psychotherapy* **8**, 468–75

Taylor JL, Robertson A, Thorpe I, Belshaw T, Watson A. (2006) Responses of female fire setters with mild and borderline intellectual disabilities to a group intervention. *Journal of Applied Research in Intellectual Disabilities* **19**, 179–90

Thornton D. (2002) Constructing and testing a framework for dynamic risk assessment. *Sexual Abuse: A Journal of Research and Treatment* **14**, 139–53

World Health Organization. (1992) *The International Classification of Diseases (ICD-10).* Geneva: WHO

Crime and Criminology

Criminology is the observational study of crime:

- A crime may be defined either by statute (an increasing proportion of offences) or by common law (e.g. murder, perverting the course of justice):
  - Many other jurisdictions have an exhaustive criminal code defining all offences in statute.
- An action is described as a crime according to socio-cultural norms and expectations, which vary with time:
  - Previously tolerated behaviours may become unacceptable (e.g. domestic violence, smoking).
  - Previously proscribed behaviours become accepted (homosexuality, swearing and suicide).
  - New criminal activity develops (Internet crime).
  - Different societies have different norms (e.g. age of consent for sexual intercourse).
- There are two criminological aspects:
  - Criminal behaviour, including who does what and why, patterns and trends of crime, victims and causes of crime.
  - Society's response to crime, encompassing societal expectations and morality and the criminal justice system.

Criminological theory has developed over several hundred years and continues to develop:

- There are many theories of crime; no single theory is adequate to explain all crime or all offenders.
- Theories often overlap and are sometimes contradictory.
- Academic thinking has been variously influenced by sociology, psychology, law, social anthropology, economics and psychiatry.
- Some theories are more influenced by psychology and psychiatry than others (e.g biological and psychological positivism).

● Criminological Theories

Some of the major theories are considered here. See Maguire *et al.* (2007) or Newburn (2007) for a more complete and detailed account.

Classicism (1700s to early 1800s)

Key figures:

- Cesare Bonesana, Marchese of Boccaria (known as Boccaria); Jeremy Bentham.

Each individual acts according to choice, as a 'rational actor', and weighs up the benefits and consequences of their actions. So they choose to commit crime:

- Previously punishment had been cruel and inconsistent. Now it was proposed that punishment should be proportional, certain and rapid, so individuals would know the consequences of criminal behaviour. Then they would be more likely to make a rational decision not to do it.
- Includes the introduction of imprisonment as punishment, rather than corporal or capital punishment.

Positivism (late 1800s to modern times)

Key figures

- Cesare Lombroso; Enrico Ferri; Raffaele Garafalo.

Observed that not all people are 'rational actors':

- The mentally ill, young people, individuals under the influence of drugs or alcohol, for example.

Posited that a criminal is born a criminal, qualitatively different from other people:

- Focused on attributes of 'the criminal', offering a scientific approach to crime, including the development of hypotheses and collection of data.
- The original theory was of its time, when scientific enquiry was de rigueur – Darwinism, for example.
- The corollary of positivism is that the consequence of crime should be treatment rather than punishment.

Two approaches may be distinguished:

- Biological positivism:
  – Facial features, phrenology (shape and contours of head), somatyping (shape of body), more recently neurotransmitters, attention deficit hyperactivity disorder (ADHD) and (molecular) genetics.
- Psychological positivism:
  – Social learning theories, application of Freud's theories of instinctual drives, Bowlby's attachment theory, Eysenck's model of personality, Piaget's cognitive development and Kohlberg's stages of moral development.

Anomie (late 1800s to 1930s)

Key figures:

- Emile Durkheim (a French sociologist rather than criminologist, in the late 1800s)
- Robert K. Merton (1930s).

Anomie refers to a lack of common social or ethical standards in an individual or a group. Durkheim's sociological theory of anomie states that the pace of societal change, originally from pre- to post-Industrial Revolution society, is too quick:

- Previously society was homogeneous, most people leading similar lifestyles and having similar views about morality and deviance. This resulted in strong social cohesion and control.
- A more sophisticated society developed after the Industrial Revolution, with greater differentiation between individuals in terms of division of labour and consequent rewards, but also morality.
- Consequently societal moral restraints became less effective at limiting individual desires; a state of anomie developed.
- Durkheim particularly related suicide to anomie.

Crime is seen as normal in society and adaptive, in that it introduces new ideas, demonstrates boundaries of acceptable behaviour, and can portray the nature of society in terms of what is considered acceptable.

Chicago School (early 1900s to 1940s)

Key figures:

- Frederic Thrasher; Edwin Sutherland; Walter Reckless; Robert Ezra Park; Erving Goffman; Clifford Shaw; Henry McKay.

Between the wars:

- Chicago saw rapid social change due to industrial development, high immigration and high crime rates.
- Chicago University had the first academic department of sociology.

Strongly influenced by Durkheim and theories of social organization, focused on crime in relation to space – where it occurred and why, using ethnographic research to determine two major findings:

- Neighbourhoods tend to be stable over decades in terms of crime rates.
- Areas of high socio-economic status have low crime rates and vice versa.

Therefore crime is linked to factors that also lead to poverty, social deprivation, delinquency, ill-health, poor environment (i.e. social disorganization), and can be considered a social problem.

Some key theories:

- Zonal hypothesis:
  - An urban area has distinct zones, including the central business district, a 'zone in transition' (area of greatest social change, immigration and social differentiation and weakest social control) and outer residential zones.
  - The 'zone in transition' was consistently found to have higher rates of crime, delinquency, mental illness and poverty.
- Cultural transmission (Shaw and McKay):
  - Behaviour is passed from generation to generation, including delinquent behaviour.
  - Considered an explanation for the observed regional stability of crime rates and contributed to young people being unable to change behavioural patterns.
- Differential association (Sutherland) and differential reinforcement (Akers):
  - Criminal behaviour is learned, and such behaviour is influenced by 'associations' (factors) that lead to either conforming to the law, or breaking the law.
  - This behaviour can be positively or negatively reinforced, leading either to further delinquent behaviour or to more conforming behaviour (differential reinforcement).

Strain theory (1930s to 1960s)

Key figures:

- Albert Cohen; Richard Cloward; Lloyd Ohlin.
- Robert Agnew (1990s).

A development of Merton's theory of anomie, which seemed not to explain juvenile delinquency:

- Hypothesized that there is competition for success in a society, but an inequality in opportunities. This leads to frustration among young people, resulting in 'strain', which leads to collaboration with others feeling the same. A delinquent subculture results.

In the 1990s Agnew revitalized this theory, suggesting that 'strain' was due to a loss of something valued (relationships, opportunities) or the presence of 'noxious' stimuli, e.g. abuse:

- This is exacerbated by a feeling of injustice, a large degree of strain, low levels of social control and chronic strain.
- Repeated exposure to strain leads to a greater probability of crime.

Subculture theories (post-1940s)

Key figures:

- Albert Cohen; Richard Cloward and Lloyd Ohlin; David Matza; David Downes.

Proposes that delinquency develops within groups that young people form in response to social disorganization and strain:

- People who cannot progress to a respectable status, due to socio-economic or family factors, develop a 'status frustration' and hostility to traditional values. Subcultures provide status and belonging.
- Also encompasses learning theory, as delinquent behaviour can be imitated or learnt, as a means to cope with frustrations, or to gain money, status or power.

Research especially looked at young, white, working-class males. Initially developed in American cities, in relation to urban gangs, but translated to the UK in studies of 'mods and rockers', 'punks', 'hippies', 'skinheads' and more recently acid house subculture.

Subculture theories have been criticized for minimizing the role of individual choice, and for being largely inapplicable to female criminality. Also tends to:

- overestimate delinquency in deprived urban areas as not all young people in these situations engage in such behaviour
- underestimate crime in other parts of society.

Control theories (1960s to 1970s)

Key figures:

- Walter Reckless; David Matza and Graham Sykes; Travis Hirschi.

A collection of related theories that consider why more people do not commit crime more often, and what controls influence individuals to conform to society rules:

- Containment theory (Reckless) proposes factors that provide resistance to crime:
  - inner containment includes having realistic goals, positive self-concept
  - outer containment relates to external positive factors, such as positive relationships.
- Social bond theory (Hirschi): the likelihood of deviant behaviour is inversely related to the strength of social bonds:
  - attachments, to family, for example
  - commitment to conforming activities such as education
  - involvement in non-deviant activities
  - belief in conventional values.
- General theory of crime (Gottfredson and Hirschi):
  - held to apply to all forms of crime
  - low self-control leads to an inability to avoid behaviours, including criminality, drug-taking, promiscuity, etc.
  - low self-control is due to poor parenting techniques in childhood.

Radical criminology

Key figures:

- Willem Bonger; Ian Taylor; Paul Walton; Jock Young.

A socio-political perspective rooted in Marxism, emphasizing differences in power and money between groups in society, and seeing crime as a social problem:

- In capitalist society laws protect the ruling classes, and crime stems from the working class's resistance to the ruling class's laws.
- A society without class differences would eventually have no crime as laws would be universally protective.

Struggles to explain white collar crime or low crime rates in some capitalist societies.

Labelling theory (1970s to 1980s)

Key figures:

- George Mead; Frank Tannenbaum; Howard Becker; Edwin Lemert; John Braithwaite.

Considers why certain people are considered to be deviant, and the reasons for social reactions to deviant behaviour:

- Rules are made by society, and applied to people; if individuals break the rules, they are considered deviant. This can result in a person becoming more deviant, as they try to live up to their name (a self-fulfilling prophesy).
- The more that a behaviour is deemed to be immoral, the more individuals are likely to behave in that way, leading to more crime.
- Associated with stigma, 'folk devils' and 'moral panics'.

John Braithwaite (1979) considered the importance of shaming, which underpins restorative justice today:

- Shaming may be disintegrative (offered in a stigmatizing or rejecting way and tending to exclude the offender from law-abiding society) or reintegrative.
- If an individual feels shame or remorse, and they can be reintegrated into the community, this will help to reduce reoffending.
- If a culture has intrinsically high expectations of its citizens, which are openly expressed, then crime control methods will be more effective than methods used by a society wanting only to give negative consequences to 'bad apples'.

Left realism (mid-1980s to 1990s)

Key figures:

- Jock Young; Roger Matthews; John Lea; Elliott Currie.

Developed in the UK and the USA in the context of a change in the political environment, which became more right wing and critical of welfare culture, had stronger views of punishment and favoured a 'free market economy':

- Traditional left-wing views tended to minimize crime, to treat offenders as 'victims'.
- Other theories excluded crime against women, such as domestic violence or sexual violence.

Young developed these ideas as a politically pragmatic criminology, seeking greater influence on policy makers than criminological theory had tended to have before:

- Crime is best seen as a function of four interdependent factors, in the so-called 'square of crime' (Young, 1997):
  - the victim
  - the offender
  - the actions (crime)
  - the reactions (of society, the criminal justice system, CJS).
- Crime control requires a comprehensive balance of interventions addressing all of these factors.
- Included a greater use of empirical evidence such as local crime surveys, leading to greater influence over local criminal justice policy development, particularly for the New Labour government of 1997 (Hopkins-Burke, 2005, pp224–7).

Feminist criminology (from the 1960s)

Key figures:

- Freda Adler; Rita Simon; Carol Smart; Pat Carlen; Frances Heidensohn.

The preceding theories are generally male-orientated, in terms of both the offenders studied and the criminologists involved:

- Female offenders and victims tended to be stereotyped (as prostitutes, for example).
- Early theories (such as biological positivism) did include women, but on the premise that women were 'more primitive' and 'less developed' than men.

Female criminologists became active in the late 1960s, and discovered that the proposed factors relating to 'male crime' (such as unemployment, antisocial behaviour, gang culture and peer group influence) were often less applicable to 'female crime'. New theories were required:

- Liberal feminist theory:
  - As women have changed their social and economic position following emancipation, they have become more like men and their propensity for crime has changed accordingly.
- Control theory in relation to women:
  - Women are often controlled, by men (through violence or other negative methods), by society expectations and in the home (historically responsible for running the house, childcare and increasingly employed in the workplace as well).
  - This means that they are less likely to commit crime.
- The proposal of 'double jeopardy':
  - When a woman commits a crime she is stigmatized both as a criminal and for behaving in a non-feminine way.
  - This leads to being dealt with paternalistically by the CJS.

Feminist criminology has also emphasized victim issues, leading to a much greater study of victims and their role within the CJS.

Contemporary classicism (1970s to current)

Key figures:

- Ron Clarke; Derek Cornish; Marcus Felson.

The rational actor model of criminality was reinvigorated, in the context of the rise of populist conservatism, and the 'nothing works' philosophy of the Home Office, which recognized that there was little evidence for the effectiveness of CJS rehabilitative interventions.

Rational choice theory (Clarke and Cornish)

- The offender is a rational actor, making individualistic choices in their self-interest, based on an appraisal of the rewards and costs of the action.
- However, they will act with 'bounded rationality', working within limits of knowledge, situation or opportunities. They will not necessarily obtain and weigh up all the facts necessary for a sensible decision.

Routine activity theory (Felson)

- Most offending is minor, acquisitive and inevitable.
- There are three key ingredients:
  - motivated individuals – mostly young men
  - appropriate targets – whether a person or property, and
  - absence of a 'capable guardian'.
- Contemporary lifestyles provide more opportunities for crime – portable computers, mobile phones and other possessions; placing people away from home.

Importantly, for both of these variants, crime prevention strategies focus on situational manipulation (locking doors, street lighting, using tokens for utility meters, etc.) rather than offenders.

A political and psychiatric context

Society has always tended to take a harsh approach to criminal justice, polls suggesting that a majority of the UK public favour reintroduction of the death penalty, for example. Unsurprisingly the utilitarian approaches of contemporary classicism have found more favour with policy makers than the sociologically based theories that went before (Reiner, 2006). This promotes:

- normalization of criminal activity, reducing the need to understand it, and legitimizing situational crime prevention measures, and
- punishment (as opposed to treatment) of the offender who is seen as having deliberately (rationally) chosen to be criminal.

In the consequent 'culture of control' (Garland, 2001), offenders are seen as qualitatively different from law-abiding citizens, and they may legitimately be punished harshly. Welfarist approaches to crime are subordinated to the management of risk and the identification of risky individuals:

- This may resonate with contemporary forensic psychiatry, in which an individual therapeutic approach is sometimes threatened by a managerial approach to risk management systems and group data.
- Those with mental disorder may be in an invidious position. The widespread prejudice that the mentally disordered are dangerous is well known, which may lead to their being categorically identified as criminal and consequently subject to the increasingly common civil powers of control that are politically justified by the contemporary criminologies.

● Recording of Crime

There are three approaches to recording crime:

- police recording of crime
- victim surveys
- offender surveys.

Police-recorded crime significantly underestimates actual crime:

- Victims do not always report crimes to the police:
  - victims do not always report incidents, due to fear or embarrassment, believing it not to be worthwhile (e.g. minor theft), having sympathy for offender or not trusting police
  - there is no victim (e.g. action between two consenting adults, such as a drugs transaction)
  - the crime is not detected, e.g. identity fraud
  - victim was involved in the offence (for example, both parties assaulted each other).
- Reported crime may not be recorded:
  - there is a lack of evidence
  - the victim does not press charges
  - the police do not pursue the matter.

The difference between actual crime and recorded crime is known as hidden crime. Victim and offender surveys may be used to estimate this. The best known example in the UK is the British Crime Survey (BCS).

Police-recorded crime

This covers all notifiable offences (i.e. notifiable to the Home Office), which are collectively known as recorded crime (Table 14.1):

- It excludes most summary offences.
- There are over 100 notifiable offences in nine categories:
  - theft and handling stolen goods
  - burglary
  - criminal damage
  - violence against the person (assault, dangerous driving, affray, attempted murder, murder)
  - sexual offences (indecent assault, rape, incest, bigamy)
  - robbery
  - fraud and forgery
  - drug offences
  - other.

British Crime Survey

The BCS is a face-to-face victimization survey carried out for the first time in 1982 which has run continuously, reporting annually, since 2001:

- Based on more than 45 000 respondents, resident in households in England and Wales, who are asked about their experience of crime in the previous 12 months.
- Since January 2009 includes a sample of 16–24 year olds and 11–15 year olds.
- Response rate is around 75 %.

Table 14.1 Police recorded crime for 2009/10 available at http://rds.homeoffice.gov.uk/rds/recordedcrime1.html

	No. of recorded offences 2009–10	Change since previous year (%)	Percentage of total recorded crime
Violence against the person with injury	**401 743**	**–5**	**9.3**
Homicide	615		
Attempted murder	588		
Driving offences leading to death	504		
Wounding with intent	22 798		
Malicious wounding	16 730		
Assault–occasional actual bodily harm	359 950		
Violence against the person without injury	**469 969**	**–3**	**10.8**
Threats/conspiracy to murder	44		
Threats to kill	9 566		
Possession of a weapon	24 380		
Public order offences	205 219		
Assault without injury	223 328		
Sexual offences	**54 509**	**+6**	**1.3**
Rape of adult female	9 102		
Rape of adult male	372		
Rape of underage female	4 889		
Rape of underage male	802		
Sexual assault of female	19 873		
Sexual assault of male	2 270		
Robbery	**75 101**	**–6**	**1.7**
Burglary	**540 655**	**–7**	**12.5**
Offences against vehicles	**494 978**	**–16**	**11.4**
Other theft, fraud and forgery	**1 189 829**	**–5**	**27.4**
Criminal damage	**806 720**	**–14**	**18.6**
Arson endangering life	3 625		
Arson not endangering life	28 954		
Drugs offences	**234 998**	**–4**	**5.4**
Miscellaneous	**70 102**	**–2**	**1.6**
Total recorded crime	**4 338 604**	**–8**	

Note: within categories, only selected offences are included, so the totals do not add up to the total for that category

Data from the BCS since 1982 shows that crime rose to a peak in 1995 and has declined since. The reported level in 2009–10 was about 50% of the level in 1995:

- This reduction in crime is mirrored in many western societies – proposed explanations for this uniform change have varied greatly among societies.

In many respects, the BCS and police-recorded crimes complement each other, and collectively offer a good coverage of criminal activity:

- Police-recorded crime has wider coverage of offences, but the BCS includes unreported/unrecorded crime.

Both methods are deficient in relation to:

- new forms of offending such as credit card fraud (credit card companies report much higher rates)
- drugs offences (where both victim and perpetrator may be involved in criminal activity).

Table 14.2 summarizes the advantages and disadvantages of the BCS.

Table 14.2 The British Crime Survey: advantages and disadvantages

Advantages	Disadvantages
Includes crimes not reported to or recorded by the police Explores victims' impressions of and fear of crime Identifies information about victims May reassure public about true rate of crime Enables development of local crime reduction policy	Based on recall and opinion, so potentially subject to bias Excludes the homeless, and those living in institutions at present Excludes businesses so may not cover white collar crime, or crimes regulated by authorities such as environmental health Does not include murder and may not be reliable for domestic violence, pornographic or paedophilic crimes due to reduced disclosure rates Respondents may be concerned about confidentiality in relation to reporting more serious crimes

Some findings from 2009–10 BCS report (http://rds.homeoffice.gov.uk/rds)

The risk of victimization varies by gender and neighbourhood:

- Young men are at greater risk of stranger violence, women at greater risk of domestic violence.
- Risk is greater in urban than rural areas, particularly in high population density areas:
  - 62% of robberies were recorded by Greater Manchester, West Midlands and Metropolitan police forces, an area containing 24% of the population.

Some 66% of respondents believed that crime had risen in recent years, though only 10% believed that they lived in a high crime area:

- This may be interpreted as suggesting that the perception of increasing crime is due to indirect knowledge derived from media reporting or politicking, rather than personal experience of crime.

Table 14.3 gives selected data from the BCS.

Table 14.3 Estimated crime in England and Wales from 2009–10 BCS

	Estimated number of crimes	Change since 2001–2 (%)
All violence	**2 087 000**	**−24**
Wounding	501 000	−23
Assault with minor injury	428 000	−40
Assault without injury	823 000	−19
Robbery	335 000	−6
All acquisitive crime	**5 427 000**	**−29**
Vandalism	2 408 000	−8
Burglary	659 000	−32
Vehicle-related theft	1 229 000	−51
Other household theft	1 163 000	−19
Theft from the person	5 25 000	−13
All BCS crime	**9 587 000**	**−24**

Within categories, only selected offences are included, so the totals do not add up to the total for that category

● Reoffending Rates

Reoffending is often taken as an outcome measure of criminal justice penalties, such that low reoffending rates imply successful penalties, but the situation is often more complex than this:

- In particular, reoffending is not the same as reconviction, which is the usual proxy measure.

There are two approaches:

- Examining the reoffending of individuals over time, to examine when individuals start and stop offending, and why.
- Examining trends among groups of offenders through official statistics, according to offence, sentence given or socio-demographic factors.

Since 2007–8, adult reoffending statistics are collated in quarterly reports giving results for each justice area:

- Available at http://www.cjp.org.uk/publications/government
- Includes convictions and police cautions for those offenders under probation supervision (either community orders or under licence):
  - therefore excludes those over 22 years released after a short sentence, and all whose period of supervision has ceased.

The rate of reoffending for this group has remained constant since 2007. In 2009–10 the rate was

- 9.71% overall:
  - 10.07% for those on community orders
  - 8.15% for those under licence.

● Correlates of Crime and Criminal Careers

The epidemiological research should be interpreted with some caution:

- Often focused on adolescent delinquency, which may be different from offending in other groups.
- Longitudinal self-report studies tend to look at less serious offending, and certain types of offence/ offender may not be included.

Key studies include:

- Graham and Bowling (1995) conducted a Home Office research study investigating self-reported offending and its correlates among 14–25 year olds in England and Wales.
- The Cambridge Study in Delinquent Development is a prospective survey of 411 males from the London area from age 8, starting in 1961 (Farrington, 1995).
- The Pittsburgh Youth Study is a longitudinal study starting in 1987, of 1517 inner city boys in the USA, in which an antisocial cohort is compared with a random sample. See http://www.wpic.pitt.edu/research/famhist/pys.htm.

It is of note that a typical offender (late teens, male, low socio-economic group) is also a typical victim.

Farrington *et al.* (2006) reported that in the Cambridge study:

- 41% were convicted of an offence (motoring convictions excluded) by age 50, and the average criminal career lasted from 19 to 28, consisting of five convictions.
- Those who began offending at a younger age gained more convictions and offended for longer.

Table 14.4 shows risk factors for offending or associated with offending.

Table 14.4 Factors associated with a general risk of offending

Risk factors for offending	Other factors associated with offending
Male gender	Large family size
Late adolescent age	Poor parental supervision
Number of previous convictions	Childhood physical abuse and neglect
Social class*	Parental conflict/loss/disturbance
Low intelligence or poor educational attainment†	Single marital status
Parental criminality	Excessive alcohol use
Impulsivity‡	Unemployment
*Evidence is mixed, depending on offence type. Antisocial crime (e.g. car theft) is more associated with lower social class †Associated with reduced empathy, difficulty in considering consequences, low self-esteem ‡Reported by teachers, parents or by self-report	

Criminal careers and typologies of offender

Longitudinal studies and recorded crime surveys consistently show a steep rise in rate of offending, peaking at mid-adolescence, falling rapidly to the mid-20s and then continuing to decline at a slower pace. This pattern is consistent across countries, across time and in different groups (men and women, for example) (Smith, 2007):

- This transient adolescent peak is due to more people engaging in criminal activity, rather than to the same people engaging in more criminal activity.

Moffit (1993) distinguishes between:

- Adolescent-limited antisocial behaviour:
  - Common and may be seen as normative and adjustive. Subjects usually have reasonable interpersonal relationships, and have developed empathy.
  - Tend to start offending later but may start with quite serious antisocial behaviour.
- Life-course persistent antisocial behaviour:
  - Antisocial behaviour starts earlier, with minor aggression, lying, hurting animals at a very young age.
  - More likely to have neurological problems and poor peer relationships, and go on to develop adult personality disorder and persistent offending.

A third group of offenders only starts offending in adulthood:

- Adult-onset offenders tend to be more neurotic and emotionally unstable than non-offenders. They are more like non-offenders at age 21, but more like adolescent-onset offenders at age 32 (Zara and Farrington, 2010).

Loeber *et al.* (1998) distinguished three developmental pathways to delinquency:

- Authority conflict:
  - Stubbornness at a young age develops into defiance (refusal and disobedience) and then into avoidance of authority (truanting, running away).
  - This pathway starts earliest, from preschool, but older boys may enter it at a late stage with staying out at night and truancy.
- Covert:
  - Lying leads on to shoplifting, property damage and then more serious property crime such as burglary.
- Overt:
  - Minor aggression and bullying develops into fighting and then violent offending.

Recently, criminal career research has increasingly focused on how protective factors interact with risk factors in determining criminality. See Piquero *et al.* (2003) for a detailed review.

References

Braithwaite J. (1979) *Crime, Shame and Reintegration*. Cambridge: Cambridge University Press.

Farrington DP. (1995) The development of offending and antisocial behaviour from childhood: key findings from the Cambridge Study in Delinquent Development. *Journal of Child Psychology and Psychiatry*, **36**, 929–64

Farrington DP, Coid JW, Harnett LM, Jolliffe D, Soteriou N, Turner RE, West DJ. (2006) *Criminal Careers up to age 50 and Life Success up to Age 48: New findings from the Cambridge study in delinquent development*. Home Office Research Study No. 299. London: Home Office

*Garland D. (2001) *The Culture of Control*. Oxford: Oxford University Press

Graham J, Bowling B. (1995). *Young People and Crime*. Home Office Research Study No. 145. London: Home Office.

Hopkins-Burke R. (2005) *An Introduction to Criminological Theory*, 2nd edn. Cullompton: Willan

Loeber R, Farrington DP, Stouthamer-Loeber M, Moffit T, Caspi A. (1998) The development of male offending: key findings from the first decade of the Pittsburgh Youth Study. *Studies in Crime and Crime Prevention* **7**,141–72

*Maguire M, Morgan R, Reiner R. (2007) *The Oxford Handbook of Criminology*, 4th edn. Oxford: Oxford University Press.

*Moffit TE (1993) Adolescence-limited and life-course-persistent antisocial behaviour: a developmental taxonomy. *Psychological Review* **100**(4), 674–701

Newburn T. (2007) *Criminology*. Cullompton: Willan Publishing

Piquero AR, Farrington DP, Blumstein A. (2003) The criminal career paradigm. *Crime and Justice* **30**, 359–506

Reiner. R (2006) Beyond risk: a lament for social democratic criminology. In: Newburn T, Rock P (eds), *The Politics of Crime Control: Essays in honour of David Downes*. Oxford: Oxford University Press

Smith DJ. (2007) Crime and the life course. In: Maguire M, Morgan R, Reiner R (eds), *The Oxford Handbook of Criminology*, 4th edn. Oxford: Oxford University Press

Young J. (1997) Left realist criminology: radical in its analysis, realist in its policy. In: Maguire M, Morgan R, Reiner R (eds), *The Oxford Handbook of Criminology*, 2nd edn. Oxford: Oxford University Press

Zara G, Farrington DP. (2010) A longitudinal analysis of early risk factors for adult-onset offending: what predicts a delayed criminal career? *Criminal Behaviour and Mental Health* **20**, 257–73

15

The Criminal Law and Sentencing

● What is the Law?

The law differs from everyday social rules and conventions because:

- it is created by institutions empowered to do so by society, that is Parliament or the courts
- there is an associated power of enforcement.

England and Wales follows the 'Common Law' legal tradition:

- There is no complete written statement of the law, which constantly evolves, usually on the basis of decisions made in the courts.
- By contrast, most European countries have the so-called 'civil' legal tradition in which there is to some extent an authoritative written statement of the law.

Sources of law

Acts of Parliament

- The primary source of law.
- Cannot be directly overturned by a UK court:
  - though could be challenged in certain circumstances, such as if Parliament is accused of itself acting illegally or if there is a conflict with European or human rights law.
- Described by subject and date, e.g. the Offences Against the Person Act 1861:
  - usually divided into numbered parts, sections and subsections, appendices called schedules
  - for example, the Mental Health Act 1983 (MHA) has 10 parts, 149 sections and 6 schedules.

Statutory instruments (SI)

- Published by Government ministers and their departments under powers delegated by Parliament.
- Provide detailed rules for applying an Act of Parliament.
- For example, the rules governing the authorization of approved mental health professionals (AMHPs) under the MHA are set out in an SI.
- Quicker and easier to publish and amend than Acts of Parliament.

Informal rules

- Created by Government departments to provide guidance for application of the law.
- They do not require formal drafting or publication and are not binding, but they should not be deviated from without very good justification.
- The MHA Code of Practice (CoP) is an example.

Courts in England and Wales

A court may deal with civil or criminal matters, and may be a trial court or an appellate court.

- Civil courts deal with law concerning the various relationships between individuals and corporations, and impose financial penalties and/or order some other remedy.
- Criminal courts deal with crimes defined by law, enforced by statutory agencies, prosecuted by the state and leading to punishment of offenders.
- Trial courts hear cases 'at first instance' and make rulings on matters of fact and law.
- Appellate courts consider the application of legal principles to a case that has already been heard at a lower court.

Judges preside over courts, and interpret the law in order to apply it to each case, taking into account:

- statute law, as laid down by Parliament and
- case law – previous interpretations by the courts in similar cases. The principle of legal precedent is that a court must follow an applicable ruling made by a higher court.

Box 15.1 Working with the law

It is not enough just to know the statute. You also need to know the relevant case law, SIs or rules. Take the Mental Health Act 1983:

- The statute has been amended many times, particularly by the Mental Health Act 2007.
- The Reference Guide to the Mental Health Act explains the main provisions of the MHA and associated and secondary legislation (Department of Health, 2008a).
- The Code of Practice (Department of Health, 2008b) provides detailed guidance on aspects of practice.
- The associated case law is summarized in the *Mental Health Act Manual* (Jones, 2010), running to over 1000 pages.

The text of all UK Acts of Parliament and Statutory Instruments, in both their original form and with any subsequent amendments, is available at http://www.legislation.gov.uk.

Judgments of the Court of Appeal are available from http://www.bailii.org. Judgments of the House of Lords and the Supreme Court are available from http://www.hmcourts-service.gov.uk/cms/judgments.htm. There are various web-based searchable databases of case law that require subscription. These are helpful if you have an institutional subscription.

● The Criminal Court Structure

Criminal courts are adversarial, such that the prosecution and the defence put forward opposing arguments and the jury is required to choose one over the other. This differs from the inquisitorial approach taken in criminal courts in some other jurisdictions, and in some English courts (for example, coroners' courts, or first tier tribunals). The inquisitorial approach seeks to investigate from a neutral position and determine the truth. Some might argue that in an adversarial system the jury is asked to decide between two arguments, neither of which is quite true.

The required standard of proof for the prosecution in criminal courts is beyond reasonable doubt. There are some matters where the burden of proof falls on the defence (for example, diminished responsibility, or when the defence raises the insanity defence), in which case the required standard is generally on the balance of probabilities.

Magistrates' court

The court sits as a 'bench' of three magistrates or sometimes one district judge sitting alone:

- Solely a trial court of first instance with no appellate function.
- Mostly a criminal court:
  - all criminal cases are first heard by the magistrates' court
  - some limited responsibility for civil issues (e.g. liquor licensing).
- Deal with summary offences and some either way offences.
- Available sentences include:
  - absolute or conditional discharges
  - community sentences
  - compensation orders of up to £5000 per offence, and fines
  - imprisonment of up to 6 months per offence, maximum 12 months overall.
- Cases may be referred to the Crown court either for trial or for sentencing:
  - defendant may elect to have their case heard in the Crown court.

Magistrates are known as Justices of the Peace:

- Mostly lay people without legal training, who are advised by a legally qualified Justice Clerk.
- A minority are full-time legally qualified magistrates, now known as district judges (previously stipendiaries):
  - In 2010 there were 28 607 magistrates sitting in 330 courts. In 2008, 184 000 trials were heard in magistrates' courts. Figure 15.1 gives an overview of the court structure.

Crown court

Crown courts are the only courts regularly sitting with a judge and jury:

- The judge decides and advises the jury on matters of law.
- The jury is the only arbiter of fact.

A Crown court is mostly a court of first instance, but also deals with appeals from the magistrates' court:

- work from 77 centres across England and Wales:
  - dealt with 97 700 trials in 2009 (Ministry of Justice, 2010).

Court of Appeal, criminal division

The Court of Appeal hears appeals from Crown courts against conviction or against sentence. It sits as a minimum of two, usually three and occasionally a 'full court' of five senior judges.

The Court may overturn convictions or alter sentences. If the Court of Appeal does not allow the appeal (i.e. agrees with the decision of the original court) the person convicted is not generally allowed to bring a further appeal.

The Court of Appeal may also receive references from the Criminal Cases Review Commission (CCRC):

- which is an independent body established in 1997 by the Criminal Appeal Act 1995
- with the purpose of reviewing possible miscarriages of justice, and where appropriate referring a case back to the Court of Appeal.

Anyone may ask the CCRC to review their case although referral back to the Court of Appeal is not guaranteed.

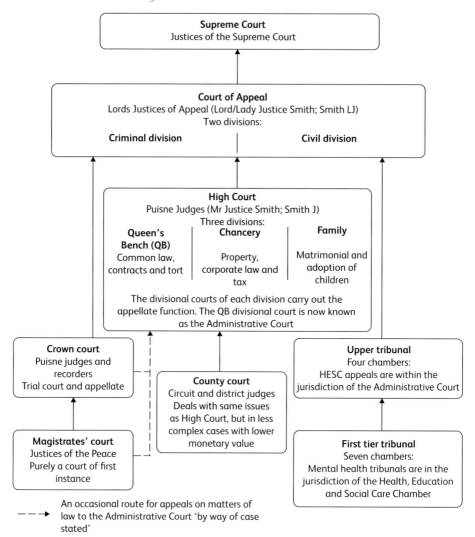

Figure 15.1 The court structure in England and Wales, the arrows representing the major lines of appeal.

The Supreme Court

The Supreme Court was created by the Constitutional Reform Act 2005 to replace the House of Lords as the final appellate court, in order further to separate the judicial and executive powers of the House of Lords:

- began operating in October 2009
- will hear only the most significant or important cases, or cases concerning points of law of general public importance.

For a more detailed account of the English legal system see Holland and Webb (2010).

● Criminal Offences

Classification of crimes

For procedural purposes, crimes may be classified as follows:

- Offences triable summarily only:
    - summary offences are more minor statutory offences, which may be tried by magistrates without a jury.
- Offences triable only on indictment:
    - offences, the seriousness of which necessarily requires a Crown court trial with a jury.
- Offences triable either way:
    - the court has discretion, considering the specific features of the case, to decide which procedure is most appropriate.

Elements of a crime – *actus reus*, *mens rea* and automatism

To be considered guilty of a crime, an individual must do an act and be to some extent responsible for their actions in terms of their state of mind. The act, or *actus reus* (literally 'guilty act'), is one of three types:

- Acts of omission:
    - a failure to engage in an action, with the result that harm is caused
    - e.g. failing to rescue a drowning child from a shallow pool.
- Acts of commission:
    - engaging in an action that directly results in harm being caused
    - e.g. punching someone in the face.
- Acts of possession:
    - although not an action as such, possession of certain items is deemed a criminal act
    - e.g. possession of firearms, illicit drugs or certain pornographic images (e.g. of children).

State of mind or *mens rea* (literally 'guilty mind') does not necessarily imply a direct motive for the crime. There are three forms of *mens rea*:

- Intention:
    - the individual does an act with a knowledge and understanding of the consequences, and a wish that they take place
    - e.g. repeatedly stabbing someone with the intention of killing them.
- Recklessness:
    - taking unjustifiable risks, by acting in the knowledge that there may be a particular consequence but not caring whether it happens or not
    - e.g. setting fire to a bin in close proximity to a row of houses.
- Negligence:
    - not acting in a way in which a reasonable person would have done
    - e.g. failing to feed and care for a child.

Some offences are partly defined by the degree of intent. There are two groups:

- Offences of basic intent:
    - the required *mens rea* is simply an intention to bring about the *actus reus*, with no need to establish any foreknowledge or intention of the eventual outcome
    - e.g. to be convicted of possession of a prohibited item (such as illicit drugs or a firearm) it is only necessary to show that the individual possessed the item and knew that they did so.

- Offences of specific intent (Allen, 2007, p73):
  - the *mens rea* must be shown to be an intention to bring about something going beyond the *actus reus*
  - to be convicted of possession of illegal drugs with intent to supply, it is necessary to prove not only that the drugs were possessed (the *actus reus*) but that this was with the intention to go on to supply them to others.

In a small group of offences (known as 'offences of strict liability') there is no need to establish *mens rea* and it is sufficient only to establish the *actus reus*. An example is driving while over the alcohol limit. These offences often relate to acts that jeopardize public safety so the public interest demands that offenders should be liable to punishment even if they were not aware of their wrongdoing or intended any harm.

Situations in which mens rea may be absent

- Intoxication with alcohol or illicit substances:
  - The basic principle that voluntary intoxication is not a defence is well established.
  - So intoxication may only be used as a defence to a crime of specific intent, reducing it to the corresponding crime of basic intent (s18 to s20 wounding, for example).
- Automatism:
  - A complex legal concept, meaning that an individual acts in an entirely involuntary manner and in doing so commits an offence.
  - Classic examples quoted include a van driver losing control of their vehicle when attacked by a swarm of bees (*per* Lord Goddard CJ, *Hill* v *Baxter* [1958] QBD).
  - To have access to a complete defence of automatism (which would result in an acquittal) it is necessary to establish that some external factor (such as the bees) has acted on the individual to cause them to act in that manner. This is a so-called 'non-insane automatism'.
  - If it is established that there was an involuntary action which was the consequence of an internal factor (including physical illness such as epilepsy) then bizarrely (and as a result of a convoluted series of legal decisions) the only defence available would be that of 'not guilty by reason of insanity', giving rise to the term 'insane automatism'.
  - Such an arbitrary division between internal and external has led to all kinds of problems, including a man with hyperglycaemia caused by non-administration of insulin only having recourse to the insanity defence (*R* v *Hennessy* [1989] 2 All ER 9), whereas another man who had become hypoglycaemic through insulin administration (thereby introducing an 'external factor') was allowed access to the complete defence of 'non-insane automatism' (*R* v *Quick* [1973] QB 910 [1973] 3 All ER 347).
  - Although the difficulties have been identified numerous times there has been no effort made to resolve them with legislation. The defence is used rarely and there remain broad variations in the approaches taken by courts.

Violent offences

Violent offences are mostly defined by common law or by the Offences Against the Person Act 1861. They are described in Table 15.1, where section numbers refer to this Act, unless otherwise specified.

Sexual offences

The current framework is mostly defined by a series of Sexual Offences Acts, most recently the Sexual Offences Act 2003. Table 15.2 describes the various types of sexual offence.

There are many other offences, relating to, for example, intercourse with a corpse or animal, exposure and voyeurism, offences relating to children (either under 13 or under 16), incest, prostitution, soliciting, and trafficking, grooming and pornography.

Table 15.1 Violent offences

Offence	Description	Maximum sentence
Murder	Where a person of sound mind unlawfully kills with intent to kill or cause grievous bodily harm ('malice aforethought')	Mandatory life imprisonment
Manslaughter	At common law, this refers to any unlawful homicide which is not murder Voluntary manslaughter is where all elements for murder are present but there is mitigation by way of: – diminished responsibility – loss of control – killing by the survivor of a suicide pact Involuntary manslaughter is an unlawful killing without intent to kill or cause grievous bodily harm; may be by an unlawful act or by gross negligence or breach of duty	Life imprisonment
Infanticide	Where a mother causes the death of her own child, who is less than 1-year-old, and (s1(1) Infanticide Act 1938) 'the balance of her mind was disturbed by reason of her not having fully recovered from the effect of giving birth to the child or by reason of the effect of lactation consequent upon the birth of the child'	Life imprisonment but custodial sentences are unusual
Wounding or causing grievous bodily harm (GBH)	Wounding means breaking the continuity of the skin. GBH implies serious harm rather than minor. Includes broken bones and probably could include psychiatric injury Section 18 wounding requires a specific intent to cause GBH Section 20 wounding is the corresponding offence of basic intent	S18 life imprisonment S20 5 years' imprisonment
Assault occasioning actual bodily harm	Actual bodily harm has its normal English language meaning, but includes psychiatric injury. Psychiatric injury, not being within the ordinary experience of a jury, requires expert evidence to be established	5 years' imprisonment
Common assault	The nomenclature of common assault and battery is confusing, their roots being in the common law An assault involves causing another person to apprehend unlawful personal physical contact or injury	6 months' imprisonment
Battery	Intentional touching of another person without consent or lawful excuse	6 months' imprisonment
Robbery	Taking another's property without consent and with force or the fear of force. The element of violence distinguishes robbery from theft	Life imprisonment

Table 15.2 Sexual offences

Offence	Description	Maximum sentence
Rape	Penetration of vagina, anus or mouth by penis where the victim at the time does not consent, and the perpetrator knows they do not consent or is reckless as to whether they consent An offence of basic intent	Life imprisonment
Assault by penetration	Intentional penetration of vagina or anus with a part of body or anything else, without consent	Life imprisonment
Sexual assault	Intentional sexual touching of another person without consent. Covers a wide range of behaviours and circumstances Accordingly it is triable either way	10 years' imprisonment
Causing sexual activity without consent	Intentionally causing another to act in a sexual way without consent, for example forced masturbation, a woman forcing a man to penetrate her or forcing sexual activity with a third party	Life imprisonment if penetration involved, otherwise 10 years

Damage to property and arson

The offence of destroying or damaging property is defined in section (1) of the Criminal Damage Act 1971, and section (3) specifies that, where the damage is caused by fire, it shall be charged as arson. The maximum penalties are life imprisonment for arson, and 10 years otherwise.

Arson is separated into three offences:

- simple arson
- arson being reckless as to whether life was endangered
- arson with intent to endanger life.

Often reckless arson and arson with intent will both appear on the indictment, enabling a jury to choose between them.

Arson is considered often to be associated with psychiatric issues:

- Psychiatric reports should be obtained before sentencing (*R* v *Calladine The Times*, December 3, 1975).
- At least for reckless arson, immediate imprisonment is warranted except in exceptional circumstances such as 'mental trouble or any recommendation for medical treatment' (*AG Reference no 1 of 1997* [1998] 1 Cr App R (S.) 54).

For further information on the criminal law see a standard textbook such as Ormerod (2008).

● Sentencing

The powers of courts in relation to sentencing are currently mostly provided by the Criminal Justice Act 2003 (CJA 2003). References to sections are to this Act unless otherwise specified. The policy background and aims include:

- reduced judicial discretion and greater political prescription of sentencing, and
- fitting sentences to the offender, rather than the offence:
  - the principle of proportionality was now to be applied to the totality of the offenders offending, rather than the instant offence
  - a prescribed menu of requirements, to be applied to the particular offender.

The purposes of sentencing are specified in s142, but there is no guidance as to how these disparate aims should be weighed up:

- the punishment of offenders
- the reduction of crime, including by deterrence
- reform and rehabilitation of offenders
- protection of the public
- the making of reparation by offenders to those affected by their offences.

Assessment of the seriousness of an offence (s143) is dependent on:

- the degree of culpability, and
- the amount of harm caused, or intended, or that was reasonably foreseeable.

Aggravating factors include:

- each previous conviction
- offences committed on bail
- offences with racial, religious, disability or sexual orientation characteristics.

The Sentencing Council was established following the Coroners and Justice Act 2009 (replacing the Sentencing Guidelines Council) to provide guidance for sentencing courts based on statutory and case law.

- Guidelines are available from http://www.sentencingcouncil.org.uk
- The Council is required to provide ranges of sentence for offences, in effect providing normal minimum sentences as well as maximum.

Statistics on sentencing are published annually and available on the Ministry of Justice (MoJ) website at http://www.justice.gov.uk/publications/sentencingannual.htm.

Pre-sentence reports (PSRs)

The CJA 2003 requires that, unless a sentencing court considers it unnecessary, it must obtain and consider:

- a probation PSR (s156)
- with respect to imposing a discretionary custodial sentence on a defendant who is or appears to be mentally disordered, a medical report by a section 12 approved registered medical practitioner (RMP) (s157).

Probation PSRs should be based on a direct interview and an offender assessment system (OASys) assessment of offending behaviour, risk of harm and risk reduction interventions. The conclusion should:

- evaluate an offender's motivation and ability to change
- state whether or not an offender is suitable for a community sentence
- make a proposal for a sentence designed to protect the public and reduce reoffending, which may include a custodial element
- recommend which requirements might be added to a community order where a non-custodial sentence is proposed
- outline the level of supervision envisaged.

Psychiatric reports for sentencing are discussed in Chapter 21.

Available sentences

Table 15.3 outlines the sentences available.

Maximum sentences are prescribed for most offences, courts otherwise having wide discretion, although they must follow precedent and the authoritative guidelines. The obvious exception is murder, which carries a mandatory life sentence. In recent years minimum sentences have started to appear on the statute book, for certain drugs trafficking offences and firearms offences.

● Community Orders and Suspended Sentences

A community order may be made for up to 3 years and includes one or more requirements, from a list of 12 defined in Chapter 4 of CJA 2003 (Table 15.4).

Mental health treatment requirement

Provided by s207 of the CJA 2003:

Table 15.3 Available sentences

No punishment	Absolute discharge	Conviction is recorded, no further sanction
	Conditional discharge	No punishment, but if a further offence is committed within a defined period (up to 3 years) they may be sentenced for both offences
	Hospital order	Under s37 MHA – see Chapter 2
Financial penalty	An order to pay a fine and/or costs	Usually payable in instalments according to the offender's ability to pay
Community sentences with requirements tailored to offending needs	Community order	Previously known as probation orders, community rehabilitation orders and community punishment orders. See below for further detail
	Suspended sentence	A term of imprisonment of up to 51 weeks, which is suspended contingent upon offender's behaviour and compliance with the requirements that are imposed. The possible requirements are the same as for community orders (see below) There are two specified time periods: • The *Supervision Period* during which the custodial sentence may be triggered by failure to comply with requirements • A longer *Operational Period* of up to 2 years, in which the custodial sentence is triggered by a further offence
Sentences of imprisonment	Determinate sentences	A prisoner is automatically released halfway through a determinate sentence of more than 12 months, or after expiry of the custody term set by the sentencing court for sentences of less than 12 months. They remain on licence and subject to recall to prison until the end of the sentence Extended sentences are determinate sentences
	Indeterminate sentences	Includes mandatory life sentences for murder, discretionary life sentences for other serious offences, and sentences of imprisonment for public protection for dangerous offenders The sentencing court sets a minimum term, after which the offender is eligible for the Parole Board to release them on life licence. See below for further detail

- The 'offender must submit, during a period specified in the order, to treatment by or under the direction of a registered medical practitioner, or a chartered psychologist, or both, with a view to improvement of the offender's mental condition'.
- Mental condition is not defined, but presumably is not necessarily the same as mental disorder in the MHA.

Treatment must be one of three types:

- as a resident patient, but not in high security
- as a non-resident patient, or
- under direction of a specified registered medical practitioner (RMP) or chartered psychologist.

Otherwise the nature of treatment may not be specified in the order.
   The court requires:

- evidence from one s12-approved RMP that 'the mental condition (i) is such as requires and may be susceptible to treatment, and (ii) is not such as to warrant a hospital order or guardianship order'
- that arrangements have been or can be made for the treatment specified
- that the offender has expressed a willingness to comply with such a requirement.

Table 15.4 Community orders and suspended sentences

1. Unpaid work	Between 4 and 300 hours Designed to make amends to the community, and help the offender develop new work-related skills
2. Activity	May include reparation
3. Programme	Participate in an accredited offender behaviour programme (see Chapter 17)
4. Prohibited activity	A ban on taking part in specified activities, either for a period of time or on specified days
5. Curfew	Requiring the offender to remain at a specified place for between 2 and 12 hours in any day. Maximum duration of 6 months. The court must include electronic monitoring unless it is considered inappropriate to do so
6. Exclusion	Prohibiting the offender from entering a defined area for not more than 2 years
7. Residence	Requiring the offender to live at a certain address, which may be approved premises
8. Mental health treatment	See below for details
9. Drug rehabilitation	Where the court, based on evidence from the probation officer, is 'satisfied that the offender is dependent upon or has a propensity to misuse drugs, and that this requires and may be susceptible to treatment' (s209(2)) Resident or non-resident, for at least 6 months Specific power for the court to review the offender's progress and the order itself
10. Alcohol treatment	Where the court is satisfied that they are dependent on alcohol Treatment may be resident, non-resident or under the direction of 'such person having the necessary qualification or experience' (s 212(5))
11. Supervision	Must attend appointments with their probation officer in order to 'promote the offender's rehabilitation' (s213(2))
12. Attendance centre	For offenders under 25 years. Provides structured group-based activities in a designated centre

Mental Health Treatment Requirements are used relatively infrequently. See Clark *et al.* (2002) for discussion of the merits of and problems associated with such sentences.

Breach and revocation of community orders

If an offender fails to comply with the requirements of their order, then the order is breached, and the offender supervisor returns the case to the Crown or magistrates' court depending on where the order was made. The court may:

- amend the order to include more onerous requirements, or
- re-sentence for the original offence, including imprisonment even if the original offence was not punishable by imprisonment.

A court may revoke a community order if it considers this to be in the interests of justice. The court may then re-sentence for the original offence.

● Custodial Sentences

Imprisonable offences carry a maximum sentence length, and occasionally a minimum sentence length:

- Minimum sentences have become more common over the last decade, as parliament has increasingly sought to limit judicial discretion and prescribe sentences.

- It is useful to look at the relevant sentencing guidelines to understand how a sentencer arrives at a sentence length.

Custodial sentences may be determinate or indeterminate:

- All custodial sentences are designed to consist of an initial period of detention in custody, followed by a period of supervision in the community.

Determinate sentences

The majority of sentences are determinate, resulting in 'fixed term prisoners'. Magistrates' courts may give sentences of up to 6 months for a single offence. If a longer sentence is thought to be warranted then the case must be referred to the Crown court for sentencing.

Extended sentences

The current version of the extended sentence is provided by ss227 and 228. It is a determinate custodial sentence with an extended licence period. It may be available where a court has decided that an offender is a dangerous offender (s229) (see below).

The total sentence must not exceed the maximum for the offence, and is made up of:

- the appropriate custodial term (if a normal determinate sentence were made)
- an extension period during which the offender is to be subject to licence in order to protect the public from serious harm resulting from further specified offences:
  - maximum of 5 years for a specified violent offence
  - maximum of 8 years for a specified sexual offence.

The law relating to sentencing dangerous offenders is discussed with reference to psychiatric evidence in Chapter 20.

Release on licence and recall

The CJA 2003 made parole automatic at the halfway point. Previously the Parole Board had discretion to release on licence, or not. The number of 'discretionary conditional release' (DCR) prisoners, i.e. those sentenced to more than 4 years pre-CJA 2003, is steadily reducing.

Section 244 provides that the Secretary of State must release a prisoner as soon as the requisite custodial period has elapsed:

- the period specified by the sentencing court (between 2 and 13 weeks for a single offence) for those serving less than 12 months
- one-half of the sentence for those serving 12 months or more
- one-half of the appropriate custodial term for extended sentence prisoners.

While on licence, a prisoner is liable to revocation of their licence and recall to prison by the Secretary of State (s254).

On recalling an offender to prison, the Secretary of State must consider whether they should be automatically released after 28 days, according to the risk to the public. If they are not automatically released, they must apply to the Parole Board for re-release. Automatic release does not apply to those who have been convicted of a specified offence in the meaning of Schedule 15 (see Chapter 20).

Indeterminate sentences

There are two forms of indeterminate sentence, which are almost identical in operation:

- Life sentence:
  - mandatory for murder
  - available for other very serious offences (discretionary life sentence).
- Imprisonment for public protection:
  - may be available where the court has decided that the offender is a dangerous offender according to the assessment set out in s229 (discussed in relation to psychiatric evidence in Chapter 20).

As with other custodial sentences, an indeterminate sentence consists of:

- a custodial term of imprisonment
  - the sentencing court is required to set a minimum term (or tariff), which is the amount of time the offender must spend in custody before becoming eligible to have their case considered by the Parole Board
- a subsequent period of conditional release on licence, with liability to recall to prison:
  - this is indefinite – so-called life licence
  - imprisonment for public protection (IPP) prisoners may apply to the Parole Board for revocation of life licence annually, starting from 10 years after release from custody.

Determining minimum terms

The procedure is described in s82A Powers of Criminal Courts Act 2000, and schedule 21 of the CJA 2003:

- Section 82A(4) provides discretion for the court not to fix a minimum term for the most serious of all offences – in other words a whole life tariff. Such an order may not be made with respect to an IPP prisoner.

The minimum term should reflect the seriousness of the offence, with the following starting points:

- Whole life for offences of exceptional seriousness:
  - e.g. murder of more than one person or a child, with planning and premeditation, abduction, sexual or sadistic conduct, to advance some cause, or by someone with a previous murder conviction.
- 30 years for offences of high seriousness:
  - e.g. killing a police or prison officer in the course of duty, using firearms or explosive, killing for gain or to obstruct justice, sexual or sadistic conduct, aggravated by racial, religious or sexual orientation issues.
- 15 years otherwise.

Then the court is required to moderate this starting point with reference to aggravating and mitigating factors, examples of which are provided in the statute.

Sentencing dangerous offenders

The powers are provided by chapter 5 (ss224–236) of the CJA 2003. Three sentences are available (but none is necessarily required) where the court decides that the offender is a dangerous offender:

- extended sentence
- imprisonment for public protection
- discretionary life sentence.

The dangerous offender provisions of the CJA 2003 are considered in Chapter 20, and in Clark (2011).

References

Allen MJ. (2007) *Textbook on Criminal Law*, 9th edn. Oxford: Oxford University Press.

Clark T. (2011) Sentencing dangerous offenders following the Criminal Justice and Immigration Act 2008, and the place of psychiatric evidence. *Journal of Forensic Psychiatry and Psychology* **22**(1), 138–55

Clark T, Kenney-Herbert J, Humphreys M. (2002) Community rehabilitation orders with additional requirements of psychiatric treatment. *Advances in Psychiatric Treatment* **8**, 281–90

*Department of Health (2008a) *Reference Guide to the Mental Health Act 1983*. London: The Stationery Office. Available at: http://www.dh.gov.uk/en/Publicationsandstatistics/Publications/PublicationsPolicyAndGuidance/DH_088162

Department of Health (2008b) *Code of Practice: Mental Health Act 1983*. London: The Stationery Office. Available at: http://www.dh.gov.uk/en/Publicationsandstatistics/Publications/PublicationsPolicyAndGuidance/DH_084597

Holland J, Webb J. (2010) *Learning Legal Rules*. Oxford: Oxford University Press

*Jones R. (2010) *Mental Health Act Manual*, 13th edn. London: Sweet & Maxwell

Ministry of Justice (2010) *Judicial and Court Statistics 2009*. Available at http://www.justice.gov.uk/publications/docs/jcs-stats-2009-211010.pdf

*Ormerod D. (2008) *Smith and Hogan Criminal Law*. Oxford: Oxford University Press

16

Psychiatry and the Police

● Pathways into Police Detention

Mentally disordered individuals may enter police detention due to:

- arrest on suspicion of committing a criminal offence
- detention under the MHA – ss18, 135, 136.

Section 135 – warrant to search for and remove patients

The warrant is issued by a magistrate:

- s135(1) – on application by an approved medical health practitioner (AMHP) where it appears that a person with mental disorder, within the jurisdiction of the magistrate:
  - has been or is being ill-treated, neglected or kept otherwise than under proper control, or
  - being unable to care for himself is living alone
- s135(2) – with respect to a patient who is AWOL from detention in hospital, on application by anyone who is authorized to re-take the patient.

The warrant authorizes a police officer to enter the premises specified in the warrant and remove the person to a place of safety:

- Under subsection 1, the police officer must be accompanied by an AMHP and a registered medical practitioner (RMP). This is not required under subsection 2.

The maximum duration of detention is 72 hours, in order to make an application for detention under Part 2 of the Mental Health Act (MHA) or 'other arrangements for his treatment or care'.

The MHA 2007 introduced a power to transfer the detainee from one place of safety to another. Place of safety is defined in s135(6) as:

... residential accommodation provided by a local social services authority, ... a hospital, an independent hospital or care home for mentally disordered persons or any other suitable place the occupier of which is willing temporarily to receive the patient ...

- The CoP (Department of Health, 2008) and the Royal College of Psychiatrists (2008) state that this is a matter for local agreement between the relevant agencies but a police station should be used 'only on an exceptional basis'.

Section 136 – mentally disordered persons found in public places

This provides a power to a police constable to remove mentally disordered persons found in public places to a place of safety. No warrant is required:

- A subjective test of presence of mental disorder – 'appears to the constable to be suffering from mental disorder and in immediate need of care or control'
- Detention must be necessary 'in the interests of that person or for the protection of others'
- A public place has been held to include the communal area of a block of flats (*Carter* v *MPC* [1975] 1 WLR 507).

The maximum duration of detention is 72 hours, but the detention is 'for the purpose of enabling him to be examined by an RMP and AMHP':

- So there is no ongoing power to detain once this has taken place.

There are no statutory forms for recording s135 or s136, so statistics on use are not readily available. However, estimated figures for England and Wales in 2005–6 are:

- 11517 people in police detention (Docking *et al.*, 2008), with evidence of considerable regional variation
- 5900 people in hospital as a place of safety (Department of Health, 2007).

● Police Detention and PACE

Figure 16.1 shows the process of police detention and charging.

Police and Criminal Evidence Act 1984

PACE provides and regulates the majority (though not all) of police powers in relation to the investigation of crime. There are eight codes of practice (Home Office, 2005):

- Code A: stop and search powers
- Code B: searching of premises, to seize and retain property
- Code C: detention, treatment and questioning of suspects not related to terrorism:
  - this is the most important for psychiatric practice
- Code D: methods used by police to identify people in investigations, and related documentation procedures
- Code E: audio recording of interviews
- Code F: visual recording guidelines
- Code G: powers of arrest amended by Serious and Organised Crime and Police Act 2005
- Code H: detention, treatment and questioning of terrorism suspects.

Code C applies to persons in a police station, whether or not they have been arrested, and including those detained under s135 or s136 of the MHA:

- does not apply to prisoners transferred from prison, or detained under immigration laws or terrorism laws.

The custody officer

This is a statutory position, at the centre of PACE procedures, in terms of both procedure and safeguards. A custody officer:

- is independent of the investigation

- is at least the rank of sergeant
- has undergone specific training
- is responsible for ensuring that all detainees are held and dealt with in accordance with PACE.

The custody officer is responsible for a series of statutory functions, including:

- deciding whether to detain following arrest
- the welfare of detained persons, including mental and physical health problems, language difficulties:
  - clinical attention must be accessed as soon as practicable for any person who appears to need it or who asks for it
- calling an appropriate adult when required to do so
- conducting a risk assessment relating to risks to the detained person or to staff:
  - guidance on the required risk assessment is provided in Code C para 3.6–3.10 and Home Office circular 32/2000
- informing the detained person of their rights, and the grounds for their detention
- compiling and maintaining a custody record
- calling and liaising with health-care professionals and liaising with solicitors

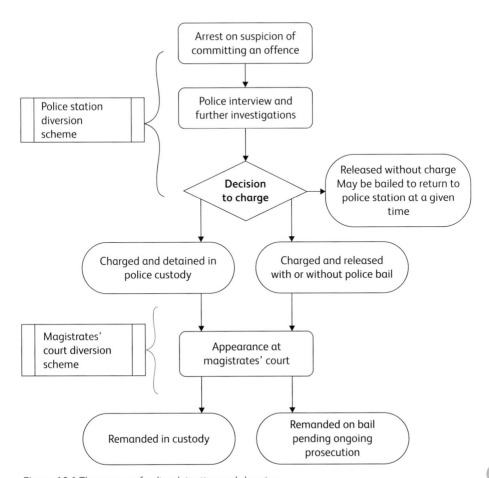

Figure 16.1 The process of police detention and charging

- deciding whether there is sufficient evidence to charge and whether they should be detained or released, with or without bail, in the meantime:
  - the Police and Justice Act 2006 transferred the authority to decide whether or not to change from the police to the CPS
- deciding whether to detain or release on bail following a charge, pending appearance at magistrates' court.

The custody officer can also request regular breaks, short interview sessions and other safe-guards that will assist in ensuring that the interview process is fair and appropriate.

Important rights of an individual detained in police custody

- Right to have someone of their choice informed of their arrest.
- Right to have free, private legal advice from a solicitor.
- Right to examine the custody record, which can be requested for up to 12 months after period of detention, and the code of practice.
- Right to an appropriate adult where appropriate.
- At least 8 hours of uninterrupted rest in any 24-hour period, not disturbed by interviews or travel. This time starts from arrest, not arrival at the police station.

Table 16.1 describes the PACE detention time limits. At the end of a period of detention the detained person must be:

- released without charge
- charged and released with or without bail, or
- charged and remanded in police custody pending a magistrates' court hearing.

Remand in custody may be justified by a risk of:

- absconding
- committing further offences while on bail
- interfering with the course of justice.

Table 16.1 PACE detention time limits

PACE clock starts	On the arrival of an arrested person at the police station, or When an individual at the police station voluntarily is arrested	Periodic reviews are conducted by an officer of rank of inspector (or above) who is not involved in the investigation. The frequency increases as the detention period becomes longer
At 24 hours	Continued detention must be authorized by an officer of rank of superintendent or above who is responsible for the police station. They must believe that: - continued detention without charge is necessary to obtain evidence (including by questioning) - the offence must be an indictable offence - the investigation is being carried out 'diligently and expeditiously' (s42(1))	
At 36 hours	This is the maximum duration of detention that can be authorized by the police Further detention requires a magistrates' warrant, up to a maximum total duration of detention, without charge for normal criminal offences (as opposed to terrorist offences), of 96 hours	

The appropriate adult

The appropriate adult without provision was introduced by PACE to provide protection for vulnerable people at a police station, whether there as a suspect or a witness. Such a person is required when dealing with anyone who is:

- mentally disordered (Code C uses the original four-part MHA classification of mental disorder)

- mentally vulnerable (has difficulty in understanding the significance of questions or their replies, for whatever reason, including problems with physical health or mental health, drugs or alcohol)
- under the age of 17.

There is a low threshold for calling an appropriate adult:

- when the 'custody officer has any doubt about the mental state or capacity of a detainee' (Code C Note 1G).

The appropriate adult may be:

- the guardian, relative or other person responsible for the person's care
- someone who has experience of dealing with mentally disordered or vulnerable people (often a mental health social worker), who is not employed by the police
- some other responsible person aged 18 or over, who is not employed by the police
- but not anyone involved in the offence or investigation:
  - this includes anyone who has received admissions from the detained person prior to attending as the appropriate adult. Sometimes this precludes a social worker from a patient's community mental health team, for example.

There is no statutory duty on local authorities (or any other body) to provide appropriate adults. There is no comprehensive description of the role of the appropriate adult, but rights include:

- private consultation
- to have information about the grounds for detention and to see the custody record
- to request legal advice
- reading of rights and interviewing must be done in the presence of the appropriate adult, and the suspect should be charged and cautioned again in their presence
- at interview the police officers must explain that the role of the appropriate adult is:
  - to advise the person being questioned
  - to observe that the interview is conducted properly and fairly
  - to assist in communication (for example, explaining words or procedures).

Investigations of practice have tended to report that appropriate adults are not called upon as often as they should be:

- A review of custody records (n = 20 805) reported that an appropriate adult should have been called in 2.3 % of cases, but was actually called in only 0.2 % (Bean and Nimitz, 1995).
- Gudjonsson *et al.* (1993) suggested that an appropriate adult was called in 4 % of cases but was justified in 15–20 %.

● The Psychiatrist in the Police Station

Practising psychiatry in a police station can be intimidating, because of the unfamiliar, restrictive and authoritarian environment. You should:

- have a sound knowledge of relevant legal rights and procedures, including PACE, MHA and the Mental Capacity Act (MCA)
- understand the roles and authority of the other individuals whom you will be working with
- be clear about the proper boundaries of your role as a psychiatrist and understand on which issues your decision is authoritative and on which you are only giving advice
- ensure that you have effective clinical supervision and know where to go for advice or discussion.

Issues that you should expect to consider include:

- fitness for detention
- fitness for interview
- risk assessment:
  - risk of self-harm or suicide, or risk of harm to others – this should be documented in the custody record, and communicated to the custody officer
- any medical advice to be given to the detained person
- any medical advice to be given to custody staff
- any requirements for periodic rousing or changes to standard observation procedures
- whether there is a need for an appropriate adult
- information about required medication
- the appropriate setting for any further psychiatric treatment that is warranted, including MHA assessment and appropriate placement.

You should not be asked about fitness to be charged. Being charged is a passive process which requires no capacity on the part of the individual being charged. A police interview is not a prerequisite to being charged.

Where you have existing knowledge of the patient, either your own knowledge or knowledge from medical notes, you need to consider how much information should be passed on to the police officers responsible for their detention:

- You should always take your medical notes away with you. If you leave them in the police station they will become part of the custody record and will no longer be confidential.

Confidentiality is dealt with generally in Chapter 4, and in relation to multi-agency public protection panels (MAPPPs) in Chapter 17.

Fitness to be detained

There is no definition of fitness to be detained. An individual is unfit when they require immediate medical investigation or treatment in hospital, and the consequences of not receiving this are serious. Examples include medical emergencies such as disturbance of level of consciousness, severe head injury, and acute metabolic or endocrine states.

It would be unusual for a psychiatric disorder to render an individual unfit for detention.

Fitness to be interviewed

This is determined by the custody officer. Health-care professionals may offer advice, and the custody officer should consider this.

Annex G of PACE Code C states:

A detainee may be at risk in an interview if it is considered that
- *Conducting the interview could significantly harm the detainee's physical or mental state*
- *Anything the detainee says in the interview about their involvement or suspected involvement in the offence about which they are being interviewed might be considered unreliable in subsequent court proceedings because of their physical or mental state*

In assessing whether the detainee should be interviewed, the following must be considered:
- *How the detainee's physical or mental state might affect their ability to*
  - *understand the nature and purpose of the interview*

      – *comprehend what is being asked*
      – *appreciate the significance of the answers that they give*
      – *make rational decisions about whether they want to say anything*
- *the extent to which the detainee's replies may be affected by their physical or mental condition rather than representing a rational and accurate explanation of their involvement in the offence*
- *how the nature of the interview, which could include particularly probing questions, might affect the individual*

Fitness to be interviewed is a dimensional and dynamic characteristic:

- Some individuals are clearly not fit, others may be considered fit so long as certain precautions or safeguards are employed.
- Some individuals are predictably unlikely to regain fitness (dementia, for example), while others (e.g. intoxication) are unfit now but will regain fitness in due course.

Suggestibility and false confessions

Gudjonsson (2003) proposes a typology of false confessions:

- Voluntary:
  - The individual actively presents themselves and confesses, due to delusions (for example, of guilt in depression), or more commonly associated with personality disorder as a way of seeking attention.
- Pressured–compliant:
  - The individual is pressurized to confess by the interview situation or associated stressors.
- Pressured–internalized:
  - A high level of suggestibility leads the confessor temporarily to believe that they are guilty. Usually occurs in association with learning disability.

The distinction between pressured–compliant and pressured–internalized may not be clear cut.

The Gudjonsson suggestibility scale (Gudjonsson, 1997) is sometimes recommended for use in assessment. However, some (Beail, 2002) consider that the scale may not be valid for this purpose because it concentrates on semantic memory rather than episodic memory (which is more important in interview situations).

The consequences of failing to follow proper procedure at interview

PACE includes safeguards in relation to the admission of evidence at trial:

- Section 76 requires a court to exclude any evidence of confession if the prosecution cannot prove that it was not obtained by oppression or in consequence of anything said or done that was likely to render it unreliable.
- With regard to 'mentally handicapped persons' s77 provides that, where a confession was made in the absence of an independent person, but is nevertheless admitted as evidence, and the prosecution case depends wholly or substantially on it, the judge must warn the jury to view the evidence with caution.
- More generally, s78 provides that the court may exclude any prosecution evidence if its admission would have an adverse effect on the fairness of proceedings.

The absence of an appropriate adult when one should have been present does not necessarily lead to evidence being inadmissible. The Court of Appeal has tended to decide cases

Box 16.1 Assessing fitness to be interviewed (adapted from Ventress *et al.*, 2008)

This is a functional test of capacity, not dependent on any particular mental disorder or diagnosis. Factors such as tiredness, emotional arousal or distress, physical pain or intoxication may constitute mental vulnerability and delay interviewing.

Before seeing the patient:

- obtain information from the forensic medical examiner (FME) and custody officer about their presentation in the police station, particularly level of intoxication, agitation, confusion, bizarre behaviour, loss of consciousness or head injury
- obtain information from the GP or mental health team about background history and pre-existing physical or psychiatric conditions
- consider potential risk of harm towards you or others during the assessment, and take appropriate measures.

On seeing the patient:

- obtain consent for the assessment, unless the person does not have capacity (in which case it is necessary to be satisfied that proceeding is in their best interests)
- attempt to take a full psychiatric history, concentrating on identifying evidence of mental disorder, learning disability, personality disorder, drug and alcohol use
- undertake a full mental state examination, including assessment of cognitive functioning as appropriate.

Consider the capacity of the individual to understand:

- why they are in the police station, and why they are to be interviewed
- the police caution and their rights
- the questions that are likely to be asked at interview, and their significance
- the significance of their answers, and the potential consequences

Consider whether the person's mental state could influence their ability to tell the truth, or to give an accurate account of events. For example:

- delusional beliefs or altered mood could lead to an exaggeration of actions
- auditory hallucinations, thought disorder or confusion could lead to the person being unable to follow conversations or to misunderstand questions
- a confession might be unreliable – look particularly for a high degree of suggestibility with a relatively low IQ and emotional distress.

Consider whether the interview process itself might lead to a significant deterioration in their condition.

Form a judgement based upon the assessment as to the impact of any symptoms of a mental (or physical) disorder upon the police interview, and the risks that this could pose (to individual's health, or to reliability of evidence given). Communicate your decision to the custody officer, and document in custody record.

Consider other recommendations:

- If the individual is currently deemed unfit for interview, would a reassessment be helpful and, if so, when?
- Do further safeguards need to be considered for the interview, such as more frequent breaks, simple language being used, or a mental health professional being present in the interview to monitor the person's mental health?
- Do further assessments need to be carried out, such as a psychological assessment, or by a specialist in old age or learning disability?

according to whether the interview evidence was actually unreliable or not, rather than whether the appropriate safeguards were used.

Appellate judgments in relation to fitness to be interviewed similarly tend to turn on the particular characteristics of the case. It would be very difficult to draw principles of clinical relevance from the judgments.

Box 16.2 Assessing suggestibility and reliability of confessions

This is usually assessed after the event, where a defence team is querying whether an interview should have gone ahead, and whether there should have been safeguards in place, and whether any confession or other statements are reliable.

Consider Box 16.1 in terms of making a retrospective assessment. In addition, you need to formulate the interviewee's suggestibility, considering:

- historical evidence of a tendency to lie, exaggerate, seek attention in other maladaptive ways – you will need a collateral history for this
- personality style, especially inadequate or histrionic types
- intelligence and strategies for coping with stress – consider a formal IQ assessment
- social skills and competence.

You will also need to assess the interview directly, by listening to tapes or viewing video. Reading the transcripts is unlikely to be adequate. Particularly look for evidence of stress expressed in an idiosyncratic way, which might not have been obvious to the interviewing police officers.

● Diversion from Police Custody

In 1990, Home Office Circular 66/90 reiterated government policy that for mentally disordered persons, 'alternatives to prosecution … should be considered before deciding that prosecution is necessary'. The policy of diversion was reinforced by the Reed Report (Department of Health and Home Office, 1992), and most recently was supported by the Bradley Report (Department of Health, 2009).

'Diversion' may imply that psychiatric treatment and criminal prosecution are mutually exclusive. In fact the relationship between the two is more complex and dynamic than that:

- where the alleged offence is trivial and the individual is floridly psychotic, then prosecution is likely to be set aside in favour of treatment
- conversely, where the offence is very serious and the individual has minor or non-acute mental health needs, psychiatric treatment is likely to give way to prosecution.

For many cases the correct path lies in between these extremes and both offending and mental health needs are properly dealt with in parallel (Figure 16.2). The key to initial management is ensuring that:

- where offending or risk require the person to remain within the criminal justice system, their mental health needs are nevertheless addressed appropriately
- where it is appropriate for him to be diverted into hospital care, his risk and offending are nevertheless addressed.

Advantages of diverting offenders out of the criminal justice system (CJS) include:

- vulnerable individuals who have committed minor crimes due to their disorder do not receive a criminal conviction
- more time is spent by police processing more serious crime
- the individual is given help and support to reduce further reoffending, rather than punishment.

Disadvantages include:

- people with a diagnosis of mental disorder may evade prosecution for serious offences
- such individuals may cause disruption if admitted to local mental health services (this was found not to be the case by James *et al.*, 2002)
- individuals who have a history of offending but who are not charged or convicted may be more difficult to manage in future, leading to further offending.

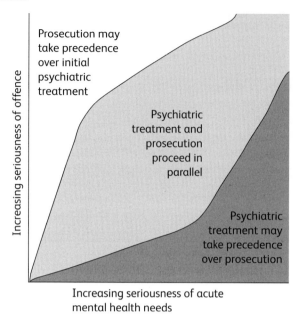

Increasing seriousness of offence

Prosecution may take precedence over initial psychiatric treatment

Psychiatric treatment and prosecution proceed in parallel

Psychiatric treatment may take precedence over prosecution

Increasing seriousness of acute mental health needs

Figure 16.2 The relationship between severity and immediacy of mental health needs, and the seriousness of the offence/risk

Diversion schemes

Diversion schemes are most often based in police stations or magistrates' courts, but may also operate in bail hostels. They recognize:

- the value of using offending and arrest as an opportunity for therapeutic intervention
- the potential vulnerability of mentally disordered individuals within the CJS.

They are often nurse-led projects, either linked with forensic mental health services, or special teams for mentally disordered offenders within local mental health services. The most successful schemes ensure good communication between mental health services (local and forensic) and the CJS, as well as availability of beds (Birmingham, 2001).

The development of diversion schemes has had no central strategic drive, so there is considerable geographical variation in provision. One of the key recommendations of the Bradley Report (Department of Health, 2009) was that all custody suites (and all courts) should have access to liaison and diversion services.

● The Police in Psychiatric Hospitals

Police liaison

Interagency working between mental health professionals and the police is important to:

- maintain safety within the hospital setting, and to address serious violence committed within the hospital
- improve public and staff confidence
- identify intelligence related to absconding or potential offences (e.g. drug offences)
- provide assistance when assessing or admitting outpatients to hospital
- provide assistance if a patient absconds from hospital.

Box 16.3 Managing mental health needs in a police station

A 32-year-old man has been arrested on suspicion of section 18 wounding. He stabbed a neighbour as he came out of the lift in their block of flats in an apparently unprovoked assault. He was arrested outside the block of flats with blood on his hand and clothes; he made an admission seeming to establish his involvement in the offence. The victim is in hospital but the seriousness of his injuries is not clear at present. The detainee has little criminal history and no previous violent offences. At the time of his arrest he was resistive, and the police officers describe him as appearing to be intoxicated. Since he has been in custody he has refused to speak to police officers, but has been noted to be agitated and muttering to himself in the cell. He looks preoccupied and sometimes frightened. The custody officer has decided that he is not fit to be interviewed and is seeking further advice on his management and mental health needs. You establish that he is not known to the local psychiatric services but he does not engage with your attempts to assess him directly. Objectively his presentation suggests that he is psychotic.

The offence is certainly very serious, although the circumstances and consequences are not yet established. The final charge may be section 20 wounding to murder. Certainly this is not a case where a prosecution should be set aside in favour of psychiatric treatment.

He also has serious and acute mental health needs, apparently being acutely psychotic. But note the following:

- While at face value it may seem likely that the offence was partly determined by his psychosis, this is not established.
- The role of intoxication in his presentation is not established; it may be that he will improve significantly with clearance of stimulant drugs.
- The offence establishes that he poses a high risk of violence to others, but there is no way to formulate this risk any further.

Given the offence, his risk and his mental health needs, it would not be appropriate for him to be released. He must be detained in custody or in hospital.

In considering admission to hospital:

- Weigh up the uncertainties mentioned above very carefully. You must be sure that his risk is manageable within a hospital setting.
- He would need to be detained under the Mental Health Act to allow effective risk management and assessment/treatment. Police bail to the hospital would not be sufficient, as this is only a requirement on the detainee to remain; no authority is conferred on the hospital or clinicians to hold him.
- Given the seriousness of the offence a medium secure bed may be required. Availability may be a problem.

If you are considering recommending that he remain in custody, and then be remanded in custody from the magistrates' court, then you must:

- consider what may be done while he remains in the police cell overnight; consider required observations, whether any medication is warranted and risk of self-harm
- liaise with the relevant court diversion scheme and the local prison to which he is likely to be remanded
- consider making an immediate referral to the relevant forensic service in order to secure as early an assessment of his need for transfer to hospital as possible.

You must constantly consider confidentiality issues and ensure that sharing of information is appropriate (see Chapter 4). Many services identify a specific liaison officer. This may enable development of a better working relationship, with better mutual understanding of roles and concerns.

- Remember that police officers have limited training in mental health issues. Their view of a situation is likely to reflect this, rather than a lack of will to assist.

Prosecuting inpatient violence

- The 'zero tolerance' policy regarding violence towards staff in the NHS (Department of Health, 1999) initially excluded mental health units.
- The NHS Security Management Service, introduced in 2003, is responsible for the protection of NHS people, property and assets.
- In 2004–5, there were over 40 000 reports of physical assaults on members of staff in mental health and learning disability settings. This was higher than other services and led to new guidelines for these services (NHS Security Management Service, 2005).

The decision to prosecute inpatient violence may be finely judged:

- The previous implied presumption against prosecution in mental health settings is wrong, many patients remaining capacitous despite their mental disorder (Behr *et al.*, 2005).

Anecdotally, many services continue to report difficulties working with the police and/or the CPS in relation to prosecuting inpatients:

- Senior police officers tend to express concerns that (Brown, 2006):
  - psychiatric patients will provide poor quality evidence
  - a prosecution is not in the public interest – the patient is already in hospital so available sanctions may be limited
  - the amount of training received by officers is inadequate.
- The CPS may request statements from responsible clinicians (RCs) about the accused's:
  - mental disorder, treatment and detention in hospital
  - other relevant information about the patient's behaviour
  - state of mind at the time of committing the alleged offence, including whether they knew what they were doing and whether it was wrong
  - fitness to plead.
- RCs should:
  - be aware that issues of fitness to plead and potential defences of not guilty by reason of insanity (NGBROI) are properly decided at court rather than at this stage
  - refer to the Code for Crown Prosecutors (see Chapter 17) in discussions with the CPS
  - emphasize that Part 3 MHA disposals may well be in the public interest, even if, for example, there is a verdict of NGBROI.

Bayney and Ikkos (2003) have provided a useful discussion of the associated issues.

Police involvement in security and drugs

Drug use is prevalent in many forensic mental health units (Durand et al., 2005). If police are to be engaged in supporting attempts to deal with this, it may be important to educate them about the particular environment of a hospital and the profound effects of cannabis on those with severe mental illness. Otherwise they may not see modest amounts of cannabis as sufficiently important.

Police contact with patients who are AWOL

Section 18 MHA provides that a detained patient who is AWOL may be taken into custody and returned by an AMHP, any member of hospital staff, a police officer or anyone with the written authorization of the hospital managers:

- A conditionally discharged patient who has been recalled to hospital is treated in the same way as one who is AWOL.

Box 16.4 Considerations in police involvement for inpatient violence

Advantages of police involvement in inpatient violence:
- may assist future risk management, ensuring that offences are recorded
- improves morale of staff, who will feel protected and valued
- may reduce adverse impact upon victim
- may improve patients' confidence in their own safety
- reduces any perception that violence is part of the job of a mental health professional
- establishes that the actions of the perpetrator have consequences.

Disadvantages of police involvement in inpatient violence:
- may adversely affect therapeutic relationship with perpetrator
- may feel punitive to perpetrator or other patients
- a low threshold for calling police may result in a reluctance to attend for more serious incidents
- prosecution may lead to adverse publicity for the hospital
- if case is not concluded, there may be dissatisfaction from victim, leading to a deterioration in the relationship between the police and mental health professionals.

If you decide to involve the police then think about the case in terms of the evidential and public interest tests described in the Code for Prosecutors (see Chapter 17), so you can have an informed discussion with the police.

The Code of Practice (CoP; para 22.12) states that the police should be involved 'only if necessary', and preferably 'only to assist' a mental health professional.

The police should be informed immediately if a missing person is (CoP para 2.14):
- considered to pose a risk to themselves or to others
- considered vulnerable in any other way
- subject to restrictions under Part 3 of the Act.

References

*Bayney R, Ikkos G. (2003). Managing criminal acts on the psychiatric ward: understanding the police view. *Advances in Psychiatric Treatment*, **9**, 359–67

Beail N. (2002) Interrogative suggestibility, memory and intellectual disability. *Journal of Applied Research in Intellectual Disabilities* **15**, 129–37

Bean P, Nimitz T. (1995) *Out of Depth Out of Sight*. Loughborough: University of Loughborough

Behr GM, Ruddock JP, Benn P, Crawford J. (2005). Zero tolerance of violence by users of mental health services: the need for an ethical framework. *British Journal of Psychiatry* **187**, 7–8.

Birmingham L. (2001) Diversion from custody. *Advances in Psychiatric Treatment* **7**, 198–207.

*Brown A. (2006). Prosecuting psychiatric inpatients – where is the thin blue line? *Medicine Science and the Law* **46**(1), 7–12.

Department of Health. (1999) *NHS Zero Tolerance Zone: We don't have to take this. Resource Pack*. London: The Stationery Office

Department of Health. (2007) *Inpatients formally detained in hospitals under the Mental Health Act 1983 and other legislation, NHS Trusts, Care Trusts, Primary Care Trusts, and Independent Hospitals, England; 1995–96 to 2005–6*. London: Office for National Statistics

Department of Health. (2008) *Code of Practice, Mental Health Act 1983*. London: The Stationery Office

Department of Health. (2009) *The Bradley Report: Lord Bradley's review of people with mental health problems or learning disabilities in the Criminal Justice System.*

Department of Health and Home Office. (1992) *Review of Health and Social Services for Mentally Disordered Offenders and Others Requiring Similar Services (The Reed Report).* Cm 2088. London: HMSO.

Docking M, Grace K, Bucke T. (2008) *Police Custody as a 'Place of Safety': Examining the Use of Section 136 of the Mental Health Act 1983.* Independent Police Complaints Commission. Available at: http://www.ipcc.gov.uk/section_136.pdf

Durand M, Lelliot P, Coyle N. (2005) *The Availability of Treatment for Addictions in Medium Secure Psychiatric Inpatient Services.* London: Department of Health

Gudjonsson GH. (1997) *Gudjonsson Suggestibility Scales.* Hove: Psychology Press

*Gudjonsson GH. (2003) *The Psychology of Interrogations and Confessions: A handbook.* Chichester: Wiley-Blackwell

Gudjonsson GH, Clare ICH, Rutter S, Pearse J. (1993) *Persons at Risk during Interviews in Police Custody: The identification of vulnerabilities.* Royal Commission on Criminal Justice. London: HMSO

Home Office. (2005) *Police and Criminal Evidence Act 1984 (s.60(1) (a), s.60A(1) and s.66(1)) Codes of Practice A–G.* London: The Stationery Office

James D, Farnham F, Moorey H, Lloyd H, Hill K, Blizard R, Barnes TRE. (2002) *Outcome of Psychiatric Admission through the Courts.* Home Office Research Development Statistics Occasional Paper No. 79. London: Home Office

NHS Security Management Service. (2005) *Protecting your NHS: Promoting safer and therapeutic services.* London: The Stationery Office

Royal College of Psychiatrists. (2008) *CR149 Standards on the use of section 136 of the Mental Health Act 1983.* Available at: http://www.rcpsych.ac.uk/publications/collegereports/cr/cr149.aspx

*Ventress MA, Rix KJ, Kent JH. (2008) Keeping Pace. Fitness to be interviewed by the police. *Advances in Psychiatric Treatment* **14**, 369–81

17
Psychiatry and the Criminal Justice System

The core criminal justice system (CJS) agencies are:

- the police (see Chapter 16)
- the Crown Prosecution Service (CPS)
- the National Offender Management Service (NOMS), encompassing:
  - National Probation Service
  - HM Prison Service (see Chapters 18 and 19)
- Youth Justice Board (YJB) and Youth Offending Teams (YOTs) (see Chapter 12):
  - the YJB is to be abolished in 2011, its functions being subsumed into the Ministry of Justice (MoJ).

Forty-two regional Criminal Justice Boards coordinate activity and share responsibility between the CJS agencies. The Parole Board is an independent body that works collaboratively with criminal justice partner agencies.

● The Crown Prosecution Service

A Government department (headed by the Director of Public Prosecutions, reporting to the Attorney General), this is the principal prosecuting authority in England and Wales, which:

- advises the police on possible prosecutions
- determines whether or not to charge
- prepares and presents cases at court.

The CPS was created by the Prosecution of Offences Act 1985 in order to separate the processes of investigation and prosecution of crime, in the interests of independence and transparency, and to reduce confirmation bias in police investigation.

The code for Crown prosecutors

Available at http://www.cps.gov.uk. A case should be prosecuted if it passes both stages of the Full Code Test:

- The Evidential Stage:
  - The evidence is such that a conviction is more likely than not.
- The Public Interest Stage:
  - A case that passes the evidential stage should normally be prosecuted unless public interest factors against prosecution outweigh those in favour (Table 17.1).

Table 17.1 Some factors to be weighed up in the public interest stage

A prosecution is more likely to be required if	A conviction is likely to result in a significant sentence
	The offence was premeditated or violent, involved a weapon or threat of violence or was committed against a person serving the public (e.g. a police officer/health-care professional)
	The offence was carried out: in breach of court order, by a group, committed in the presence of a child, motivated by any form of discrimination or committed in order to facilitate more serious offending
	The suspect took advantage of: the victim's vulnerability, a marked difference in ages of suspect and victim, a marked difference in levels of understanding of suspect and victim or a position of authority or trust
	The victim was corrupted or the suspect was a ringleader
	Previous convictions are relevant to the present offence
	A prosecution would positively impact on community confidence. There is a risk the offence will be repeated
A prosecution is less likely to be required if	The court is likely to impose a nominal penalty, or the seriousness and consequences can be appropriately dealt with by an out-of-court disposal
	The suspect played a minor role, has put right the loss or harm, or has been subject to regulatory proceedings or a civil penalty
	The loss or harm is minor or the offence was committed as a result of a genuine mistake or misunderstanding
	There has been a long delay between the offence and trial (with various caveats). A prosecution is likely to have an adverse effect on the victim's physical or mental health
	The suspect is or was suffering from significant mental or physical ill health at the material time
	A prosecution may require details to be made public that could harm the sources of information, international relations or national security

Prosecutors:

- will take into account views expressed by victims, but must form an overall view of the public interest
- select charges that:
  - reflect the seriousness of the offence
  - give the court adequate powers to sentence.

● The Parole Board

Parole, as introduced by the Criminal Justice Act (CJA) 1967, was intended to promote rehabilitation, while maintaining the deterrent of recall to custody for transgressions. Now, protecting the public and managing risk may be the preferred focus, reflecting contemporary socio-political preoccupations.

The Parole Board is an independent, executive, non-departmental public body, which was sponsored by HM Prison Service from 1996, by the Home Office from 2003 and by the Ministry of Justice since 2007:

- A recent consultation document (Ministry of Justice, 2009a) notes that the Board's role has changed from an advisory body to a more 'court-like' decision-making body, and suggests options for future organization and sponsorship.

In addition to a chair, chief executive and members of the secretariat, in March 2010 there were 73 judicial members, 30 psychiatrists, 10 psychologists, 10 probation members and 90 independent members.

Some important case law principles:

- *Thynne* v *UK* (1991) EHRR 666:
  - Discretionary life sentence prisoners were entitled to be considered for release at an oral hearing by an independent court-like body.
- *Stafford* v *UK* (2002) 25 EHRR 32:
  - Post-tariff mandatory lifers were only entitled to be detained if necessary for public protection.
  - Justification for their continued detention had to be considered at an oral hearing, at regular intervals, by a court-like body with the power to direct release.
- *R* v *Parole Board* [2005] UKHL 1:
  - A determinate sentence prisoner on licence is entitled to an oral hearing to consider his recall where there are significant disputes of fact.

The CJA 2003 made parole automatic for prisoners serving standard determinate sentences of >12 months whose offence was committed on or after 4 April 2005. Therefore the Board now considers whether or not to release:

- indeterminate sentence prisoners who are post-tariff or who have been recalled to prison
- discretionary conditional release (DCR) prisoners (pre-CJA 2003, see Chapter 15) or extended sentence prisoners who have completed their minimum term of imprisonment
- recalled determinate sentence prisoners.

The statutory test for the release of indeterminate sentence prisoners is that:

- The Board is satisfied that it is no longer necessary for the protection of the public that the prisoner should be confined.
- If a prisoner is not to be released:
  - 'risk must mean dangerousness … it must mean there is a risk of Mr. Benson repeating the sort of offence for which the life sentence was originally imposed; in other words risk to life and limb' (*R* v *Secretary of State for the Home Department ex parte Benson (no.2)*, *The Times*, 21 November 1988)
  - To justify post-tariff detention, the risk should be 'substantial … not merely perceptible or minimal … unacceptable in the judgment of the Parole Board' (*R* v *Parole Board ex parte Bradley* [1991] 1 WLR 134).

The test for release differs for determinate sentence prisoners.

Parole Board hearings

The Board sits as a one-, two- or three-member panel, reviewing suitability for release in paper hearings and oral hearings. Paper hearings are used:

- to consider cases in which a DCR prisoner is applying for parole:
  - these are becoming less frequent now that parole is automatic
- to serve as the initial hearing where a prisoner has been recalled from release on licence.

Oral hearings normally take place in prisons, considering suitability for release from indeterminate sentences:

- Chaired by a sitting or retired judge for life sentence prisoners, and often by an experienced independent member for imprisonment for public protection (IPP) prisoners.
- Specialist members are included in those cases where psychiatric or psychological factors are important.

Box 17.1 The oral hearing

Before the hearing, the panel will familiarize itself with a dossier containing reports from the offender manager, offender supervisor, prison staff and any specialist reports.

A public protection advocate may submit (written or oral) evidence on behalf of the Secretary of State, and seeks to represent the views of the victim. Since 2007, victims/victims' families have been able to attend (part of) the hearing.

The prisoner's representative will be invited to make an application, and panel members adopt an inquisitorial role to test the evidence of witnesses. Hearings are as informal as possible; the order of questioning and witnesses varies. Witnesses almost always include:

- the offender manager
- any other professionals involved in the risk assessment and management of the prisoner.

The decision

A majority decision is sufficient. The panel chair drafts the written reasons for the decision, for agreement by co-panelists.

Decisions are issued within 14 days of the hearing. A decision to release is binding on the Secretary of State; a recommendation to transfer to open conditions is not binding.

Data from 2009–10 (Parole Board, 2010) shows that:

- 24 204 cases were considered:
  - 2974 oral hearings
  - 2202 determinate sentence paper panels
  - 13 423 recall cases.
- The rate of release has declined:
  - 18% of DCR cases were granted parole (24% in 2008–9)
  - 11% of life sentence prisoners were released (15%)
  - 5% of IPP cases were released (8%).
- The rate of recall to custody has remained constant:
  - 50 determinate sentence prisoners were recalled, a rate of 4%, the same as in 2008–9
  - 90 out of 1797 life sentence prisoners under active supervision in the community were recalled (a rate of 5%, compared with 5.4% in 2008–9).

Psychiatric reports for Parole Board hearings

The task of a psychiatrist instructed to provide a report for a Parole Board hearing is to provide an assessment of risk, and the risk of serious harm in particular. Treating psychiatrists, such as those who provide regular clinical sessions to the prison, should consider carefully whether to provide parole reports:

- Information gathered while treating the patient is subject to medical confidentiality.
- As a patient, the prisoner will have provided medical information without expecting it to be shared.
- If they believe a treating psychiatrist will share information with the body that will decide whether to release them, a prisoner may be less likely to engage in a therapeutic relationship and provide information that will allow modification of risk.

It may be preferable for reports to be separately commissioned by the relevant primary care trust or the prisoner's legal representative.

Box 17.2 Writing a report for the Parole Board in relation to an indeterminate sentence prisoner

Before agreeing to provide a report for the Board, psychiatrists must obtain fully informed and valid consent for the disclosure of medical information. The body of the report will be similar to a psychiatric report for courts or tribunals.

Ensure that you have all the information you need. This will include:

- The parole dossier, which contains information about conduct in prison, sentence progression and participation in offending behavior programmes (OBPs).
- Prison medical records and (if applicable) previous psychiatric records.

It is important to give a clear structure and to use headings. Reports will usually include:

- An introduction detailing your sources of information.
- Background information encompassing the usual sections of a psychiatric history.
- An analysis of the index offence, discussing any relevant psychiatric issues.
- Analysis of the offender's response to offending behaviour work.
- A summary of psychiatric treatments received during prison sentence.
- A mental state examination.
- A risk assessment.
- A summary of the recommendations of other report writers, particularly the offender manager and supervisor. Are they recommending release or transfer to open conditions?
- An analysis of the proposed risk management plan – is it viable? Outline additional psychiatric needs; how they should be addressed and by whom.
- Opinions and recommendations.

The risk assessment for a parole report should, in particular, consider:

- How the prisoner's mental disorder relates to their risk.
- Risk factors identified by CJS agencies, and any risk assessment instruments that have been used. Do they have face validity? Are there psychiatric factors that may make them less accurate for this individual than for non-mentally disordered offenders?
- Are there additional psychiatric factors that need to be taken into account?
- State clearly whether the risk is more than minimal to life and limb.

The recommendation section should give a clear statement as to whether you are in a position to support release:

- You can recommend release only where you have determined that the risk is no more than minimal to life and limb.
- Alternatively, would you support a transfer to open conditions? If so, comment on the risk of absconding.
- Provide a rationale for your recommendation, based on both the assessed risks and the viability of proposed risk management plans.

● National Offender Management Service

Created in response to Lord Carter's unpublished 2003 review of correctional services, NOMS is an executive agency of the MoJ that brings together the administrative organization of HM Prison Service and the National Probation Service:

- It aims to deliver 'end-to-end management' of offenders throughout the offender pathway.
- By introducing a new approach to offender management.

The Offender Management Approach (National Offender Management Service, 2005)

Having originally been a welfare-orientated service, by the 2000s the priority of the Probation Service was public protection. A single offender manager (OM) 'manages' an offender throughout their contact with NOMS, whether in custody or the community. Management is more rigid, systematized and programmatic than before:

- The offender management process involves (ASPIRE):
  - Assessment
  - Sentencing planning
  - Implementation
  - Review
  - Evaluation.
- The OM is responsible for the supervision of the offender:
  - directly in the community
  - by delegation to a prison officer or another probation officer in custody.
- The 'four Cs' offer the best chance of achieving reform and rehabilitation:
  - Consistency – of message and behaviour, over time and across staff.
  - Commitment – of staff to offenders. Success is more likely when this is reciprocated.
  - Consolidation – turning new learning into routine and instinctive behaviour through positive reinforcement.
  - Continuity – to improve engagement.
- Four offender management approaches, allocated on basis of risk and need:
  - Tier 1: Punish
  - Tier 2: Punish and help
  - Tier 3: Punish, help and change
  - Tier 4: Punish, help, change and control.

The 'resources follow risk' principle means offenders at Tiers 3 and 4 will be subject to higher levels of supervision and support, often via a multi-agency approach.

A meta-analysis suggested that correctional work is most effective when offenders are involved in their own assessment and are active collaborators in the implementation of their sentence plan (Dowden and Andrews, 2004).

Assessment of risk and OASys

Criminal justice agencies rely on the Offender Assessment System (OASys) and Risk Matrix 2000 (RM2000) risk assessments.

OASys is the principal risk assessment and management system used by NOMS in England and Wales, providing a structured approach to examining the following areas of criminogenic need, with defined thresholds for intervention:

- offending history
- analysis of offence – with an emphasis on risk of serious harm
- accommodation
- education, training and employability
- financial management and income – and how this relates to offending
- lifestyle and associates – examining how peers influence behaviour
- relationships – including history of violence/domestic abuse
- drug misuse – and relationship to offending
- alcohol misuse – and relationship to offending

- emotional wellbeing
- thinking and behaviour – assessing the offender's reasoning ability and consequential thinking skills
- attitudes – towards offending and supervision.

Offenders are assessed at the pre-sentence stage to inform sentence planning, at regular intervals throughout sentences and at the end of interventions as a means of monitoring change.

The outcome commonly used, particularly in relation to a multi-agency public protection panel (MAPPP), is risk of serious harm (ROSH):

- Serious harm means 'an event which is life threatening and/or traumatic, from which recovery, whether physical or psychological, can be expected to be difficult or impossible' (National Offender Management Service, 2009).

The levels of ROSH used by OASys are:

- Low:
  - current evidence does not indicate the likelihood of causing serious harm.
- Medium:
  - there are identifiable indicators of serious harm
  - the offender has the potential to cause serious harm, but is unlikely to do so unless there is a change in circumstances, for example failure to take medication, loss of accommodation, relationship breakdown, drug or alcohol misuse.
- High:
  - there are identifiable indicators of risk of serious harm
  - the potential event could happen at any time and the impact would be serious.
- Very high:
  - there is an imminent risk of serious harm
  - the potential event is more likely than not to happen imminently and the impact would be serious.

OASys also indicates the likely subject of harm: the public, prisoners, a known adult, children, staff and self.

An evaluation of the second pilot of OASys (Howard, 2006) found:

- The most frequent areas of need were:
  - education, training and employability
  - thinking and behavior.
- The risk of serious harm was assessed as:
  - low for 53%
  - medium for 36%
  - high for 11% of offenders.
- 2-year reconviction rates of:
  - 26% for those rated as low likelihood of reconviction
  - 58% for medium likelihood
  - 87% for high likelihood.

Analysis of OASys data has led to the development of actuarial tools, which differentially weight OASys factors to generate percentage risks of reoffending over 1 and 2 years:

- OASys Violence Predictor (OVP)
- OASys General re-offending Predictor (OGP)
- Offender Group Reconviction Scale (OGRS) – based on age, gender, current offence and previous offending.

Proponents describe them as demonstrating good predictive accuracy (Howard, 2009) and they are routinely quoted in pre-sentence reports, though whether they are useful in relation to those with mental disorder is not established. Certainly they do not take into account psychiatric treatment for severe mental illness as a dynamic factor.

RM2000 is an actuarial risk assessment instrument which includes subscales for sexual violence, non-sexual violence, and overall violence. Actuarial risk assessments is discussed further in Chapter 6.

Offending behaviour programmes

Offending behaviour programmes for use in custody and the community should be centred on these principles (Mackenzie, 2006):

- based on an explicit model of the causes of crime
- target criminogenic needs
- responsive
- based on a cognitive–behavioural approach.

OBPs aim to:

- understand the reasons for offending
- facilitate risk assessment
- reduce future offending and help manage risk.

There are 22 OBPs accredited for the prison setting and 18 for the community (Table 17.2), but availability varies between regions and prisons. Attendance at OBPs forms part of an offender's sentence plan, and failure to attend may lead to breach proceedings.

Evaluations of OBPs tend to show inconsistent and modest effect sizes on reoffending. In some cases early reductions are not sustained on longer follow-up:

- Completers do better than non-starters; non-completers do worst of all (Harper and Chitty, 2004).
- Wilson *et al.* (2005) found a mean effect size of 0.32 (a moderate effect) on reoffending rates for various cognitive–behaviourally based OBPs.
- Enhanced Thinking Skills (ETS) led to a reduction in self-reported impulsivity, reduction in prison security reports, and improvements in measures of locus of control, attitudes to offending and cognitive indolence (McDougall *et al.*, 2009).
- Meta-analysis of 16 studies in 4 countries suggested a 14% reduction in recidivism for participants in Reasoning and Rehabilitation compared with controls (Joy Tong and Farrington, 2006).
- The Sainsbury Centre for Mental Health (2008) estimated that, overall, OBPs lead to 10–24% reduction in reoffending.

● Victim Liaison Units

Victim liaison units (VLUs) sit within local probation trusts, and seek to represent the interests of victims of crime in the CJS. Over the last 10 years the rights of victims have gained an increasingly prominent place in sentencing and offender management.

Section 69 of the Criminal Justice and Court Services Act (CJSCA) 2000 placed victim work on a statutory footing for the first time, requiring, in relation to violent or sexual offenders who receive 12 months or more custody, probation boards to:

- Ascertain whether the victim(s) wishes to:
  - make representations about restrictions or requirements on release, or

Table 17.2 Some commonly available offender behaviour programmes

General offending	Thinking Skills Programme (TSP; previously Enhanced Thinking Skills, ETS)	20 sessions over 4–10 weeks, looking at interpersonal problem-solving skills and emotional self-management The most commonly delivered programme in prison
	Think First	22 sessions delivered over up to 3 months, in a community setting
	Reasoning and Rehabilitation	Similar to TSP and delivered in prison for prolific offenders, particularly those with sexual, violent or drugs offences 38 sessions over 9–18 weeks
	Cognitive Skills Booster Programme	A short enhancement for those who have already completed a general offending behaviour programme
Aggression and violence	Controlling Anger and Learning to Manage it (CALM)	24 sessions aiming to help male prisoners monitor and understand their emotions Not suitable for those who use violence instrumentally or those convicted of domestic violence
	Aggression Replacement Training	Social skills, anger management and improved moral reasoning 28 sessions, for medium to high risk of harm offenders
	Cognitive Self-change Programme	For offenders over 24 years with a lifespan history of violence and some motivation to change Examines violence promoting cognitive style and individual risk factors. Five modules delivered in prison, the last after release
Domestic violence	Community Domestic Violence Programme	Community-based programmes for male perpetrators of domestic violence
	Integrated Domestic Violence Programme	Teach non-controlling behaviour strategies and enhanced victim empathy Take around 6 months to complete
	Healthy Relationships Programme	For prisoners with a history of violence in relationships
Sex offending	Sex Offender Treatment Programme (SOTP)	A family of programmes for sex offenders, including an adapted version for those with learning disability, and a pre-release booster programme Available in prison and in the community
	Internet Sex Offender Group Programme	For adult male non-contact Internet offenders. Core modules challenge offending, impulse control and emotional management skills to improve victim empathy
Substance use	Offender Substance Abuse Programme	For men and women who are sufficiently stable, motivated and whose offending is linked to substance use 26 sessions over 12–24 weeks
	Drink-impaired drivers	Men and women whose drinking is stabilized
	Programme for Individual Substance Misusers (PRISM)	An individual programme delivered over 50 hours in 10–20 sessions

- receive any information about such restrictions or requirements.
- Pass such information to or from the victim as appropriate.

The Domestic Violence, Crime & Victims Act (DVCVA) 2004 extended this duty to victims of mentally disordered offenders subject to restrictions.

The Mental Health Act (MHA) 2007 further extended this duty to the victims of patients who receive unrestricted hospital orders.

Restricted patients

The DVCVA 2004 requires the Justice Secretary and/or the First Tier Tribunal to notify probation:

- when a patient applies for a tribunal
- if a patient is to be discharged
- whether the discharge will be conditional or absolute
- of the conditions of the discharge in so far as they relate to contact with the victim
- if restrictions are lifted
- when a section 47/49 patient is remitted to prison.

Mental Health Unit (MHU) practice is to notify the VLU:

- when a patient is transferred to another hospital
- when leave is granted to a patient (on the basis that the victim will not be given details of the leave)
- when a patient previously unfit to plead is remitted for trial
- when a conditionally discharged patient is recalled to hospital.

The MHU may:

- inform the VLU when a patient has absconded if there is a perceived risk to the victim
- seek information from the VLU when considering leave applications.

Unrestricted patients

VLUs should relay the wishes of the victim to the hospital managers who will pass on representations to the responsible clinician (RC). RCs must inform managers if they are considering:

- discharging a patient from detention
- discharging a patient onto a community treatment order (CTO)
- varying the conditions of a CTO (in so far as they relate to contact with the victim)
- discharging a patient from a CTO.

Box 17.3 Disclosing information to victims

Disclosure is intended to reduce the risk of harmful confrontations between patients and victims:

- There is no statutory requirement for clinicians to disclose information directly to victims.
- Aside from the information to which victims are entitled, there is no statutory duty to break patient confidentiality.

Having considered all aspects of the case, clinicians should consider whether to liaise directly with victim liaison officers prior to making decisions about leave, or at other important stages of a patient's rehabilitation:

- It is often helpful for the clinical team to be made aware of the views of the victim at an early stage of a patient's care pathway.

You should always inform and seek consent from the patient when sharing information about their case. Explain that disclosures may reassure victims and improve the prospects of a patient's successful rehabilitation into the community:

- Patient consent is not required for the disclosures specified in statute.
- Valid and fully informed consent is required for more extensive disclosures.

RCs and approved mental health practitioners (AMHPs) should consider any representations made by the victim when deciding on conditions (e.g. exclusion zones) for supervised community treatment (SCT):

- But the purpose of restrictions must be those defined in s17B MHA.

● Multi-agency Public Protection Arrangements (MAPPAs)

The legal framework

Sections 67 and 68 of the CJCSA 2000 placed a statutory duty on police and probation (the responsible authority [RA]) to 'establish arrangements for the purpose of assessing & managing the risks' posed by violent and sexual offenders in their area. HM prison service was incorporated into the RA by the CJA 2003.

A number of agencies have a 'duty to co-operate' with the RA, including social care, housing, education and health. Each of the 42 MAPPA areas has a:

- strategic management board (SMB) responsible for monitoring and developing MAPPA
- MAPPA coordinator with responsibility for oversight of the local arrangements.

The key functions of MAPPA:

- Identification of MAPPA offenders
- Assessing the risks posed by offenders
- Managing the risks posed by offenders
- Sharing information about offenders.

The desired outcome of MAPPA is effective risk management (Kemshall, 2003):

- Zero risk can never be achieved
- Risk management should be based on:
  - a rigorous risk assessment
  - defensible decision-making.

Identification of offenders

There are three formal categories of MAPPA eligible offender:

- Category 1 – registered sex offenders (RSOs)
- Category 2 – violent or other sex offenders:
  - sentenced to 12 months' imprisonment or longer, or
  - sentenced to a hospital order or guardianship under the MHA.
- Category 3 – other offenders, 'who, by reason of offences committed by them ... are considered by the RA to be persons who may cause serious harm to the public':
  - although this category is intentionally broad, most of these offenders are likely to be people who have committed serious sexual or violent offences prior to the introduction of the legislation.

Many police forces have also agreed local protocols relating to a fourth category:

- Potentially dangerous offenders:
  - those without a criminal conviction or caution to place them in any category above, but whose behaviour gives reasonable grounds for believing that there is a present likelihood of them committing an offence that will cause serious harm.

An MDO will remain eligible for MAPPA for a defined period as shown in Table 17.3.

Table 17.3 Multi-agency public protection arrangement eligibility period

Category	Transferred prisoner	s37	s37/41
1	For the period specified at the time of sentence	Required to remain on sex offender register for 7 years	For life
2	Until expiration of licence	Until discharged from hospital or from community treatment order	Until absolute discharge
3	When a level 2 or 3 MAPP meeting decides that the risk of harm has reduced sufficiently and the case no longer requires multi-agency management		
Offenders whose supervision has ended may be included as a category 3 offender			

On 31 March 2009 there were 44 761 MAPPA cases (Ministry of Justice, 2009b)

- 32 336 category 1
- 11 527 category 2
- 898 category 3.

Notification of MAPPA-eligible offenders

The responsibility for identifying MAPPA-eligible offenders falls to each agency with a statutory role in their care or supervision, including health.

Relevant offenders for mental health are MAPPA eligible offenders:

- who are subject to a conditional discharge from a restricted hospital order made under the MHA or equivalent legislation
- who are discharged by the RC under a CTO made under s17 of the MHA
- whose conditional discharge is planned within the next 6 months
- who are required to register with the police and whose discharge is planned within the next 6 months.

Box 17.4 Notification of MAPPA-eligible patients

Clinical teams must maintain an awareness of which of their patients are MAPPA (multi-agency public protection arrangement) eligible, and routinely consider at what point in the care pathway liaison with MAPPA is appropriate.

The 2009 MAPPA Guidance (National Offender Management Service, 2009) recommends that:

- the MAPPA coordinator be notified of offenders already in the community for whom notification had not taken place, and that
- there is a process in place to identify all MAPPA-eligible offenders within 3 days of sentence/admission to hospital (and on every fresh admission or transfer)
- MAPPA form F/G is submitted to the relevant MAPPA coordinator within 10 days of the relevant point, i.e. 6 months prior to the planned release/discharge or with as much notice as possible.

Appendix 4 of the 2009 MAPPA Guidance contains a MAPPA document set, which includes

- Form A: allows any professional involved in the management of a MAPPA-eligible offender to make a referral to a level 2 or 3 meeting.
- Form G: for the Initial Notification of MAPPA mental health patients.

The completed forms should be sent to the relevant MAPPA coordinator. Most mental health trusts will have protocols for the sharing of relevant information with MAPPA.

Risk management

MAPPA-eligible offenders are managed at one of three levels (Table 17.4).

Table 17.4 Levels of MAPPA (multi-agency public protection arrangement) management

Level 1	Ordinary agency management	Risks posed by an offender can be managed by the agency responsible for supervision/care of the offender Offender has been assessed as presenting a low or medium risk of serious harm (ROSH); or, if high risk, a robust risk management plan is in place Represents the highest proportion of offenders Does not preclude the sharing of information between agencies Cases should be reviewed every 4 months In health, level 1 patients will be managed under care programme approach arrangements
Level 2	Active multi-agency management	Offender assessed as posing a significant ROSH – usually high or very high on Offender Assessment Systems Requires active involvement and coordination of interventions from other agencies to manage risk Has previously been managed at level 3 and the seriousness of risk has diminished and/or the complexity of multi-agency management of risk has been brokered and a MAPPA risk management plan has been established Cases will be reviewed every 8–12 weeks
Level 3		The offender is assessed as presenting a high or very high ROSH. Present risks can only be managed by a plan that requires close cooperation at a senior level due to complexity or the need for unusual resource commitments Although not assessed as high risk, there is a high likelihood of media scrutiny and/or public interest Cases will be reviewed every 4–6 weeks

Guidance from the Royal College of Psychiatrists (2004) recommends the following level of clinical representation:

- Strategic management board – consultant psychiatrist
- Level 3 meeting – consultant forensic psychiatrist
- Level 2 meeting – consultant forensic psychiatrist or consultant general psychiatrist with special training in, or experience of, the interface between psychiatry and the CJS.

MAPPP meetings produce a risk management plan, the minutes of which will be produced and distributed within:

- 5 days for level 3 cases
- 10 days for level 2 cases.

Between April 2008 and March 2009 there were 10 924 cases (24% of the total) being managed at multi-agency level (Ministry of Justice, 2009b):

Category of offender	Level 2	Level 3
1	4 408 (10%)	424 (1%)
2	3 891 (9%)	320 (0.7%)
3	1 701 (4%)	180 (0.4%)
Total	10 000 (22%)	924 (2%)

Outcomes for offenders managed at multi-agency level in 2008–9 (Ministry of Justice, 2009b):

	Returned to prison for breach of licence	Returned to prison for breach of SOPO	Charged with serious further offence*
Level 2	1297 (11.87%)	58 (0.53%)	40 (0.37%)
Level 3	117 (1.07%)	10 (0.09%)	8 (0.07%)
*A serious further offence is defined as homicide or attempted homicide, rape or attempted rape, and other serious violent or sexual offences with a maximum penalty of 14 years imprisonment or more Percentages are of the total level 2 and 3 populations SOPO, sex offending prevention order			

Box 17.5 Attending a MAPPP meeting

MAPPP meetings vary considerably in their attitude to mentally disordered offenders, their understanding of psychiatric issues and their acceptance of medical confidentiality.
- In some cases, excellent relationships have developed which allow effective collaboration.
- But sometimes you may be the only health-care professional in a large group of CJS workers, and this can be intimidating.
- The other attendees may form an initial evaluation of the case based on the offending history, not taking into account the role of mental illness and the intervening period of psychiatric treatment and rehabilitation.
- Sometimes this leads to a MAPPP making unreasonable requests, perhaps related to covert observations or restrictions on leave, or information about every leave that is taken.

Before attending, consider:
- What information is appropriate to disclose.
- What you are hoping to achieve from the meeting. This might include gaining further information or might be to reduce risk-related anxiety among CJS agencies.
- What requests might be made by a MAPPP meeting and how you will deal with them.

Discuss the meeting with the patient, in order to:
- gain permission for the disclosure of the appropriate amount of information
- reassure the patient about continued CJS involvement, and explain that it is often helpful to work with CJS agencies.

At the meeting:
- Bear in mind your aims and the parameters that you have set around information sharing.
- Be prepared politely to decline to give undertakings or assurances, pending further discussion at the hospital and a subsequent MAPPP meeting.

Make sure that you keep careful notes of the meeting, including what information was disclosed and what information was gained.

If the patient refuses consent to share information you must consider whether or not disclosure is warranted in the public interest:
- The usual rules and guidance apply to this – see Chapter 4.
- Remember that it is for the doctor to determine whether or not release of medical information is justified in the public interest.
- OASys assessments are indicative only.
- Always ensure that you make comprehensive notes of your deliberations, to record how you weighed up the issues in terms of the professional guidance available.

Information sharing and confidentiality

The MAPPA 2009 Guidance (National Offender Management Service, 2009) requires that the process of information sharing between agencies:

- has lawful authority
- is necessary, proportionate and done in ways that are:
  - accountable
  - ensure the safety and security of the information shared.

The CJA 2003 requires the cooperation of health, which 'may include the exchange of information'. However:

- there are no new powers allowing the release of medical information
- there is no change in the threshold for release of information without consent
- it does not over-ride:
  - the Common Law Duty to protect patient confidentiality
  - the Data Protection Act 1998
  - Article 8 of the European Convention on Human Rights.

References

Dowden C, Andrews DA. (2004) The importance of staff practice in delivering effective correctional treatment: a meta-analysis of core correctional practices. *International Journal of Offender Therapy & Comparative Criminology* **48**, 203–14

Harper G, Chitty C. (2004) *The Impact of Corrections on Re-offending: A review of what works.* Home Office Research Study No. 291. London: Home Office

Howard P. (2006) *Findings 278: The Offender Assessment System: An evaluation of the second pilot.* London: Home Office

Howard P. (2009) *Improving the Prediction of Re-offending using the Offender Assessment System. Research Summary 2/09.* London: Ministry of Justice

Joy Tong LS, Farrington D. (2006) How effective is the 'reasoning and rehabilitation' programme in reducing reoffending? A meta-analysis of evaluations in four countries. *Psychology, Crime and Law* **12**(1), 3–24

Kemshall H. (2003) The community management of high-risk offenders. *Prison Service Journal* **March**

Mackenzie DL. (2006) *What Works in Corrections: Reducing the criminal activities of offenders & delinquents.* Cambridge: Cambridge University Press

McDougall C, Perry AE, Clarbour J, Bowles R, Worthy G. (2009) *Evaluation of HM Prison Service Enhanced Thinking Skills Programme: Report on the outcomes from a randomised controlled trial.* Ministry of Justice Research Series 3/09

Ministry of Justice. (2009a) *The Future of the Parole Board. Consultation Paper 14/09.* Available from: http://www.justice.gov.uk

Ministry of Justice. (2009b) *National Statistics for Multi-agency Public Protection Arrangements Annual Reports 2008–9.* London: Ministry of Justice

National Offender Management Service. (2005) *The NOMS Offender Management Model.* London: Home Office

*National Offender Management Service. (2009) *MAPPA Guidance 2009 Version 3.0.* Available at: http://www.probation.homeoffice.gov.uk

Parole Board. (2010) *Annual Report and Accounts the Parole Board for England and Wales 2009/10.* London: The Stationery Office

*Royal College of Psychiatrists. (2004) *Psychiatrists & Multi-agency Public Protection Arrangements: Guidelines on representation, participation, confidentiality & information exchange.* London: Royal College of Psychiatrists

*Sainsbury Centre for Mental Health. (2008) *A Review of the Use of Offending Behaviour Programmes for People with Mental Health Problems.* London: Sainsbury Centre for Mental Health

Wilson DB, Bouffard LA, Mackenzie DL. (2005) A quantitative review of structured, group-orientated, cognitive behavioral programs for offenders. *Criminal Justice and Behaviour* **32**, 172–204

18

Prisons and Prisoners

● The Size of the Prison Population

In February 2010, the total prison population in England and Wales was 83 925 (data available from monthly bulletins, available at: http://www.hmprisonservice.gov.uk/resource centre/publicationsdocuments/):

- This represented 110% of the uncrowded prison capacity.
- 79 701 (95%) were men; 4224 women.
- 70 116 (84%) were sentenced; 4494 (5%) were convicted but unsentenced; 8271 (10%) were untried.
- 72 596 (86.5%) were adults; 9633 were young adults (18–20 years); 1696 were 15–17 years.
- The prison turnover in the UK is 140 000–150 000 per year.
- At the end of March 2008, 10 911 prisoners were serving indeterminate sentences. Of these 4170 were serving imprisonment for public protection (IPP) or detention for public protection (DPP) and the rest life imprisonment.

The average resource cost in England and Wales is £39 000 per prisoner per year:

- 2.5% of the gross domestic product is spent on the criminal justice system (CJS).

 Rate of imprisonment in December 2008 (Figure 18.1; data from Walmsley, 2009):

- UK – 153/100 000 population
- average for western Europe and Scandinavia – 95/100 000:
  - highest was Spain – 160/100 000
  - lowest was Andorra – 37/100 000
- The United States had the highest prison population rate in the world, 756 per 100 000 of the national population, followed by Russia (629) and Rwanda (604).

Prison population trends

The prison population in the United Kingdom has been increasing for the last several decades (Figure 18.2). The rate of change has increased particularly since the 1990s, reflecting a more punitive political approach to law and order:

- 1997–2007 – the number of prisoners increased by 30%
- 1996–2006 – the number of people found guilty remained constant; more use of custodial sentences
- 1997–2009 – the number of women in prisons increased by 60%.

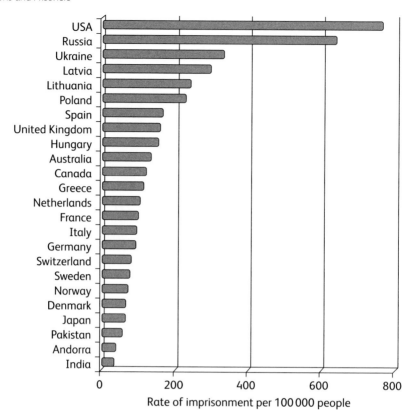

Figure 18.1 Rate of imprisonment of selected countries per 100 000 of the population (data from Walmsley, 2009)

Age

Over half of all prisoners are between the ages of 20 and 34, the sentenced population being somewhat older than the remand one. In February 2010, there were:

- 1696 15–17 year olds in prison (2 % of the total population)
- 9633 young adults (18–20 years) in prison (11 % of the total)
- 7358 prisoners were over 50 years (9 %):
  - of these, 518 were over 70 years.

Ethnicity

Black and minority ethnic (BME) groups are greatly over-represented in prison (Ministry of Justice, 2009):

Ethnic grouping	Prison population (Ministry of Justice, 2009) (%)	General population (2001 census) (%)
BME	26	7.9
Black	15	2
Asian	7	4
Mixed	3	1.2
Chinese/other	2	0.8

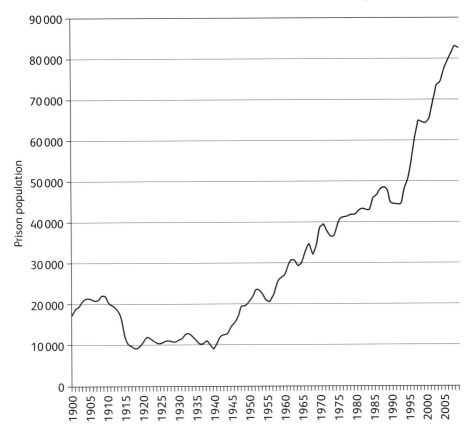

Figure 18.2 Prison population in England and Wales from 1900

- 14 % of the male, 23 % of the female, and 38 % of the BME prison population were foreign nationals.
- Excluding foreign nationals, the rate of imprisonment (based on 2001 general population figures) was:
  - 1.3/1000 for white
  - 3.7/1000 for mixed
  - 6.8/1000 for black
  - 1.8/1000 for Asian
  - 0.5/1000 for Chinese or other.

Stewart (2008) surveyed 1457 newly sentenced prisoners from 49 prisons. The proportion of non-white prisoners serving sentences of more than 1 year was greater than for white prisoners. This difference was not accounted for by offence category.

Prisoners and low IQ

Among young offenders, 23% had an IQ below 70, 36% were between 70 and 79, and 23% were between 80 and 89 (Harrington and Bailey, 2005). Mottram (2007) found an average IQ ranging from 83 to 87 in three prisons. Twenty-five per cent of adult prisoners had an IQ less than 80 and 7% had IQ less than 70.

Socio-economic factors

Of sentenced prisoners (Social Exclusion Unit, 2002):

- approximately 50% of sentenced prisoners ran away from home as a child (five times the normal population)
- 27% were taken into care as a child (compared with 2% general population)
- 48% had a reading ability, and 65% a numeracy ability, below level 1 (the level expected of 11 year olds); the comparable rate for both in the general population was 23%
- 49% males and 33% females had been excluded from school (2% general population)
- 32% were homeless prior to imprisonment.

In a survey of newly sentenced prisoners (Stewart, 2008):

- 40% had been permanently excluded from school
- 13% had never been employed
- 62% had been on benefits in the year prior to custody
- 61% were single
- 46% had no qualifications.

Physical health and deaths in prison custody

Fazel and Baillargeon (2011) note the high rates of infectious diseases among prisoners worldwide, as well as higher than expected rates of hypertension, diabetes, asthma and arthritis in US studies. In contrast to previous assertions, the prevalence of epilepsy seems not to be increased (Fazel *et al.*, 2002).

In 2009, there were 168 deaths in prison:

Self-inflicted	60
Non-self-inflicted	101
Homicide	0
Awaiting classification	5
Other non-natural causes	2

● Psychiatric Morbidity in Prisons

The prevalence of psychiatric morbidity among remand and sentenced prisoners in UK prisons was established in a series of studies in the 1990s. More recently, research has turned its focus on to particular subgroups of the prisoner population. All studies demonstrate much higher rates of mental disorder than in the general population. This research effort has mostly taken the form of cross-sectional prevalence studies. There has been little research into psychiatric processes within prisons, perhaps with the exception of reception screening, and virtually no longitudinal studies. Consequently empirical research has yet to establish the effect of imprisonment on severe mental illness, or whether imprisonment causes psychosis.

The Institute of Psychiatry studies

These two studies of random samples from the male prisoner population gave the prevalence rates shown in Table 18.1.

Office for National Statistics (ONS) survey of psychiatric morbidity among prisoners

A survey commissioned by the Department of Health and the High Security Psychiatric Services Commissioning Board, carried out between September and December 1997 by Singleton *et al.* (1998):

- initial sample size – 3563 prisoners in England and Wales (5.7 % of the total prison population).

The research included interviews in two stages. In stage 1 all randomly selected prisoners were asked to take part in an initial interview covering all topic areas. In stage 2 a random subsample of 1 in 5 of the stage 1 respondents were interviewed clinically for psychotic disorders (using SCAN v 1 and CIS-R) or personality disorders (using SCID-II):

- response rate – 88 % for stage 1; 76 % for stage 2.

This is the most widely quoted study of psychiatric morbidity in prisons, for the following reasons:

- The number of subjects was higher than for other studies.
- It used a comparable methodology to the ONS General Household Survey, enabling direct comparison with the general population.
- It suggests even higher rates of morbidity than other studies.

Table 18.1 Institute of Psychiatry studies of prison psychiatric morbidity

	Brooke *et al.* (1996)	Gunn *et al.* (1991)
	Unconvicted male prisoners randomly selected from 16 adult prisons and 9 YOIs Semi-structured clinical interview making diagnoses according to ICD-9 criteria	Sentenced male prisoners randomly selected from 13 adult prisons and 3 YOIs Semi-structured clinical interview making diagnoses according to ICD-10 criteria
n	1478 adults, 406 young offenders	544 adults, 206 young offenders
Psychosis	4.8 %	1.9 %
Neurosis	25.6 %	5.9 %
Personality disorder	11.2 %	10 %
No psychiatric diagnosis	37.5 %	63 %

An often-quoted headline is that this study showed that fewer than 1 in 10 prisoners had no mental health needs (Tables 18.2–18.4):

- Sleep problems (67 % (male) and 81 % (female) of the remand population) and worry (58 % and 67 %) were the most commonly reported symptoms.

Table 18.2 Point prevalence of neurotic symptoms (i.e. score of 12 or more on CIS-R at lay interview)

	Remand	Sentenced	General population*
Male	58 %	39 %	12 %
Female	75 %	58 %	18 %
*Data from contemporaneous General Household Survey (Jenkins *et al.*, 1997)			

Table 18.3 Prevalence of functional psychosis in the past year

Disorder	Male sentenced	Male remand	Female (remand and sentenced)
Schizophrenia	1%	2%	3%
Other non-organic psychotic disorders	4%	7%	10%
Manic episode	1%	1%	1%
Severe or recurrent depression and psychosis	1%	1%	1%
Any functional psychosis	7%	10%	14%
In the General Household Survey, the prevalence of psychosis was 0.4%			

Table 18.4 Personality disorders (PDs) among prisoners

Disorder	Male sentenced	Male remand	Female
Antisocial PD	49%	63%	31%
Paranoid PD	20%	29%	16%
Borderline PD	23%	23%	20%
Any PD	64%	78%	50%

Brugha *et al.* (2005) compared a random sample (*n* = 3142) of remand and sentenced male and female prisoners, with a random sample (*n* = 10 108) of household residents:

- This methodology sought to avoid sampling and ascertainment biases that might have affected previous studies.
- The weighted prevalence of probable functional psychosis was:
  - 0.45% among the household residents
  - 5.2% among the prisoners.

Psychiatric morbidity in prisons worldwide

A systematic review of 62 surveys across 12 countries (Fazel and Danesh, 2002) covered 22 790 prisoners, with a mean age of 29 years. The prevalence of psychiatric disorder is shown in Table 18.5.

Table 18.5 Prevalence of psychiatric morbidity in prisons worldwide

Disorder	Male	Female
Psychotic illnesses	3.7%	4%
Major depression	10%	12%
Personality disorder	65%	42%
Antisocial PD	47%	21%

Substance misuse in UK prisons

Earlier studies indicated that substance misuse (Table 18.6) in unconvicted male prisoners was 38% (Brook *et al.*, 1996) and in sentenced male prisoners was 23% (Gunn *et al.*, 1991).

Table 18.6 Prevalence of substance misuse in the year prior to prison

	Hazardous drinking		Any evidence of drug dependence	
	Remand	Sentenced	Remand	Sentenced
Male	58%	63%	51%	43%
Female	36%	39%	54%	41%

The ONS survey (Singleton *et al.*, 1998) showed:

- 1 in 4 women and 1 in 10 men who were dependent on drugs reported having methadone replacement treatment in the month before coming into prison.

Liriano and Ramsay (2003) demonstrated differing rates of drug use by age, as shown in Table 18.7:

- Overall, 73 % of respondents had taken an illegal drug in the 12 months prior to imprisonment, nearly half (47 %) having used heroin or cocaine (crack or powder).
- Other studies have found similar figures – 60–70 % (Burrows *et al.*, 2001) and 63 % (Swann and James, 1998).
- The general population use of illicit drugs was 9.3 %.
- The most frequently used drugs were cannabis (65 % overall) and heroin.

Table 18.7 Recorded drug use in the year prior to imprisonment

Drug	17–24 years (n = 747)	25–59 years (n = 1089)
Cannabis	80 %	54 %
Cocaine	37 %	28 %
Crack	33 %	29 %
Ecstasy	43 %	21 %
Heroin	32 %	31 %

A systematic review of 13 studies (n = 7563) published between 1966 and 1994 showed that (Fazel *et al.*, 2006):

- prevalence rates of alcohol abuse/dependence in male prisoners ranged from 17.7 % to 30.0 % (seven studies) and among female prisoners 10.0 to 23.9 % (five studies)
- prevalence rates for drug abuse/dependence in male prisoners ranged from 10.0 to 48.0 % (eight studies) and among female prisoners 30.3 to 60.4 % (six studies)
- limitations include marked heterogeneity in the sample, different prevalence rates depending on the assessors and 88 % of the sample from US prisons.

● Prison Structure and Organization

There are 139 HM Prison Service establishments in England and Wales. Prisons may be:

- closed (where security measures aim to prevent escape), or
- open (where prisoners have more freedom within the prison and may go out of the prison to engage in community-based employment)
- local (primarily housing unsentenced prisoners, or those serving short sentences), or
- training (where there is greater availability of interventions aimed at reducing offending).

All local prisons are closed. Training prisons may be closed or open.

A remand or newly sentenced prisoner will be housed in a local prison. Those who receive longer sentences will in due course be allocated to a training prison. Local prisons have induction procedures for new prisoners, and many have a first night centre, where prisoners are housed initially, before moving to a wing.

High security prisons house prisoners who are category A or B.

Categories of prisoner

Prisons are often described with reference to the security category of prisoner that they predominantly house. There are four security categories for adult male prisoners:

- Category A prisoners are those whose escape would be considered highly dangerous to the public, or a threat to national security.
- Category B prisoners are those for whom escape must be made very difficult.
- Category C applies to prisoners who cannot be trusted in open conditions.
- Category D prisoners can be reasonably trusted in open conditions.

Unconvicted adult prisoners will generally be treated as category B prisoners.

Female prisoners are not categorized in the same way, only category A being distinguished, and defined in the same way as for men. Women's prisons may be:

- closed, for prisoners who are not trusted in an open prison
- semi-open, for those who can be trusted to stay in a semi-open prison, or
- open, for those who can be trusted to stay in an open prison.

Unconvicted adult female prisoners will be held in closed conditions.

Young offenders are categorized as category A, Restricted, Closed or Open.

Prison structural organization

- Gatehouse: checking the ID and maintaining a record (Gate Book) of anyone going in or out of prison. Following this, visitors may have to go through security checks which will vary according to the category of prison.
- Reception: all receptions and discharges go through this area. Responsible for the roll of the prison along with the gatehouse. The reception procedure involves collection of personal details, recording of personal property, allocation of a prison number, review of health needs and mental health screen.
- House block/accommodation: prisoners live in cells or occasionally in dormitories. Cells are usually shared. House blocks are usually divided into separate units or wings.
- Visitors' centre.
- Health-care centre: the level of service varies between prisons – see Chapter 19. Prisoners can see a GP, optician, dentist, psychiatrists or other health professionals according to need.
- Segregation unit: the purpose of the segregation unit is to maintain safety, order, discipline and respect for human dignity. It can also be used for vulnerable individuals to keep them safe from others if a specialist or vulnerable unit is not available.
- Vulnerable prisoners' wing: most prisons have a designated wing where prisoners who are at risk of becoming a victim of violence from others are housed, to separate them from the general prison population. The most common group is those charged with or convicted of sexual crimes, particularly against children. Prisoners choose to be housed here, under Prison Rule 45.
- Education and training centre.
- Chaplaincy.
- Gymnasium.

Close supervision centres

These are effectively segregation units within high security prisons, which hold the most difficult and challenging male prisoners. In comparison to segregation units in other prisons, often prisoners are held here for longer periods.

Grades of prison staff

Uniformed staff include the following:

- Operational support grades (OSG), who are employed in various duties around the prison.
- Instructional officers, who provide vocational training for prisoners.

- Prison officers, whose primary duty is custodial, ensuring the safety and security of the prison. Duties are wide ranging, including locking and unlocking doors, counting prisoners, searching cells, prisoners and visitors, escorting prisoners around the prison.
- Senior officers, who have responsibility for a group of prison officers, or some aspect of prison functioning.

Managerial positions, otherwise known as governors, include:

- Operational managers (Grades G to E), who may, for example, have responsibility for a particular houseblock, or for health care
- Senior managers (Grades D to A). The governor of a prison is often known as the 'Number One Governor'.

Prisons are strictly hierarchical. It is important to remember this when working within a prison.

Some prison officers act as personal officers, having a particular responsibility for the treatment of one or more prisoners. They may contribute to sentence planning, resettlement and otherwise support an individual's rehabilitation. In some prisons these roles are taken on by probation officer offender managers. The interface for offender managers, personal officers and other staff is flexible.

The prison regime

Prisons provide a rigid, routine-based structure, in which all is subordinate to good order and discipline. The regulatory framework for the treatment of prisoners in England and Wales is provided by The Prison Rules 1999, a statutory instrument which is frequently amended. While there are some minimum standards and requirements, these are often couched in flexible terms such as 'so far as reasonably possible'. Therefore there is considerable local variation in the regimes provided in different prisons, authority for this lying within the local hierarchical structure.

Most prisoners are housed in shared cells, and are required to maintain their cell in a clean and tidy state, subject to inspection by prison officers. The property allowed in cells varies among prisons.

All prisoners, including those subject to restricted regime for discipline reasons, should be allowed at least 1 hour of fresh air every day. Association periods allow prisoners on a wing to mix and socialize recreationally.

Unsentenced prisoners are distinguished from sentenced prisoners in a number of ways. They may generally wear their own clothes, they may receive more visits, and they are not required to work or attend education or training, though those who exercise their right not to do so may be ineligible for certain privileges.

Prisoners may buy items from the prison shop, known as the canteen. Money may be sent in by friends or relatives, or earned through working. A set maximum amount may be spent each week, any excess being saved until release.

Incentives and earned privileges

There are three levels of regime: basic, standard and enhanced. Prisoners are allocated to a level depending on their behaviour and conduct. Privileges include:

- the amount of money a prisoner may spend
- frequency of visits
- own clothes
- amount of association.

Discipline and punishment

The range of offences against prison discipline includes:

- fighting or other violence, hostage-taking, escaping or absconding
- obstruction of an officer in the execution of his duty, being disrespectful to an officer
- disobeying an order, rule or regulation
- consumption of alcohol
- possessing, selling or delivering an unauthorized article
- intentionally failing to work properly.

The alleged offence is considered at an adjudication, usually chaired by a Governor. Punishments include removal of privileges, confinement to cell or serving more of the sentence in custody.

See the Prison Discipline Manual, available on the HM Prison Service website, for further information.

Visitors

The number and frequency of visits allowed to a prisoner vary among prisons, according to local facilities. Generally, convicted prisoners should be allowed a minimum of one hour-long domestic visit a fortnight. Unconvicted prisoners are allowed more visits than sentenced prisoners. The prisoner sends a visiting order to prospective visitors, enabling them to visit.

Work, vocational training and education

Provision varies among prisons. In training prisons, prisoners are expected to engage in some form of activity. Common work opportunities include working as a wing cleaner, in the laundry, on the servery at meal times or as a gardener, as well as various types of industrial workshop.

Roll checks

Checks tend to occur before or after meal times, or when prisoners return to wings following activity sessions. Each section of the prison counts its prisoners, feeding their total back to a central point. While a roll check is taking place, and until it is correct, the prison may be on stand fast – limiting movement of prisoners, but also staff and visitors.

Release on temporary licence (ROTL)

Prisoners may be allowed leave from the prison either on compassionate grounds or for resettlement purposes.

Prison therapeutic communities

These prisons, or units within prisons, aim to provide a therapeutic environment based on therapeutic community (TC) principles and psychological treatment. For example:

- HMP Grendon (Buckinghamshire):
  - The most well-established prison TC, with places for up to 235 residents of category B status. Each of six wings operates as an autonomous therapeutic community.
  - Criteria for reception:
    - Prisoners must be serving a sentence that will let them stay at Grendon for at least 24 months.
    - Prisoners cannot be on psychotropic medication.
    - Need to evidence some degree of motivation or reflectivity about their offending.

- HMP Dovegate (Staffordshire):
  - 200-bed TC.
  - Criteria for reception:
    - Sentenced, category B or C.
    - No open assessment, care in custody and teamwork (ACCT) for 6 months.
    - Not category A or E list for 6 months.
    - No psychotropic- or codeine-based medication.
    - No positive mandatory drug test for 6 months, more than 18 months to parole eligibility date (PED).
    - Volunteer for therapy.
    - PCL-R scores to be less than 25.

Dangerous and severe personality disorder services within prisons

There are two prison-based units for male prisoners with dangerous and severe personality disorders, which complement the dangerous and severe personality disorder (DSPD) units at Rampton and Broadmoor high secure hospitals:

- HMP Frankland – 86 places
- HMP Whitemoor – 70 places.

The Primrose Project is a 12-bed pilot DSPD service for women, based at HMP Low Newton. The DSPD programme is discussed further in Chapter 9.

Box 18.1 Booking a visit in prison

Know whether you are booked in to health-care or legal visits. The former is preferable as the medical notes are more likely to be available and there may be health-care staff to act as informants.

If a prison insists on booking you in to legal visits, ensure that you will have a private room available for the interview and ask in advance to see the medical notes. Ensure that you know who booked the visit, when and with whom, in case you are asked at the gate.

Make sure that you are aware of contraband items. The list will vary among prisons:

- Carry the minimum equipment with you and if you need to bring any contraband items with you (a Dictaphone perhaps) ensure that permission is granted in writing and in advance.
- Find out in advance if you can leave your phone or other items at the gate. If not, leave them in your car.

Schedule in the time it may take to pass through the security procedures and waiting for someone to pick you up. It is often helpful to arrive at times of shift changeovers so staff coming into the prison can escort you through.

Have the internal extension at hand as sometimes there are phones in the waiting areas which may be useful if you have been waiting for a long time.

Regulation of prisons

Prison and probation ombudsman

- Investigates:
  - complaints from prisoners, people on probation and immigration detainees held at immigration removal centres
  - deaths of prisoners.
- The ombudsman is appointed by the Secretary of State for Justice and is independent of the Prison Service, the National Probation Service and the Border Agency.

Her Majesty's Inspectorate of Prisons

- An independent inspectorate, which reports on conditions for and treatment of those in prison, young offender institutions and immigration detention facilities.

There are three categories of inspection:

- Full inspections:
  - each establishment holding adults and young adults is inspected once every 5 years, and those holding juveniles once every 3 years
  - an announced inspection, which lasts for at least one week
  - inspection findings are reported back to the establishment's managers and reports are published within 16 weeks of inspection
  - the establishment is expected to produce an action plan, based on the recommendations made within the report, within a short period following publication.
- Full follow-up inspections:
  - unannounced and proportionate to risk
  - assess progress made with particular focus on areas of serious concern identified in the previous full inspection, particularly on safety and respect.
- Short follow-up inspections:
  - unannounced, conducted where the full inspection suggested fewer concerns.

The Inspectorate also carries out thematic inspections, across establishments, focusing on particular groups of prisoner, interventions or services.

All inspection reports, thematic reports and research publications are freely available on the Inspectorate website at: http://www.justice.gov.uk/inspectorates/hmi-prisons.

Independent monitoring board

Every prison and immigration removal centre has its own independent monitoring board (IMB), made up of volunteer lay people, which aims to monitor day-to-day standards of prison functioning in the interests of care and decency.

IMB members have unrestricted access to the prison and to prisoners on scheduled visits and can respond to confidential requests from prisoners.

● Reducing Reoffending in Prisons

Offending behaviour programmes

Offending behaviour programmes (OBPs) are CBT-based interventions, mostly delivered on a group basis, which aim to develop understanding of the reasons for offending and modify thinking styles and behavioural patterns that contribute to offending.

There is a menu of accredited OBPs available in prison and in the community. These are discussed further in Chapter 17.

Drug treatment in prisons

Addiction and problematic drug use is seen as a paramount criminogenic need among the imprisoned population. It is accepted that, if an intervention is effective in treating drug addiction, then it will also have an impact on reoffending rates.

There are a number of treatment approaches provided across the prison estate.

Counselling, assessment, referral, advice and throughcare service (CARATs)

- Established 1999, now well-established across the prison service.
- Provides:
  - initial assessment following referral
  - advice to prisoners with substance misuse problems
  - liaison with health care both in prison and in the community
  - care plan assessments
  - drawing up a care plan for the prisoner
  - one-to-one counselling and groupwork services
  - assessment for intensive treatment programmes in prison
  - throughcare linking with community drug treatment services
  - ensuring, where required, that prisoners are offered post-release support for up to a maximum of 8 weeks.

Prison addressing substance-related offending (P-ASRO)

- CBT-based group work programme.
- Aims to address drug dependence and related offending in prisoner.
- 20 sessions over 5 weeks.
- Four modules:
  - Motivation to Change
  - Personal Scientist, focused on identifying triggers for use and coping strategies
  - Relapse Prevention
  - Lifestyle Change, including developing skills such as problem-solving and negotiation.

Rehabilitation of the addicted prisoners' trust (RAPt)

- Based on the 12-step Minnesota model, lasts 16–20 weeks, and often delivered on a drug-free wing.
- Includes group sessions, community meetings, community activities, peer evaluation, with many of the counsellors being in recovery from addiction themselves.
- The long-term goal is abstinence.
- A phased programme, continuing after release:
  - motivational enhancement therapy
  - primary phase – first 5 steps of the 12-step programme
  - relapse prevention – recognizing high-risk situations and developing skills to cope with them
  - post-custody treatment, on residential or day treatment basis.
- Early evaluations (Martin *et al.*, 2003) showed:
  - 48 % referred completed the programme
  - 95 % of those completing the programme remained abstinent in prison
  - post-release reconviction at 1 year was 25 % (vs 38 % in control group); reconviction at 2 years was 40 % (vs 50 % for the control group).

Integrated Drug Treatment System (IDTS)

- The most recent initiative, rolled-out across 49 prisons so far.
- Aims to integrate the various treatment services available within a prison, including primary care, mental health care and CARATs, and improve continuity of care for users in prison (McSweeney *et al.*, 2008).
- No evaluation available.

● The Effectiveness of Imprisonment: Absconding, Escaping and Reoffending

The aims of imprisonment include retribution, deterrence, incapacitation and rehabilitation. Retribution and deterrence are achieved by the process of imprisonment itself. Incapacitation is achieved by containment, success being measured by the rate of escapes and absconds, an abscond being defined as an escape that does not involve overcoming a physical security measure (mostly from open prisons):

- In 2008–9, there were 362 absconds, 1 escape from prison and 4 escapes from a prison escort. These figures represent a dramatic decrease over recent years (Figure 18.3), probably following the introduction of key performance indicators for prisons in the 1990s.

The socio-political debate about the success of imprisonment as a method of crime reduction tends to centre on reconviction rates, although rehabilitation might be measured in other ways too.

Reconviction rates, at one year post-release, are:

- 47% for all prisoners
- 60% of those released after serving less than 12 months of sentence
- 76% for those having at least 10 previous custodial sentences
- 75% of children group (<18 years).

An estimated one million crimes per year (or 18% of recorded, notifiable crimes) are committed by ex-prisoners at a cost of £11 billion pounds (Social Exclusion Unit, 2002).

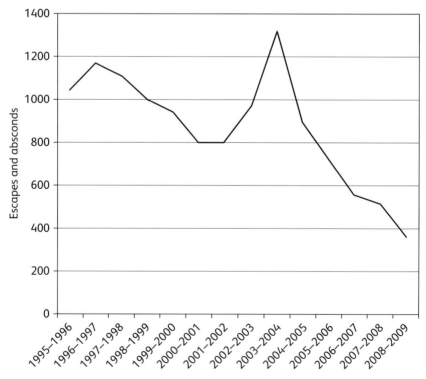

Figure 18.3 Trends in escape and absconding from prison (data from HM Prison Service website)

The strongest predictors of reoffending for men released from prison were (Motiuk, 1998):

- unemployment
- substance misuse
- criminal associates
- single status
- personal or emotional problems.

Multiple logistic regression analysis of data from three surveys of about to be released prisoners, matched with reoffending data from the Police National Computer (May *et al.*, 2009), suggested that the following factors were associated with increased risk of reoffending:

- greater number of previous convictions
- younger age
- drug problems
- shorter sentence
- employment and accommodation problems
- having no visits from a partner or family member
- offence type:
    - theft and handling associated with increased reoffending
    - drug offences (in contrast to having drug problems) were associated with lower risk of reoffending; this replicates previous research (Cunliffe and Shepherd, 2007)
    - fraud and forgery and sex offences were also associated with a relatively lower risk of reoffending.

References

Brook D, Taylor C, Gunn J, Maden A. (1996) Point prevalence of mental disorder in unconvicted male prisoners in England and Wales. *British Medical Journal* **313**, 1524–7

*Brugha T, Singleton N, Meltzer H, Bebbington P, Farrell M, Jenkins R, *et al.* (2005) Psychosis in the community and in prisons: a reports from the British national survey of psychiatric morbidity. *American Journal of Psychiatry* **162**(4), 774–80

Burrows J, Clarke A, Davison T, Tarling R, Webb S. (2001). *Research into the Nature and Effectiveness of Drugs Throughcare*. Occasional Paper 68. London: Home Office

Cunliffe J, Shepherd A. (2007) *Reoffending of Adults: Results from the 2004 cohort*. Home Office Statistical Bulletin 06/07. London: Home Office

Fazel S, Baillargeon J. (2011) The health of prisoners. *The Lancet* **377**, 956–65

Fazel S, Bains P, Doll H. (2006) Substance abuse and dependence in prisoners: a systematic review. *Addiction* **101**, 181–91

*Fazel S, Danesh J. (2002); Serious mental disorder in 23 000 prisoners: a systematic review of 62 surveys. *The Lancet* **359**, 545–50

Fazel S, Vasos E, Danesh J. (2002) Prevalence of epilepsy in prisoners: systematic review. *British Medical Journal* **324**, 1495

Gunn J, Maden A, Swinton M. (1991) Treatment needs of prisoner with psychiatric disorders. *British Medical Journal* **303**, 338–41

Harrington R, Bailey S. (2005) *Mental Health Needs and Effectiveness of Provision for Young Offenders in Custody and in the Community*. Youth Justice Board. Available at: http://www.yjb.gov.uk/publications/Resources/Downloads/MentalHealthNeedsfull.pdf

Jenkins R, Lewis G, Bebbington P, Brugha T, Farrel M, Gill B, Meltzer H. (1997) The National Psychiatric Morbidity Surveys of Great Britain – initial findings from the Household Survey. *Psychological Medicine* **27**, 775–89

Liriano S, Ramsay M. (2003) Prisoners' drug use before prison and links with crime. In: Ramsay M (ed.), *Home Office Research Study 267: Prisoners' drug use and treatment: seven research studies*. London: Home Office

Martin C, Player E, Liriano S. (2003) Results of evaluations of the RAPt drug treatment programme. In: Ramsay M (ed.), *Home Office Research Study 267: Prisoners' drug use and treatment: seven research studies*. London: Home Office

May C, Sharma N, Stewart D. (2009) *Factors Linked to Reoffending: A one-year follow-up of prisoners who took part in the Resettlement Surveys 2001, 2003 and 2004*. Ministry of Justice Research Summary 5. London: Ministry of Justice

McSweeney T, Turnbull PJ, Hough M. (2008) *The Treatment and Supervision of Drug-dependent Offenders: A review of the literature prepared for the UK Drug Policy Commission*. London: UK Drugs Policy Commission

Ministry of Justice. (2009) *Statistics on Race and the Criminal Justice System 2007/08*. London: Ministry of Justice

Motiuk L. (1998) Using dynamic factors to better predict post-release outcome. *Forum on Corrections Research* **10**, 12–13

Mottram PG. (2007) *HMP Liverpool, Styal and Hindley Study Report*. Liverpool: University of Liverpool

*Singleton N, Meltzer H, Gatward R, Coid J, Deasy D. (1998) *Psychiatric Morbidity among Prisoners. Summary report*. London: Office for National Statistics

Social Exclusion Unit. (2002) *Reducing Re-offending by Ex-prisoners*. London: Social Exclusion Unit

Stewart D. (2008) *The Problems and Need of Newly Sentenced Prisoners: Results from a national survey*. Ministry of Justice Research Series 16/08. London: Ministry of Justice

Swann R, James P. (1998) The effect of the prison environment upon inmate drug taking behavior. *Howard Journal* **37**(3), 252–265.

*Walmsley R. (2009) *World Prison Population List*, 8th edn. London: International Centre for Prison Studies

19

Mental Health Care in Prisons

● Health-care Services in Prisons

Until recently health-care services in prisons were run by the Home Office (as it then was) and the NHS had no responsibility for the health care of prisoners. This separation was criticized from the 1960s by the Royal College of Physicians (RCP), the Royal College of Psychiatrists and Her Majesty's Inspectorate of Prisons (HMIP). A momentum for change began to gather in the mid-1990s with a series of critical reports:

- The principle of equivalence was stated in 1997 (Healthcare Advisory Committee for the Prison Service, 1997):
  – Prisons 'should give prisoners access to the same quality and range of healthcare service as the general public receives from the NHS'.
- The National Health Service Reform and Health Care Professions Act 2002 provided for the funding for prison health care to be transferred to the NHS and imposed a duty of partnership between the NHS and the Prison Service.
- Since April 2006, commissioning of health-care services in prisons has been the responsibility of the NHS through primary care trusts (PCTs).

The facilities provided vary greatly among prisons, depending on the size of the prison and its purpose. Local remand prisons, for example, tend to need more comprehensive health-care services, particularly psychiatric, than open prisons. Often there are informal arrangements in place whereby prisoners are transferred from a prison without 24-hour nursing cover to a nearby prison which has this.

According to Brooker *et al.* (2008):

- The expenditure on prison mental health care was £306 per head of prison population per annum (11% of total prison health-care spend).
- Estimated spend in the community is between £42 and £79 per head per annum, depending on what services are included.
- So spending in prison is between 3.9 and 7.3 times greater than in the community.
- The psychiatric morbidity is around 20 times greater in prison.

Categories of health-care centre

- Type 1 prison health-care services: daytime cover, generally by part-time staff (no inpatient facilities).
- Type 2 prison health-care services: daytime/24-hour cover, generally by full-time staff (no inpatient facilities).

- Type 3 prison health-care services: healthcare centre with 24-hour nurse cover, usually with inpatient facilities.
- Type 4 prison health-care services: as type 3 but also serving as a national or regional assessment centre, used by other prisons.

Mental health in-reach teams

In 2001, a strategy document (Department of Health, 2001) perceived that prison mental health care was too focused on the health-care centre and visiting clinicians. In-reach teams, analogous to community mental health teams (CMHTs) in the community, were to be developed, enabling prisoners with mental health problems to remain on ordinary location and receive, as it were, treatment in the community:

- By 2008 there were 350 mental health in-reach workers in post (exceeding the Government's target of 300).
- A deliberate policy of non-prescription, allowing services to develop according to local need, led to a lack of focus and consistency, expanding case loads and complaints of understaffing (Brooker *et al.*, 2008).

Primary care mental health teams

In pursuit of the principle of equivalence, some PCTs have developed primary mental health-care teams within prisons:

- Models of care for prisons are not consistent, but the essence of these teams is that prisoners can access them directly, and the teams concentrate on supporting and treating common mild and neurotic disorders.
- The corollary is that the in-reach teams can concentrate on 'severe and enduring mental illness'.

Models of care that adopt some degree of functionalization need to account for the differences between the prison environment and prisoner population, and the general community. Severe neuroses and personality disorders are particularly common within the prison environment, both because they are more common within the prisoner population, and because the prison environment precipitates crises. Such prisoners may not fulfil the criteria for the in-reach team, but may require more intensive support than the primary care team can provide.

Recommended psychiatric staffing

The Royal College of Psychiatrists (2006) recommends the following complement:

- Category B local remand prison of 500 places:
  - 0.5 whole-time equivalent (wte) consultant (general adult or forensic)
  - 0.5 wte non-consultant grade
  - plus 0.2 wte addiction specialist sessions.
- Category A local remand prison of 500 places:
  - 0.75 wte consultant (general adult or forensic)
  - 0.5 wte non-consultant grade
  - plus 0.2 wte addiction specialist sessions.
- Category B dispersal prison of 500 places:
  - 0.5 wte (forensic or forensic rehabilitation)
  - 0.5 non-consultant grade.
- Category C and D dispersal prison:
  - unlikely to require full psychiatric team so perhaps 0.3 wte per 500 places but with same access to specialist services through a mental health trust.

● Psychiatric Assessments in Prisons

Carrying out a psychiatric assessment in prison follows the same principles as in other settings. Assessment of suicide risk is of particular importance in all cases.

Although there is little empirical evidence about the pathoplastic effect of imprisonment (Hassan *et al.*, 2011), at face value prison is not a good environment in which to treat mental disorder. For some, coming to prison is part and parcel of their lifestyle. For others, reception into custody is profoundly stressful:

- It leads to a sudden and complete interruption of the prisoner's life.
- They are separated from family and support structures in the community.
- They may feel that they have an uncertain future, certainly in the short term, possibly in the long term.
- They may be concerned about the fidelity of their spouse, loss of job, financial instability, loss of house/accommodation/possessions.
- They may find the prison an unfamiliar, hostile, even threatening environment.
- They may experience discrimination or bullying.
- They may have difficulty coming to terms with the crime that they have committed.

So it is unsurprising that imprisonment often precipitates neurotic mental illnesses and also, in those with a predisposition to it, psychosis.

Always be aware of personal safety:

- Consider placement of furniture in the room.
- Note where the alarm button is located and where the nearest staff are.
- Ask prison staff about the patient you are seeing, to gauge level of risk.

Remember that prisoners on remand are often in an acutely stressful situation which will change over time:

- They may have recently come into prison and might be withdrawing from drugs or alcohol.
- They may have a trial or sentencing hearing approaching.
- Consider the relationship of any symptoms to appearances in court, visits from family or other significant events.

Box 19.1 Assessing depression in prison

It is difficult to assess depressive symptoms in prison, leading to a risk of both over- and under-diagnosis:

- Following remand or sentencing, prisoners may experience depressive symptoms, as part of an adjustment disorder.
- Anhedonia – there is often little to find pleasure in within the prison environment.
- Disturbed sleep is usual among prisoners.
- Negative cognitions, such as guilt, may be linked to their offence.
- Limited opportunities for activity often lead to lack of motivation.

It can be helpful to focus on the biological symptoms and objective symptoms of depression.

- It is important to enquire about a past history of depression as being imprisoned may precipitate a recurrence.

Reception screening

- A health screen, using the revised F2169 document, takes place before the prisoner's first night to detect:

- immediate physical health problems
- immediate mental health problems
- significant drug or alcohol problems
- risk of suicide and/or self-harm.

- Each prison should have protocols to address the identified immediate health needs
- Non-urgent general health assessments should be completed in a week.
- The reception screen has 15 questions and takes approximately 5–10 minutes to deliver.
- A positive score on any of the following four specific questions within the screen can identify 82 % (Birmingham *et al.*, 2000) to 86 % (Grubin *et al.*, 2002) of those with serious mental illness:
  - a charge of murder or manslaughter
  - previous treatment by a psychiatrist outside prison
  - previous prescription for antipsychotic or antidepressant medication
  - a history of self-harm outside prison.

Box 19.2 Assessing a newly remanded prisoner charged with murder

The stressors listed above are often seen most acutely in newly remanded prisoners charged with murder because:

- The offence is exceptionally serious, and qualitatively different from other offences.
- The deceased may have been well known to the prisoner, perhaps their spouse or a friend, killed in rage or intoxication. There may be a complex mixture of guilt, shame, remorse and bereavement.
- The killing may have directly affected the dynamics of their support structures.
- They are facing a very long prison sentence, with complete loss of their established lifestyle.

Such prisoners are often very distressed on reception into custody with a characteristic constellation of symptoms:

- Poor sleep, with racing thoughts; usual preoccupations of the deceased and family.
- Re-experiencing symptoms relating to the alleged offence, including intrusive thoughts, memories and recurrent nightmares; flashbacks may occur but are less common.
- Low mood and anxiety, tearfulness.
- Severely impaired concentration.
- Suicidal thoughts.

Typically this syndrome gradually improves over a period of several weeks with supportive treatment. Pharmacological treatment is not usually necessary. In some cases a persistent depressive episode develops, which should be treated accordingly.

Ganser syndrome

A syndrome of:

- approximate answers
- clouding of consciousness
- conversion symptoms
- hallucinations
- abrupt resolution with amnesic gap.

This only warrants mention because it was described, in 1898, as a reaction to imprisonment. The original description was based on a series of three patients. Its nosological status is dubious and it is not described in contemporary classifications of mental disorder.

Usually the term is used to describe a dissociative state, as Ganser intended it. Sometimes it is used to imply malingering. The ICD-10 differential diagnosis of such a patient is likely to encompass:

- malingering
- schizophrenia and other psychoses
- a dissociative disorder, perhaps primary, but more likely to be secondary to depression
- pseudo-dementia.

The diagnosis of Ganser syndrome is best avoided.

Box 19.3 Distinguishing psychosis in prison

Personality disorder and other neuroses are common, and often present with complaints suggestive of psychosis. On the other hand, because of underlying neuroses, psychosis may present atypically. It is especially important:

- to be rigorous in classifying psychopathology, and
- to concentrate on delineating characteristic syndromes, rather than being too focused on a particular symptom.

The most common such combination of symptoms is paranoid sensitive ideas of reference and auditory verbal pseudo-hallucinations. This combination is more likely to be due to a paranoid disposition coupled with the environment of prison, than to psychosis.

It is important to consider observations of others, but note:

- the prisoner may be in their cell most of the day and not observed as they would be in hospital even if they are on health care, so psychosis may go unnoticed
- alternatively, non-psychiatric staff may assume that paranoia and voices are due to psychosis
- the assessment of prison staff may lack objectivity and be coloured by attitudes to particular types of offender or offence.

Be aware of the possibility that prisoners may feign or exaggerate symptoms in order:

- to gain medication, which may be abused or traded within the prison
- to mitigate their offence
- to gain a hospital transfer.

● Psychiatric Treatment in Prison

The principles of psychiatric treatment in prison are no different from elsewhere, but a prison is an inadequate environment for the treatment of severe mental illness and psychosis. Usually prisoners located on health-care wings are in single cells, and they may have less opportunity for exercise, association and activity than other prisoners. Spending long periods of time alone and unoccupied tends to exacerbate psychosis.

Prison health-care centres are not recognized as hospitals for the purposes of the Mental Health Act (MHA) 1983:

- Treatment cannot be provided in prison under the MHA 1983.
- The Mental Capacity Act (MCA) 2005 may be used for the treatment of prisoners who lack capacity, but where the prisoner is suffering from a mental disorder transfer to hospital under the MHA 1983 is preferred.

Before prescribing, ask about local policies and procedures relating to:

- timing of medication rounds
- having medication in possession or under supervision.

Care planning in prisons

The care programme approach (CPA) applies to those in prison in the same way as it does in the community. For existing patients of mental health services CPA responsibility should remain with existing community teams, certainly for those on remand or serving short sentences. Effective care planning is more difficult in a prison environment, particularly in local remand prisons because of:

- rapidly changing population
- diverse and multiple mental health needs
- resistance from mental health teams in the community to maintain contact with patients/accept referrals
- difficulty in planning for release
- more difficult to involve families or carers.

The work of in-reach teams often involves liaison with community teams or hospitals more than face-to-face contact with patients (Brooker *et al.*, 2008).

Transfer of prisoners between prison and hospital

- To hospitals – see Chapter 2.
- From hospitals – see Chapter 3.

Food refusal and other extreme behaviours

Food refusal is a common protest behaviour in prison. Physical management is described in recent Department of Health (2010) guidance.

There are four broad categories:

- Those suffering from acute mental illness:
  - Most common diagnoses are severe depression, non-affective psychosis, or less commonly an acute stress reaction.
  - Accurate diagnosis is the first priority. Many will require urgent transfer to hospital, though some with a more acute, situationally determined stress reaction may respond to supportive care within prison.
  - Those with a psychosis are likely to have delusional ideas about the nature of the food provided or the intentions of those preparing or serving it. Sometimes providing sealed food (sandwiches, for example) is helpful in the short term.
- Those with paranoid personality traits/disorder:
  - Tend to be engaged in an oppositional struggle with authority, perhaps making some specific demand, but sometimes without making an explicit demand.
  - This may be seen as a dynamic clash between a stubborn, self-important prisoner and a rigid, controlling prison regime.
  - In most cases the prisoner will cease food refusal of their own accord eventually, perhaps spuriously rationalizing this to avoid loss of face, or moving on to some other oppositional behaviour.
  - The only way to expedite this is to enable some face-saving manoeuvre for the prisoner. This requires careful mediation between the inflexible prisoner and the similarly inflexible prison.
- Those who are making an apparently genuine demand, such as to move to a different prison, or to have some privilege:
  - These cases require support and counselling to persuade them to pursue their demand in a more appropriate way. In most cases these food refusals are short-lived.

– Food refusal among immigration detainees seeking to avoid repatriation is relatively common and may be of this type, though the food refusal may be particularly persistent.
• Those who are prepared to starve themselves to death, usually to make some political point:
  – An uncommon group. The prisoner will have an established history of activism and commitment to the cause. Their offending may well be related to this.
  – This group pose a very serious ethical challenge to prisons and health-care workers. Occasionally such protesters have succeeded in martyring themselves.

Important legal principles

• *Leigh* v *Gladstone* (1909): Home Office had a duty to preserve the health of the prisoners, even to the extent of forcibly feeding them. This principle has been superseded by
• *The Secretary of the State* v *Robb* [1995] 2 WLR 722: held that an individual's right to self-determination outweighed any other countervailing interests of the state. Although R was of sound mind and understood what he was doing, and although he persisted in his refusal, it was lawful to abide by his wishes and withhold nutrition and hydration.

Principles of health care

Food refusers are likely to require a psychiatric assessment. Management of health-care needs should be carried out jointly by mental health staff and physicians:

• Assessment:
  – Full psychiatric assessment to establish presence of acute mental illness.
  – Assess and clearly document capacity to decide to refuse food and/or fluids.
  – Conduct a thorough nutritional status assessment (e.g. food and fluid intake, weight, BMI, oedema).
  – Conduct relevant laboratory investigations (FBC, U&Es, Mg^{2+}, Ca^{2+}, PO_4^{3-}, CRP, ESR, glucose and LFTs).
• Management:
  – Document the presence or absence of an advance refusal.
  – Regular physical reviews – weekly (including blood tests) if drinking fluids, more frequently if abnormalities develop.
  – Consider offering food supplements.
  – Involve independent mental capacity advocate if appropriate.
  – Transfer to general hospital if the prisoner becomes dehydrated, weak, oedematous or develops significant biochemical abnormalities.

Re-feeding syndrome

A potentially fatal complication of re-feeding:

• The risk is negligible if fast of less than 5 days, with BMI >18.5 kg/m^2.
• The risk is high in presence of either one major risk factor or two lesser risk factors:

Major risk factors	Lesser risk factors
BMI < 16 kg/m^2	BMI < 18.5 kg/m^2
Weight loss > 15%	Weight loss > 10%
Little or no nutritional intake for more than 10 days	Little or no nutritional intake for more than 5 days
Low K$^+$, Mg^{2+} or phosphate levels before the onset of re-feeding	History of alcohol abuse or use of some drugs including insulin, chemotherapy, antacids or diuretics

See Department of Health (2010) for further guidance on management of re-feeding syndrome.

Dirty protesting

This is usually a strategy to achieve some gain and/or associated with paranoid personality disorder. The prisoner defecates and/or urinates in their cell, smearing faeces on the walls and often on their body and clothing.

There are well-established prison procedures for dealing with this. Clearly there are health risks for the prisoner and for the staff dealing with them, but the need for input from physical or mental health-care staff is less than in food refusal. Psychiatric assessment is often necessary as sometimes very florid psychosis may lead to similar behaviour, but the diagnosis is usually evident.

Self-harm

Deliberate self-harm (DSH) to relieve distress and subjective tension is a relatively common behaviour in prison. There is little research evidence to guide management.

Of 1741 male sentenced prisoners, drawn from 25 prisons (Maden *et al.*, 2000):

- 17% of men reported DSH on at least one occasion during their life.
- Self-harm was more common among white than non-white prisoners.
- More white men in the medium and long-term sentence group than in the short-term sentence group gave a history of DSH.
- DSH was associated with alcohol dependence but not with drug addiction.
- Neurotic and personality disorders were more commonly diagnosed in the DSH group.

Extreme and persistent self-harm

This small group of prisoners taxes the prison system, because they are difficult to care for in prison, just as they are elsewhere. Many show the expected clinical features: high levels of impulsivity and emotional instability, other features of borderline personality disorder, a history of abusive experiences in childhood, disturbed early attachments, early onset of conduct disorder, drug/alcohol abuse to cope with emotional distress.

But they are a heterogeneous group. Motivations are often complex and may be obscure, being an admixture of:

- relief of subjective negative emotion
- exerting control over environment and custodians
- a deliberate strategy to achieve a gain.

Clinical management is very difficult and can be demoralizing for those staff involved. Often mental health teams provide intense input as a reaction to a period of self-harm and then, as the behaviour wanes, withdraw having been exhausted. It is probably helpful to maintain some consistency in the support provided, perhaps by differentiating between two roles:

- Staff who will respond to crises by providing more intense support and participating in assessment, care in custody and teamwork (ACCT) reviews.
- Staff, perhaps a visiting clinician, who will provide regular, consistent supportive treatment, both at times of crisis and in between them.

Suicide

The rate of suicide:

- Prison population - 133/100 000
- Remand prison population – 339/100 000
- General population – 9.4/100 000.

A national survey of suicides in prison between 1999 and 2000 (Shaw *et al.*, 2004) found that, of 172 self-inflicted deaths:

- 49% were of prisoners on remand
- 32% occurred within 7 days of reception into prison
- 92% were by hanging or self-strangulation
- 72% had a history of mental disorder.
- The commonest (27%) primary diagnosis was drug dependence
- 57% had symptoms suggestive of mental disorder at reception into prison
- 24% had an F2052SH* open at the time of death
- 51% had had an F2052SH* open at some during sentence.

(*At the time of data collection, the form F2052SH was the record of observations opened on prisoners who were considered at risk of self-harm. It has since been superseded by ACCT.)

Table 19.1 A typology of prison suicide (Liebling, 1995)

	Young prisoners with poor coping skills	Older prisoners facing long sentences	Those with psychiatric illness
Proportion of total (%)	30–45	5–0	10–22
Motivation	Fear/helplessness Distress/isolation	Guilt; hopelessness	Alienation/loss of self-control fear/helplessness
Importance of their situation	Acute	Chronic	Varied
History of previous suicidal behaviour	Common	Less common	Varied

There are significant differences between those prisoners who had attempted suicide and controls (Liebling, 1995):

- Protective factors:
  - involvement in PE
  - job in prison
  - active in cell.
- Risk factors:
  - bullied at school
  - childhood sexual abuse
  - previous self-injury
  - difficulties with other prisoners
  - receiving few letters
  - no release plans
  - high hopelessness score
  - persistent sleeping problems.

Managing risk of suicide in prison

ACCT – assessment, care in custody and teamwork

A system for monitoring and protecting prisoner at risk of serious self-harm or suicide. The approach aims:

- to encourage all staff to work as a team to recognize and manage suicide risk
- to alter the balance from watching and preventing self-harm, to engaging the prisoner in working collaboratively to deal with their problems.

Box 19.4 Assessing suicide risk in prison

This should follow the same principles as assessing suicide risk in the community. Assessment for the presence of mental illness is obviously very important, but not all prisoners who complete suicide were mentally ill. With respect to the prison environment you should particularly consider the following.

Have they been in prison before?
- If so how did they cope then? Is this time any different to last time?

Have they a previous history of self-harm in the community or in prison?
- It is important to consider both environments because they are very different, and suicidal behaviour may be situationally determined.

Are they vulnerable to being bullied?
- Ask about experiences of bullying in prison, or any other interpersonal problems with prisoners or with staff.
- Ask if they were bullied at school or in employment.

Ask about the offence:
- While a remand prisoner may legitimately be cautious about discussing their charge, it is important to gain an understanding of their associated feelings and emotions. In the context of suicide, shame is perhaps particularly important.
- What are their expectations of their court case? What are the prospects for a prison sentence? It is common for prisoners to feel that they would not be able to cope if they were to receive a long sentence. This must be distinguished from feeling currently overwhelmed or hopeless.

What support structures are available to them?
- Ask about frequency of visits, telephone calls and letters.
- Do they have any friends within the prison?
- Are they religious? Do they use the prison chaplaincy services?

How do they spend their time in prison?
- Are they working or attending education? Do they use the gym?

Remember that sleep problems are very common. So while impaired sleep may be an important and distressing symptom for an individual, it may not discriminate well.

Useful practical advice about the process is available in the HM Prison service guidebook, *The ACCT Approach: Caring for people at risk in prison*, available from: http://www.hmprisonservice.gov.uk/assets/documents/10000C1BACCTStaffGuide.pdf:

- Any member of staff can open an ACCT plan.
- The unit manager, in collaboration with other staff, will formulate an immediate action plan to keep the prisoner safe.
- A trained assessor will carry out an assessment within 24 hours, and this should be followed by:
  - the first case review, where an individualized CAREMAP (Care and Management Plan) is drawn up
  - further case reviews are carried out according to individual need.
- Closure of the ACCT should be planned, and is followed by a post-closure review.

Other sources of support within prison

- Peer support schemes:
  - The Listeners scheme is the most well established. Prisoners may be designated as a Listener, and receive training and supervision from the Samaritans. Listeners are available on the wings to support and counsel fellow prisoners.
  - This provides an excellent source of support for some. Other prisoners find it difficult to place trust in another prisoner.

- Personal officer.
- Chaplaincy.
- Mental health in-reach or primary care teams.

References

Birmingham L, Gray J, Mason D, Grubin D. (2000) Mental illness at reception into prison. *Criminal Behaviour and Mental Health* **10**(2), 77–87

Brooker C, Duggan S, Fox C, Mills A, Parsonage M. (2008) *Short Changed: Spending on prison mental health care.* London: Sainsbury Centre for Mental Health

Department of Health. (2001) *Changing the Outlook: A strategy for developing and modernizing mental health services in prisons.* London: Department of Health

Department of Health. (2010) *Guidelines for the Clinical Management of People Refusing Food in Immigration Removal Centres and Prisons.* London: Department of Health

Grubin D, Carson D, Parsons S. (2002) *Report on the New Prison Reception Health Screen and the Results of the Pilot Study in 10 Prisons.* London: HM Prison Service

Hassan L, Birmingham L, Harty M, Jarrett M, Jones P, King C, *et al.* (2011) Prospective cohort study of mental health during imprisonment. *British Journal of Psychiatry* **198**, 37–42

Healthcare Advisory Committee for the Prison Service. (1997) *The Provision of Mental Health Care in Prisons.* London: HM Prison Service

*Liebling A. (1995) Vulnerability and prison suicide. *British Journal of Criminology* **35**, 173–87

Maden A, Chamberlain S, Gunn J. (2000) Deliberate self harm in sentenced male prisoners in England and Wales: some ethnic factors. *Criminal Behaviour and Mental Health* **10**(3), 199–204

Royal College of Psychiatrists. (2006) *College Report 141: Prison Psychiatry: Adult prisons in England and Wales.* London: Royal College of Psychiatrists

*Shaw J, Baker D, Hunt IM, Moloney A, Appleby L. (2004) Suicide by prisoners: national clinical survey. *British Journal of Psychiatry* **184**, 263–7

20

Psychiatric Issues in Criminal Courts

● Fitness to Plead and be Tried

The legal test

Originally formulated in *R v Pritchard* (1836) 7 Car & P 303 KB, a case involving a deaf and dumb defendant, as consisting of three elements:

- 'Whether the prisoner is mute of malice or by visitation of God':
  - a defendant might have refused to enter a plea as a strategy to avoid their estate being claimed by the Crown following conviction and execution.
- 'Whether he can plead to the indictment or not':
  - an illiterate deaf–mute, for example, had no way of communicating their plea.
- 'Whether he is of sufficient intellect to comprehend the course of proceedings on the trial, so as to make a proper defence – to know that he may challenge any of you to whom he may object, and to comprehend the details of the evidence ...'

In *R v John M* [2003] EWCA Crim 3452, the Court of Appeal approved the trial judge's more contemporary explication of the *Pritchard* criteria, which required that the defendant was capable of:

- understanding the charges and deciding whether to plead guilty or not
- exercising their right to challenge jurors
- instructing solicitors and counsel, which involves being able to:
  - understand the lawyers' questions, apply their mind to answering them and convey their answers intelligibly
- following the course of proceedings, which means that they are able to:
  - understand what is said by witnesses and counsel to the jury, to communicate to their lawyers
- giving evidence in their own defence, which includes being able to:
  - understand the questions they are asked, apply their mind to answering them, and convey their answers intelligibly to the jury.

Note also the Strasbourg Jurisprudence:

- Article 6(1) ECHR provides the right to participate effectively in the criminal trial process.
- Effective participation was expanded on in *SC v UK* [2005] 40 EHRR:

  ... does not require the ability to understand every point of law or evidential detail ... effective participation ... presupposes that the accused has a broad understanding of the nature of the trial process and what is at stake for him or her, including the significance of

any penalty which may be imposed. It means that he or she, if necessary with the assistance of, for example, an interpreter, lawyer, social worker, or friend, should be able to understand the general thrust of what is said in court. The defendant should be able to follow what is said by the prosecution witnesses, and, if represented, to explain to his lawyers his version of events, point out any statements with which he disagrees, and make them aware of any facts which should be put forward in his defence

- Domestically, *R v Miller* [2006] EWCA Crim 2391, confirmed that 'the bottom line ... is that every defendant should have a fair trial', and that this requires 'effective participation'.

Note that fitness to plead and be tried is a single issue only. Strictly speaking a defendant cannot be fit to enter a plea but unfit to be tried (*R v Sharp* [1957] CrimLR 821):

- This sometimes causes practical difficulty, and is a particular area of dissatisfaction for some (The Law Commission, 2010)

The Court of Appeal has avoided establishing that any specific problem of itself renders an individual under disability. This includes:

- amnesia for the offence (*R v Podola* (1959) 43 Cr.App.R. 220)
- a conclusion that the defendant is highly abnormal (*R v Berry* (1978) 66 Cr.App.R. 156)
- delusions about evil influences in the proceedings (*R v Moyle* [2008] EWCA 3059).

The procedure

This is provided by the Criminal Procedure (Insanity) Act 1964, (which was amended by the Criminal Procedure (Insanity & Unfitness to Plead) Act 1991, and then by the Domestic Violence, Crime and Victims Act 2004).

Under the title 'finding of unfitness to plead', the Act refers to 'fitness to be tried', and the state of being 'under a disability'. This loose terminology is unhelpful and there is no established difference between these various terms. The courts have also tended to use the terms interchangeably (e.g. *R v Ghulam* [2009] EWCA Crim 2285).

The issue may be considered at any time up until the opening of the defence case:

- If raised by the defence it must be proved on the balance of probabilities (*R v Robertson* (1968) 52 Cr.App.R. 690).
- If raised by the prosecution it must be proved beyond reasonable doubt (*R v Podola* (1959) 43 Cr.App.R. 220).
- It is decided by the judge, on the basis of the written or oral evidence of two registered medical practitioners (RMPs), one of whom must be section 12 approved.

A finding of disability must be followed by a trial of the facts, in which:

- A jury determines whether or not they 'did the act or made the omission' that constitutes the offence:
  - if the jury is not satisfied beyond reasonable doubt, then they are acquitted
  - otherwise, the court proceeds to disposal.
- The trial of the facts protects a mentally ill defendant who has done nothing wrong from being made subject to an order of a criminal court.
- However, some argue that the trial of the facts is itself not compatible with Article 6 rights (see for example, Bartlett and Sandland, 2007, pp226–30).
- Although the statute requires a trial of the facts to follow a finding of disability, *R v Hasani* [2005] EWHC 3016 (Admin) provides authority for a second trial of issue to take place, where a defendant regains fitness to plead before the trial of the facts takes place.

Box 20.1 Assessing fitness to plead and stand trial

There are no standardized instruments for assessing fitness to plead:

- The first such tool described in a UK setting showed unconvincing reliability and validity (Akinkunmi, 2002). Dependent on a full psychiatric examination, this is a cross-sectional assessment of capacity. Therefore where an advance opinion in writing concludes that the defendant is under disability, this must be followed up by a further assessment and opinion as close as possible to the trial of issue in court.

Consider these issues:

- Can the defendant explain to you the charges against them in simple terms?
- Can they give an account of what factors would lead them to decide on a guilty or not-guilty plea?
- Do they have a basic understanding of the people who will be in the court room and their roles? If you explain an aspect of this to them, can they assimilate it?
- Ask them what they would do if they knew someone on the jury, or someone on the jury did not like them.
- Can they discuss the events that led to their charges, and give an account of themselves?
- How well can they participate during the course of a psychiatric interview? Is there any evidence of distractedness or distractibility, poor short-term memory, agitation or other impairment?

Cognitive deficits:

- Simple objective tests of cognitive ability, such as a serial 7s and registering and recalling a name and address, may be helpful. But they are not determinative, being rather different to the task required in a court room.
- Where dementia or other cognitive disturbance is suspected, an MMSE is useful but remember that this is a screening test for dementia, not a capacity test for the courtroom. Similarly further cognitive testing (e.g. MEAMS, CAMCOG) or brain imaging may support a conclusion that they are unfit, but are not essential to the capacity assessment.
- In suspected learning disability formal IQ assessment may be important supportive evidence, but a low IQ does not necessarily lead to being under disability.

The following psychiatric symptoms commonly interfere with fitness to plead:

- Auditory hallucinations may distract the patient, preventing them from following evidence or giving evidence – consider the frequency, intensity and degree of insight. Look for objective evidence that the patient is distracted, during your examination, for example. Less commonly, somatic hallucinations or passivity may have a similar impact.
- Psychotic disorganization symptoms, such as perplexity and thought disorder, are likely, if present, to render a defendant under disability.
- Depression may affect the patient's ability to attend to, concentrate on and remember the evidence. Such cognitive deficits may be evident on simple testing. Evidence of psychomotor retardation, irrepressible tearfulness or an intense preoccupation with depressive cognitions may be important.
- Hypomania may affect attention and concentration, and short-term memory. A patient who is sufficiently disturbed to be considered manic will almost certainly be under disability.
- Delusions are most likely to affect fitness to plead when they relate to the court procedure. So if a patient is deluded that, for example their defence team is conspiring against them, or that the court is in some other way fixed, they may not be able to instruct council and participate in the trial properly.

Try not to adopt too dichotomous an approach to the clinical decision-making. You should consider what measures might be put in place to enable a fair trial to take place. This might include measures such as:

- more frequent than usual breaks
- having a friend or intermediary with them in the dock
- giving evidence by video link rather than in person
- pointing out to the court how any further deterioration in mental state might be recognized and managed.

Fitness to plead is an issue only at Crown court. A magistrates' court, if satisfied that he did the act charged, may either adjourn for inquiry into the offender's condition and most appropriate disposal, or make a hospital order under s37(3) of the Mental Health Act (MHA).

● Not Guilty by Reason of Insanity (NGBROI)

The legal test of insanity

Insanity at the time of committing an offence is one circumstance in which the *mens rea* is lacking, and may be a defence to any offence where *mens rea* is an issue.

The M'Naghton Rules were formulated by the House of Lords in a majority ruling to establish the law *after* Daniel M'Naghton had been found not guilty by reason of insanity. It is often said that ironically M'Naghton would not have fulfilled his own criteria:

> *To establish a defence on the ground of insanity, it must be clearly proved, that, at the time of committing the act, the party accused was labouring under such a defect of reason, from disease of the mind, as not to know the nature and quality of the act he was doing, or, if he did know it, that he did not know it was wrong*

Defect of reason

Defect of reason may be temporary or permanent (*R v Sullivan* (1983) 77 Cr.App.R. 176), but does not include:

- momentary absent-mindedness in context of depression in a case of shoplifting (*R v Clarke* (1972) 56 Cr.App.R. 225)
- uncontrollable impulse (*R v Kopsch* (1927) 19 Cr.App.R. 50).

Disease of the mind

Disease of the mind includes 'The major mental disorders which doctors call psychoses, such as schizophrenia ... any mental disorder that manifests itself in violence and is prone to recur' (*Bratty v Attorney-General for Northern Ireland* 1963).

Mind means 'mental faculties of reason, memory and understanding' and it does not matter whether 'the aetiology of the impairment is organic ... or functional' (*R v Sullivan* (1983) 77 Cr.App.R. 176).

It has been held to include:

- arteriosclerosis (*R v Kemp* (1956) 40 Cr.App.R. 121)
- psychomotor epilepsy (*Bratty v Attorney General for Northern Ireland* (1962) 46 Cr.App.R. 1)
- sleepwalking (*R v Burgess* (1991) 93 Cr.App.R. 41), where it was held further that the danger of recurrence of a mental disorder manifesting in violence may go towards categorizing it as a disease of the mind, rather than as an automatism due to external cause

but not:

- where a diabetic recklessly fails to take food, thus causing hypoglycaemia (*R v Bailey* (1983) 77 Cr.App.R. 76).

It must be of internal cause, rather than external (compare with non-insane automatism, Chapter 15):

- In *R v Hennessey* (1989), hyperglycaemia due to diabetes was a disease of the mind.
- In *R v Quick* (1973) 57 Cr.App.R. 722, hypoglycaemia due to administered insulin to a diabetic was not a disease of the mind, non-insane automatism being the proper defence.
- Non-insane automatism remains a possibility where temporary impairment results from some external physical factor such as a blow to the head causing concussion (*R v Sullivan*, above).

- A defence of non-insane automatism may be allowed where external factors (prescribed drugs and alcohol) operate on an underlying mental condition (mixed personality disorder), if the underlying disorder would not in itself produce a state of automatism (*R* v *Roach* [2001] EWCA Crim 2698).

According to Memon (2006) the courts have adopted a broad interpretation of disease of the mind and a restrictive interpretation of defect of reason.

Nature and quality of the act

A unitary construct, which refers to 'the physical character of the act' and which does not encompass issues of morality (*R* v *Codere* (1916) 12 Cr.App.R. 21).

Did not know it was wrong

This is legally wrong, as opposed to morally wrong (*R* v *Windle* [1952] 36 Cr.App.R. 85). In *R* v *Johnson* [2007] EWCA Crim 1978, the Court of Appeal was obliged to follow this strict interpretation, but acknowledged that courts had sometimes been more flexible and encouraged a further appeal to the House of Lords. See also MacKay *et al.* (2006).

Box 20.2 Not guilty by reason of insanity (NGBROI) in practice

Hypothetical case examples illustrate the difficulty in interpreting clinical cases in the terms of the M'Naghton rules. For clinicians, the problem tends to be in the nature and quality and legal wrongness aspects of the defence, rather than in what constitutes a disease of the mind.

The case of a man who assaults another individual because he delusionally believes that the victim is about to attack him is likely to satisfy the criterion of not knowing that his actions are legally wrong, because, in his mind, he is acting in self-defence:

- If the attack is not believed to be imminent, then this defence becomes weaker.
- If he assaults someone whom he delusionally believes has sexually abused his children, he might not satisfy this criterion, because even if his delusion were true it would be legally wrong to resort to violence.

A woman who kills her child because she is deluded that the child is about to be abducted, tortured and slowly killed nevertheless knows that her actions are legally wrong. It may be difficult to argue that she did not understand the physical character of her acts.

- It might be argued that her delusions alter the nature and quality of the act, such that in her deluded state she is saving the child from a worse fate, rather than acting to kill it.

Procedure for a defence of NGBROI

The issue may be raised by the defence (on balance of probabilities), the prosecution (beyond reasonable doubt) or the court itself (standard of proof unclear). In contrast, where the issue is automatism not due to disease of the mind, then the onus is on the prosecution to prove its absence beyond reasonable doubt.

The verdict must be returned by a jury on the written or oral evidence of two registered medical practitioners (RMPs) (one s12 approved). A plea of NGBROI cannot be accepted by the court without trial.

● Disposal Options Following the Special Verdict or a Finding of Disability

There are three disposal options following either a finding of NGBROI, or of unfitness to be tried and that they did the act:

- Hospital order under s37 MHA 1983 with or without a restriction order:
  - The criteria are exactly as for a hospital order following conviction, except that there is no requirement for the hospital managers to confirm availability of a bed. Rather, it is the duty of the hospital managers to admit them in accordance with the order. This reflects the lack of any custodial alternative for the court (in contrast to a convicted defendant).
  - A restriction order must be made where the alleged offence was murder.
  - If a restriction order is made, then s5A(4) provides that the Secretary of State may, if satisfied by the responsible clinician that they can properly be tried, remit the person for trial, either to court or to prison.
- Supervision order:
  - Defined in schedule 1A of the CPIA 1964 as requiring the individual to be under the supervision of a social worker or probation officer for a maximum of 2 years. An order may also include requirements of residence or of medical treatment.
  - The court must be satisfied that the proposed supervising officer is willing to undertake the supervision, and that arrangements are in place for the treatment that is specified.
  - There is no sanction for any failure to comply by the supervised person. A magistrates' court may revoke or amend, but not extend, the order.
- Absolute discharge.

A supervision order may include a requirement to 'submit … to treatment by or under the direction of an RMP with a view to the improvement of his mental condition':

- Requires written or oral evidence from two RMPs (one ss12 approved) that he has a mental condition that requires and may be susceptible to treatment, but which does not require a hospital order.
- The treatment may be specified only as:
  - non-resident treatment, or
  - treatment under the direction of an RMP.
- However, it may be arranged subsequently for part of the treatment to be given as a resident patient.

Prior to disposing of the case, ss35, 36 and 38 MHA 1983 are also available.

A guardianship order under s37 is not available in these circumstances, and neither is a hospital direction under s45A.

Box 20.3 Disposals following findings of unfit to plead or NGBROI

When working as an expert witness, your first duty is to the court, but you should also deal with the patient's clinical need. It is always preferable for a clinical service to make its own decisions about admission of patients.

- In cases of disability or NGBROI, the court requires medical evidence that a hospital order is appropriate but does not require confirmation of bed availability.
- It is essential that, as a clinician, you make it your business to ensure that the responsible clinical service is aware of the patient, and is involved in the case at as early a stage as possible.
- You should make the referral yourself; it is poor practice simply to advise solicitors to do so and leave what will ultimately be a clinical matter in the hands of non-clinicians.

● Unfitness to Plead and NGBROI in Practice

The use of NGBROI and unfitness to plead increased dramatically following the Criminal Procedure (Insanity and Unfitness to Plead) Act 1991, which introduced discretion into disposal for the first time, detention in hospital previously being inevitable. Kearns and Mackay (2000) and Mackay *et al.* (2006, 2007) reviewed court data between 1987 and 2001 (Figure 20.1).

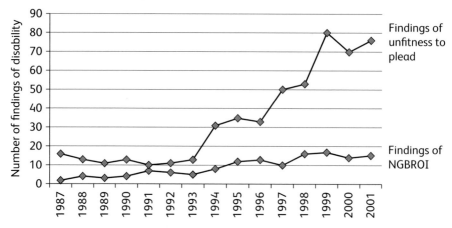

Figure 20.1 Annual frequency of findings of disability in England and Wales (NGBROI – not guilty by reason of insanity)

Between 1997 and 2001:

- schizophrenia and mental impairment each accounted for about one-third of the findings of unfitness to plead (Mackay *et al.*, 2007)
- schizophrenia accounted for half the findings of NGBROI and other psychoses about 11%. Other diagnoses included depression and anxiety disorders, epilepsy and hypomania (Mackay *et al.*, 2006).

Table 20.1 shows disposals following findings of disability and NGBROI for the years 1997–2001.

Box 20.4 Criticisms of the Pritchard criteria and M'Naghton Rules

These rules date back to the mid-1800s, and many consider them overdue for substantive, statutory update:

- The Law Commission published a consultation paper in relation to fitness to plead in October 2010, and is scheduled to publish a consultation on the insanity defence in summer 2011.
- It is likely that the law in this area will change over the coming years.

The Pritchard criteria:

- are often considered to be weighted too heavily on the cognitive capacity of the defendant, rather than on a capacity assessment within the spirit of the Mental Capacity Act (MCA) 2005
- do not allow a disjunctive consideration of fitness to plead and fitness subsequently to participate in a trial
- may be applied inconsistently by psychiatrists
- bear little relation to the statutory test of capacity in the MCA 2005.

See Rogers *et al.* (2008, 2009) for a critical review favouring a more systematized assessment process, and the Law Commission (2010) generally.

The M'Naghton Rules:

- are out of date in relation to contemporary psychiatric thinking
- are sometimes confusing in relation to non-insane and insane automatisms
- are interpreted by experts inconsistently, and they are different from the law (Mackay *et al.*, 2006)

The requirement not to know the physical character of the act or not to know that it was legally wrong forms a very high standard. Experience suggests that trial courts often show more flexibility than the rules explicitly contain.

Table 20.1 Disposals following findings of disability and not guilty by reason of insanity (NGBROI) 1997–2001 (data from Mackay *et al.*, 2006, 2007)

	Unfit to plead (n = 329)	NGBROI (n = 72)
	Percentages of total *n*	
Detention in hospital	63	47
restricted	39	38
unrestricted	24	10
Community supervision	24	43
Absolute discharge	4	10
Unknown	9	0

● Diminished Responsibility and Loss of Control

For offences committed on or after 4 October 2010, the three partial defences to murder, which reduce the conviction to manslaughter, are provided by the Coroners and Justice Act 2009. Expert psychiatric evidence is required for diminished responsibility because it is founded on the existence of a recognized medical condition. It may sometimes be admissible in relation to loss of control, and in rare cases of killing by the survivor of a suicide pact.

Diminished responsibility

This partial defence, which must be proved by the defence on the balance of probabilities, is provided by s52 of CJA 2009. It requires that the defendant was suffering from:

- an abnormality of mental functioning, which arose from a recognized medical condition, and:
  - the Ministry of Justice (MoJ) guidance (Ministry of Justice, 2010) mentions ICD-10 and DSM-IV but also states that 'there is scope for conditions not specified in such a list' to satisfy this criterion
- substantially impaired ability to do one or more of the following:
  - understand the nature of his conduct
  - form a rational judgement
  - exercise self-control, and
- 'Provides an explanation for D's acts and omissions' in relation to the killing, in that it 'causes or is a significant contributory factor in causing, D to carry out that conduct':
  - this explicit requirement for a causal link may sometimes be difficult to satisfy, and for some commentators is likely to make the defence too restrictive.

The term 'mental functioning' probably does not substantively differ from 'mind' in the previous definition of diminished responsibility. So the guidance in *R v Byrne* (1960) 44 Cr.App.R. 246 remains applicable:

A state of mind so different from that of ordinary human beings that the reasonable man would term it abnormal ... wide enough to cover the minds activities in all its aspects, not only the perception of physical acts and matters, and the ability to form a rational judgment whether an act is right or wrong, but also the ability to exercise will power to control physical acts in accordance with that rational judgment.

'Substantial' will continue to mean its usual English language meaning: more than trivial or minimal but short of total. The relationship between intoxication and diminished responsibility is considered below.

Other aspects of this new defence will be refined further by the Court of Appeal in due course.

Loss of control

The common law defence of provocation is replaced with the partial defence of 'loss of control' (s54 of CJA 2009). Where there is sufficient evidence to raise the defence (decided by the judge), then the burden of proof is on the prosecution to prove that it is not satisfied. This partial defence is available where all of three criteria are satisfied:

- The acts or omissions in relation to the killing resulted from loss of control:
  - the loss of control may or may not be sudden (s54(2)), so there 'may be a delay between the incident which was relevant to the loss of control and the killing' (Ministry of Justice, 2010, para 18), but presumably not between the loss of control itself and the killing
  - this delay allows cumulative provocation, as in prolonged domestic abuse, to constitute a qualifying trigger.
- The loss of control had a qualifying trigger, attributable to either or both of:
  - a fear of serious violence from the victim to the defendant or another (a subjective test)
  - things said or done which 'constituted circumstances of an extremely grave character and which caused the defendant to have a justifiable sense of being seriously wronged' (an objective test)
  - things said or done need not be said or done by the deceased, though they must cause the defendant to feel wronged.
- A person of the same sex and age, with a normal degree of tolerance and self-restraint and in the circumstances of the defendant, might have reacted in the same or similar way:
  - the circumstances of the defendant refers to all his circumstances except those whose only relevance is that they bear on his general capacity for tolerance or self-restraint
  - so, for example, a dispositional tendency to lose one's temper cannot in itself satisfy this criterion.

The partial defence of loss of control is not available where:

- the act is committed in a considered desire for revenge (s54(4)), or
- the defendant incited the qualifying trigger in order to use violence (s55(6)):
  - the defence is excluded if the purpose of the defendant's actions was to justify violence, but the fact that he caused a reaction in others which in turn caused him to lose self-control does not necessarily exclude the defence
- sexual infidelity in itself cannot constitute a qualifying trigger (s55(6)):
  - this reflects the tendency of the Court of Appeal to be unsympathetic to infidelity as a provoking factor, but it is likely to generate appellate court judgments.

Psychiatric evidence may be relevant to an understanding of the 'circumstances of the defendant'.

● Intoxication as a Defence

Most authorities deal with alcohol; generally the principles will apply to drugs too. The starting point is that, where the necessary *mens rea* is proved to have existed, it is no defence that it only existed because of intoxication, whether the intoxication is voluntary or involuntary. A drunken intent is still an intent (*R v Kingston* [1995] 2 A.C. 355):

- Intoxication may be involuntary where drinking is the result of an irresistible craving for or compulsion to drink. Alcohol dependence is usually required to satisfy this. It is acknowledged that even a severely dependent drinker may nevertheless sometimes choose to delay his next drink, so a degree of control is not inconsistent with involuntary intoxication.
- Ignorance of the strength of an alcoholic drink does not make subsequent intoxication other than voluntary.

For crimes of basic intent or where recklessness is sufficient *mens rea*, unawareness of risk due to self-induced intoxication is no defence (*DPP* v *Majewski* (1976) 62 Cr.App.R. 262):

- So, for manslaughter, assault, s20 wounding, reckless arson or criminal damage, rape and sexual assault, intoxication is mostly irrelevant.
- An exception may be where it is reasonable to suppose that the defendant did not know that the drug would have such an effect. In these cases it must be established whether the taking of the drug was itself reckless.

But for a crime of specific intent, the jury should take into account the drunkenness when deciding, in the round, whether or not they did have the requisite intent:

- Psychiatric expert evidence is sometimes called in relation to whether the defendant had the capacity to form the required intent. This is a very difficult judgement to make and back up with evidence. In any case, for the jury the issue is simply whether they did have the requisite intent, drunk or not.
- Drinking in order to offend (Dutch courage) does not provide a defence for a crime of specific intent.

Intoxication and diminished responsibility

There is considerable case law relating to alcohol and diminished responsibility, which applies to the previous construct of diminished responsibility. But much of this remains applicable post Coroners and Justice Act 2009 (Richardson, 2010):

- Where an abnormality of mind is present, the fact that he would not have killed if he had not also been drunk does not necessarily prevent the defence being available (*R* v *Dietschmann* [2003] UKHL 10).
- Where alcoholism has reached the stage that the defendant's brain has been injured by repeated insults from intoxicants so that there is gross disturbance of judgement and emotional responses, this may constitute an abnormality of mind (*R* v *Tandy* (1988) 87 Cr.App.R. 45), and probably would constitute an abnormality of mental functioning arising from a recognized medical condition:
  - this does not depend on there being demonstrable brain damage (*R* v *Wood* [2008] EWCA Crim 1305)
  - but alcohol dependence syndrome does not necessarily constitute an abnormality of mind (*R* v *Stewart (James)* [2009] EWCA Crim 593).
- In *R* v *Stewart* (above) the court suggested that, in considering a defence of diminished responsibility based upon alcohol dependence or involuntary intoxication, the jury might consider, *inter alia*:
  - the extent and seriousness of the defendant's dependency on alcohol
  - the extent to which his ability to control his drinking or to choose whether to drink or not, was reduced
  - whether he was capable of abstinence from alcohol, and for how long, and
  - whether he was choosing to drink for some particular reason, such as a birthday celebration.
- Presumably, following *Stewart*, a jury may find that an irresistible craving for or compulsion to drink constitutes an abnormality of mental functioning arising from the recognized medical condition of alcohol dependence syndrome.

● The Need for a Restriction Order

A restriction order, provided by s41 MHA 1983, is available at the discretion of the sentencing Crown court:

- where a hospital order under s37 MHA 1983 has been made, and
- where 'It appears to the court ... that it is necessary for the protection of the public from serious harm'.

Whether or not it is necessary is decided with regard to:

- The nature of the offence
- The antecedents of the offender
- The risk of him committing further offences if set at large:
  - not the seriousness of the risk that the defendant will reoffend, but the risk that if he does so the public will suffer serious harm … the potential harm must be serious, and a high possibility of minor offences will no longer be sufficient (*R* v *Birch* (1989) 11 Cr.App.R. 202).

The court must hear oral evidence from one of the RMPs who has recommended the hospital order, but it is not required for this evidence to recommend a restriction order.

The effects of a restriction order are dealt with in Chapters 3 and 5.

Box 20.5 Giving oral evidence in relation to restriction orders

It is unusual for a court not to make a restriction order where the psychiatric evidence is that it is warranted. Over the years, the threshold for imposing a restriction order has reduced. If the court has required you to attend, clearly it has a restriction order in mind. Persuading a court not to make a restriction order is likely to be a harder task than the reverse.

The effect of the advent of supervised community treatment (SCT) is uncertain in this regard:
- It might be that psychiatrists are increasingly comfortable with the notion of coercion in the community, and consequently recommend s41 more often.
- On the other hand, there may be patients whose risks can now be managed civilly, with a community treatment order (CTO), and therefore an s41 is not necessary.

You should explicitly consider the alternatives of an s41 now, or a CTO later:
- Section 41 is a more onerous and secure measure for the court to make, which may be attractive for the sentencer and for public confidence.
- The future involvement of the MoJ in management can be useful, enabling the clinical team to take a more neutral position, separate from the 'stick' of MoJ sanctions.
- A CTO is less restrictive and allows more clinical flexibility in the future, but an approved medical health practitioner (AMHP) will have to agree to its imposition and subsequent renewals.

The nature of the offence may be considered in terms of the seriousness of the harm actually caused, or the potential harm that may have been caused.
- Also consider issues such as motivation and intent, planning, weapon use, excessive or extreme violence, contributory situational factors, intoxication.

Antecedents of the offender include previous convictions but may also include established previous risk behaviours that have not been prosecuted

Risk of further offences implicitly means further offences that are likely to result in serious harm:
- So the fact that an offender is highly likely to reoffend at a high frequency but in a relatively minor way, would not justify a restriction order.

● The Assessment of Dangerousness under s229 CJA 2003

Protection of the public from serious harm has always been considered a legitimate aim of sentencing, courts using common law powers to impose longer sentences than required by the seriousness of the offence.

A series of statutory measures for dealing with offenders deemed to be dangerous were used sparingly by the courts. But the current dangerous offender provisions provided by chapter 5 of Part 12 of the CJA 2003, amended by the Criminal Justice and Immigration Act 2008, have been used frequently. The statutory framework, associated case law and issues of use have been reviewed by Clark (2011).

For the purposes of the Act, an offender is dangerous if:

- he has committed a specified offence, and
- there is a significant risk of further specified offences, and
- there is a significant risk that such offences will lead to serious harm to the public.

There are over 150 specified violent and sexual offences listed in schedule 15 of the CJA 2003, some of which are shown in Table 20.2. These may be further categorized as 'serious specified offences' where the usual maximum sentence is 10 years or more imprisonment.

Table 20.2 Some common specified violent and sexual offences listed in schedule 15 of CJA 2003

Attempted, conspiring, incitement to murder, manslaughter, infanticide	Rape, assault by penetration, sexual assault, indecent assault
s20 and s18 wounding, actual bodily harm, threats to kill	Various sexual offences against minors
Kidnapping, false, imprisonment, child cruelty	Exposure and voyeurism
Robbery, aggravated burglary or vehicle taking	Possession of indecent photographs of children
Arson, criminal damage, causing death by dangerous driving	Offences related to sexual activity with individuals with mental disorder

'Significant risk of serious harm'

- 'Significant' means its usual English meaning, and does not equate to any numerical probability. In particular the actuarial OASys-based tools used by the probation service, while instructive, are not determinative of this risk judgement.
- 'Serious harm' means 'death or personal injury whether physical or psychological' (s224(3)).
- Repetitive low level violent or sexual offending is not sufficient to satisfy the test, even where it is possible that future victims may be harmed more seriously than those who have gone before (*R* v *Lang* [2005] EWCA Crim 2864).

In considering this issue, the court:

- must take account of available information about the offence
- may take into account available information about:
  - previous offences
  - any pattern of behaviour of which the offences form a part
  - the offender.

There is no statutory requirement for psychiatric evidence beyond the usual requirement when making a custodial sentence in relation to a defendant who appears to be mentally disordered:

- However, psychiatric evidence may be relevant to these domains of enquiry and it is commonly sought.
- The Court of Appeal has tended to support this as good practice where, for example, 'the danger is due to a mental or personality problem' (*R v Fawcett* (1995) 15 Cr.App.R.(S.) 55).

Box 20.6 Assessing dangerousness for the purposes of section 229 of the Criminal Justice Act 2003

This single dichotomous assessment should be contrasted with the dimensional repetitive risk assessments of clinical practice. The tendency of psychiatrists to overestimate risk has even greater potency where there is no prospect of review. The conservatism of clinical practice should not be carried into the court room.

It is probably helpful to adopt the familiar strategy of clinical risk assessment to delineate circumstances in which risk of reoffending will go up and when it will go down.

The significant risk criterion may be considered satisfied:

- where there seems to be a high risk of reoffending regardless of situational factors, or
- where high-risk situations are so common in ordinary life that they are bound to occur at a high frequency.

Psychiatric issues are less relevant to the likelihood of serious harm criterion:

- While future victims may be more seriously harmed than past victims, a high likelihood of relatively minor offending does not constitute dangerousness even where more serious harm is possible (but not likely).

The nature and circumstances of the offence:

- Consider premeditation and planning, use of violence more extreme or sustained than required, evidence of sadism or sexually motivated violence, the circumstances and nature of the provocation, weapon use and weapon carrying.

Previous convictions and past patterns of behaviour:

- Previous violence that has not led to conviction may be taken into account.

Information about the offender:

- Consider particularly the nature of any mental illness or personality disorder and its relationship to violence.
- Relevant characteristics may include emotional instability, impulsivity, dispositional paranoia, pro-criminal or pro-violent attitudes, alcohol and drug misuse.

Sentencing options for dangerous offenders

Previously the statute required imprisonment for public protection (IPP) where the offender was considered 'dangerous'. The Criminal Justice and Immigration Act 2008 reintroduced judicial discretion into sentencing, so, while there are still prescribed qualifying criteria, IPP and extended sentences become available when they are satisfied rather than inevitable (Table 20.3).

Table 20.3 Available sentences for dangerous offenders

Discretionary life sentence	Available where the offence is a serious specified offence, and the nature and circumstances of it justify a life sentence A life sentence cannot be justified on the grounds of risk because risk is equally well managed by the (slightly) less onerous IPP
Imprisonment for public protection (IPP)	Available at the judge's discretion for a serious specified offence where: – the notional custody time is more than 2 years*, or – he has a previous schedule 15A conviction†
Extended sentence	Available at the judge's discretion for any specified offence where: – the notional custody time is more than 2 years*, or – he has a previous schedule 15A conviction†
Sentencing as usual	Available at judge's discretion for any offence that does not justify a life sentence

*The notional custody time refers to the amount of time that the prisoner would spend in custody after sentencing, and equates to a determinate sentence of 4 years or a minimum term of 2 years.
†Schedule 15A convictions include: attempt, conspiracy or incitement to commit murder; manslaughter; wounding with intent; possession of firearm with intent to endanger life; robbery using a firearm; various sexual offences carrying a liability to life imprisonment; rape or attempted rape; intercourse with a girl under 13; assault by penetrations.

References

Akinkunmi AA. (2002) The MacArthur competence assessment tool – fitness to plead: a preliminary evaluation of a research instrument for assessing fitness to plead in England and Wales. *Journal of the American Academy of Psychiatry and the Law* **30**, 476–82

Bartlett P, Sandland, R. (2007) *Mental Health Law: Policy and practice*, 3rd edn. Oxford: Oxford University Press

Clark T. (2011) Sentencing dangerous offenders following the Criminal Justice and Immigration Act 2008, and the place of psychiatric evidence. *Journal of Forensic Psychiatry and Psychology* **22**(1), 138–55

Kearns G, Mackay RD. (2000) An upturn in unfitness to plead: disability in relation to the trial under the 1991 Act. *Criminal Law Review* **July**, 532–46

Law Commission, The. (2010) *Unfitness to Plead. A consultation paper*. Available at: http://www.lawcom.gov.uk/unfitness_to_plead.htm

Mackay RD, Mitchell BJ, Howe L. (2006) Yet more facts about the insanity defence. *Criminal Law Review* **May**, 399–411

Mackay RD, Mitchell BJ, Howe L. (2007) A continued upturn in unfitness to plead – more disability in relation to the trial under the 1991 Act. *Criminal Law Review* **July**, 530–45

Memon R. (2006) Legal theory and case law defining the insanity defence in English and Welsh law. *Journal of Forensic Psychiatry and Psychology* **17**(2), 230–52

Ministry of Justice (2010) Circular 2010/13. Available at: http://www.justice.gov.uk/publications/bills-and-acts/circulars/2010/index.htm

Richardson J. (2010) *Archbold 2011: Criminal pleading evidence and practice*. London: Sweet & Maxwell

Rogers TP, Blackwood NJ, Farnham F, Pickup GJ, Watts MJ. (2008) Fitness to plead and competence to stand trial: a systematic review of the constructs and their application. *Journal of Forensic Psychiatry and Psychology* **19**(4), 576–96

Rogers TP, Blackwood NJ, Farnham F, Pickup GJ, Watts MJ. (2009) Reformulating fitness to plead: a qualitative study. *Journal of Forensic Psychiatry and Psychology* **20**(6), 815–34

21

Providing Expert Evidence to Criminal Courts

This chapter considers the role of the expert in criminal courts. Many of the principles also apply to civil and family courts, but there are important differences. If necessary, familiarize yourself with the family procedure (adoption) rules, civil procedure rules, or the Coroners' Rules (all available from the Ministry of Justice website, http://www.justice.gov.uk). See also Rix (2008) in relation to civil cases and St John-Smith *et al.* (2009) for Coroners' Courts.

● Psychiatry and Criminal Law

There are three categories of witness:

- Witnesses of fact, who give evidence about events that they have observed directly.
- Professional witnesses, for example a doctor giving factual evidence about the treatment that they have provided for a patient.
- Expert witnesses, who provide courts with opinion based on expertise in some specific scientific field.

There is a high-order tension between law and psychiatry:

- The law deals in dichotomous, categorical certainty.
- Psychiatry deals in diverse, dimensional probability.

Consequently, psychiatric expert evidence is at risk of being appropriated by either side, or ridiculed as vague and unhelpful. Psychiatric experts must:

- be acutely aware of this dynamic
- ensure that their opinions are sound and defensible on the facts
- be robust in defending their opinions
- accept some responsibility for ensuring that their opinions are not misappropriated.

The admissibility of expert evidence

An expert witness is distinguished from an ordinary witness by having some particular knowledge or experience that goes beyond that of most people:

- The 'Bonython criteria' have been adopted into the Common Law by the Court of Appeal:
  - 'whether a [non-expert] person ... would be able to form a sound judgment on the matter without the assistance of [an expert]'
  - 'Whether the matter forms part of a ... reliable body of knowledge or experience', such that an expert opinion would be 'of assistance to the court'

— 'whether the expert has acquired by study or experience sufficient knowledge ... to render his opinion of value ...'.

- With regard to psychiatry, an expert's opinion is admissible to furnish the court with scientific information which is likely to be outside the experience and knowledge of a judge or jury ... Jurors do not need psychiatrists to tell them how ordinary folk who are not suffering from mental illness are likely to react to the stresses and strains of life (*R* v *Turner* [1974] 60 Cr.App.R. 80)

An expert's evidence must be relevant and within their field of expertise, in order to be admissible:

- An opinion on a matter that is ultimately for the jury to decide (diminished responsibility, for example) may be admissible. See *R* v *Stockwell* (1993) 97 Cr.App.R, 260, a case involving identification experts.
- Some argue that psychiatrists should refrain from addressing the ultimate issue because it may involve interpretation of facts which themselves may be challenged in court.
- For others it is unhelpful to justify not giving an opinion by stating that it is a matter for the jury. All matters of fact are for the jury; the expert is simply giving their opinion, and the jury is not bound by it.

According to Kenny (1984), a discipline may be called a science if:

- it is consistent, that is, different experts would generally give the same answers to questions that are central to the discipline
- it is methodical, such that there is agreement on appropriate, replicable procedures for gathering information
- the body of knowledge is cumulative, such that established knowledge may be used reliably as a basis from which to develop new knowledge, and
- it is predictive and falsifiable, allowing the not-yet-known to be predicted from the already-known.

Some question whether psychiatry, as practised in the courtroom, can satisfy these criteria (Coles and Veiel, 2001; Rogers, 2004). A reflective psychiatrist may acknowledge that, if these criteria define the parameters of what is scientific, then an expert psychiatric witness is sometimes pressed to go beyond them.

Hearsay evidence and psychiatry

In general, the facts on which an expert bases their opinion should be proved by admissible evidence, i.e. not hearsay. The Criminal Justice Act (CJA) 2003 preserves certain common law exceptions to this (s118), including that:

- an expert witness may draw on the body of expertise relevant to their field
- a statement is admissible if it relates to a physical sensation or mental state.

The strict position is:

- A doctor may not state what a patient told him about past symptoms as evidence of the existence of those symptoms because that would infringe the rule against hearsay, but he could give evidence of what the patient told him in order to explain the grounds on which he came to a conclusion with regard to the patient's condition. (Tapper, 2010, p542)

In practice courts are sometimes more flexible:

- Archbold (Richardson, 2011, at para 199-77) notes that 'as a concession, doctors are sometimes allowed to base their opinion on what the defendant has told them without those matters being proved by admissible evidence'.

The dual agent role of psychiatric expert witnesses

In the UK, in contrast to some other jurisdictions such as the USA, psychiatrists often act as 'dual agents' (Stone, 1984), acting on behalf of:

- the patient in the interests of care and treatment
- the court to inform sentencing.

O'Grady (2002) suggests that UK psychiatrists should adopt a mixed ethical framework encompassing:

- medical ethics of beneficence and non-maleficence
- justice ethics of truthfulness, respect for autonomy and respect for human rights of others.

This is often necessary when working within the UK system, particularly when dealing with severely ill defendants who perhaps require a hospital disposal. But psychiatrists should retain a high sensitivity to potential conflicts, and separate their roles when necessary:

- For example, it is difficult for a visiting psychiatrist to a prison to treat a prisoner and also provide objective expert evidence to a court.

Independence of expert witnesses

Instructions for expert psychiatric reports mostly come from the defence, with fewer from the Crown Prosecution Service or directly from the Court.

As an expert you have a professional duty to those instructing you, to carry out your work diligently, in a timely manner and to a high standard. But your over-riding duty is to assist the court to achieve its objective of dealing with the case justly. Accordingly your report is independent, unbiased and objective; you would write the same report regardless of who instructed you:

- Roscoe *et al.* (2009) reviewed psychiatric reports on perpetrators of homicide in England and Wales between 1996 and 2001. The agreement on diagnosis between defence and prosecution reports was significantly lower than between reports prepared for the same side:
  - All psychiatrists should be aware of the possibility of an unwitting bias towards the instructing side.

Remember that, where the instruction is from the defence, your report may or may not be disclosed and used in court. Where your report is prepared for the prosecution, it will be disclosed. Consequently a prosecution expert sometimes becomes a defence witness; the reverse is less likely.

● Criminal Procedure Rules

The Criminal Procedure Rules, available from http://www.justice.gov.uk, govern the practice and procedure to be followed in the criminal division of the Court of Appeal, Crown courts and magistrates' courts.

There are 76 Parts. All expert witnesses must be familiar with Part 33 which relates to expert evidence. This Part:

- defines an expert as 'a person who is required to give or prepare expert evidence for … criminal proceedings, including … [in relation to] fitness to plead or … sentencing'
- defines the expert's duty to the court and includes requirements for the content of the report (see 'Writing the Report' below)

- includes rules regarding introducing expert evidence in a case
- provides for the court to direct that experts discuss the case and 'prepare a statement for the court of the matters on which they agree and disagree':
    - if an expert does not comply with such a direction, then their evidence may not be introduced
- provides for the court to direct that a single joint expert be instructed by more than one defendant:
    - applies where a number of defendants all wish to introduce expert evidence on some issue
    - does not apply to the appointment of a single expert for defence and prosecution; this would compromise the adversarial nature of a criminal trial
    - rarely relevant to psychiatric evidence, which is necessarily defendant-specific.

Agreeing to provide a psychiatric report: accepting instructions

The quality of instruction varies from a general request for a 'full psychiatric report' to a tailored list of issues specific to the particular case.

The General Medical Council (GMC) guidance emphasizes that 'you must ensure that you understand exactly what questions you are being asked to answer' (General Medical Council, 2008):

- A telephone conversation may be helpful.
- In practice, some issues are contingent on other issues, so it may not be possible to generate a complete list of questions at the start.
- Therefore you should use your professional discretion to consider issues that you think are relevant, but do not go too far without checking with those instructing. For example, you may not be thanked for giving your opinion on diminished responsibility where the issue on which you have been instructed was fitness to plead.

Consider your expertise and competence. You must be satisfied that you are able to answer the questions asked. If you are not, try to suggest an alternative expert with greater experience in the particular area.

You must also ensure that you have sufficient indemnity cover for your fee-paying work.

Sources of information

Consider what documents you require. For most criminal cases this will include:

- witness statements
- transcript of interviews (sometimes tapes or videotapes)
- custody record
- proof of evidence
- previous convictions and cautions
- previous medical records (GP and psychiatric or general hospital records).

In some cases, particularly cases of murder, you should ensure that you receive the 'unused material':

- In serious cases there is often a wealth of evidence gained from witnesses, some of which is not required to prove the prosecution case. This unused material often contains psychiatrically relevant information about the defendant and their circumstances.

Ask the solicitors to get the medical records for you in advance of seeing the patient. It is best to read all the paperwork before seeing the patient. This allows a much more focused and revealing psychiatric examination.

You should always note what documents you have not obtained that you would have liked to obtain. You must form your opinions with any such evidence gap in mind, and state this clearly in your report.

Fees and information governance

Defence solicitors are required to gain prior authority from the Legal Services Commission (LSC) for expert fees exceeding £100. This allows solicitors to receive payment from the LSC, and pass it on to the expert, prior to conclusion of the case:

- You will need to provide an estimate of the maximum fee that you think you will charge, based on an hourly rate and the maximum number of hours' work required.
- If the case turns out to require more work than you thought, the solicitors can apply for an extension of funding.
- It is reasonable to charge for assessing the defendant, reading the relevant papers, interviewing necessary informants, and for formulating your opinion.
- You should not charge for researching clinical or legal issues that might be required for you to come to an opinion; as an expert you are expected to know this already. Similarly it is not reasonable to charge for the time you spend preparing and improving a series of draft reports or for supervision time.

The CPS does not need to gain prior authority, but will wish to agree your fees in advance in much the same way.

Information governance is as important for court reports as for other clinical work. You should use encrypted storage media, and take proper precautions in relation to electronic communication.

Ensure that you keep accurate time records of the work undertaken. The LSC requires solicitors to instruct only those professionals who keep such records and make them available to the LSC on reasonable notice.

Once you have completed the report the instructing solicitors will have ownership of the report, and you should not disclose it without their permission. However, where you have concerns about a defendant's acute mental health needs or associated risks, you still have a professional duty of care. You must ensure that these are communicated to the appropriate people.

The assessment

Introduction and gaining consent

Ensure that the defendant understands:

- That you are not acting in a therapeutic capacity, but to inform the court whether there are any psychiatric issues that are relevant to the case.
- That although their solicitors (or the CPS) have asked you to see them, you are independent of the defence (or prosecution).
- That in contrast to most medical consultations what they tell you is not confidential. The instructing side will certainly see the report, the judge may well see it and it may be read out in open court.
- What will happen to the report and paperwork after conclusion of your work, where it will be held and under what circumstances it may be accessed in the future.

A full psychiatric history and mental state examination

This follows the standard scheme. In comparison to a general psychiatric history there may be a particular emphasis on:

- behavioural problems in childhood, to understand the genesis of offending behaviour
- the development or course of any mental illness, and its relationship to offending or risk behaviours
- dispositional factors relevant to offending.

Detailed accuracy is important:

- The history you collect needs to be internally consistent. Ensure that dates or timeframes do not conflict.
- But remember that a self-report history is only as good as the defendant's recollection and engagement allows. So always be aware that there may be inaccuracies in what you have been told and tailor your conclusions accordingly:
  - For most clinical issues, detailed dates and times are not crucial.
  - Beware spending so much time and attention on a detailed episodic history that you forget to think about the defendant's emotional state or subjective experiences.

The mental state examination follows the standard procedure, bearing in mind issues such as fitness to be tried where relevant.

The current alleged offence

You should include both a summary of the evidence contained in the prosecution papers and a report of the defendant's account to you. The amount of detail required varies from case to case, generally dependent on the importance of mental state at the time of the offence. For example:

- Relatively little detail is required in the case of a habitual thief charged with a series of thefts, who happens to have developed a psychosis while on remand. Here the crucial issues are their current mental state, in relation to their fitness to be tried and the need for a psychiatric disposal.
- By contrast where you are considering a defence of not guilty by reason of insanity or diminished responsibility, considerable detail is necessary.

As with most history taking it is important to use as high a proportion of open questions as possible. Use the following ways of encouraging recall:

- Find a point in time prior to the alleged offence that the defendant remembers well and work forward step by step.
- When recall apparently fails, use prompts from the witness statements to remind them of innocuous aspects of the situation.
- Ask about different mental functions specifically and sequentially: what did they see or hear? How did this make them feel? What thoughts came into their mind?

Remember to ask about actions after the offence. Sometimes these are seen in court as important indicators of motivation or intention, so your opinion must take them into account.

Closing the interview

Ensure that you have their permission to contact any necessary informants.

Explain what will happen next and how long it will take to complete your report. Consider how much of your opinion to feed back to them straightaway.

Ensure, particularly in custodial settings, that you communicate any concerns about acute needs or risks appropriately. If possible make a brief entry in the prison medical record, to document that you have carried out an assessment.

Further information

Now collect any additional sources of information, including a collateral history, and write your report.

● Writing the Report

Accuracy and internal consistency are important. Inaccuracies and errors, even typographical errors, may be used to undermine an expert in court.

Use normal English language as far as possible. Some psychiatric terminology is necessary but it should always be adequately explained, probably in parentheses.

Occasionally a solicitor will ask you to change your report after you have submitted it:

- You should not agree to alter your opinion.
- If the solicitor is pointing out a typographical error or minor factual issue then it may be reasonable to issue a revised version.
- If there is some new information to be considered, it is better to prepare a brief addendum.

A suggested macro-structure

Use sub-headings and number your paragraphs. This will make it much easier to navigate around the report when giving oral evidence.

The precise structure will vary between cases and experts. But all reports should include:

- an introductory section
- the body of the report, in which the evidential information is set out
- a final section including a summary and opinions.

An introductory section

This should contain:

- A list of the sources of information used, and a note of any wanted sources that have been unobtainable.
- A brief account of the defendant's situation, including, for example:
  - the charges against them and the dates on which they are alleged to have occurred
  - the stage that the case has reached and important forthcoming hearing dates
  - whether they are in custody or on bail.
- A statement in relation to informed consent, making specific reference to confidentiality, and subsequent storage of the report and associated paperwork.

It may contain three other requirements of the Criminal Procedure Rules. These are all required in every report, though their placement may vary:

- 'details of the expert's qualifications, relevant experience and accreditation' (rule 33.3(1)(a))
- 'a statement that the expert understands his duty to the court, and has complied and will continue to comply with that duty' (33.3(1)(i)):
  - The 'expert's duty to the court' is defined in three parts at 33.2: (1) 'to help the court achieve the overriding objective by giving objective unbiased opinion on matters within his expertise'; (2) 'this duty overrides any obligation to the person from whom he receives instructions or by whom he is paid'; (3) 'an obligation to inform all parties and the court if the expert's opinion changes from that contained in a report served as evidence or given in a statement.'
  - The over-riding objective of the court is defined at 1.1 as 'that criminal cases be dealt with justly', and some characteristics of a just process in this context are listed.
- 'the same declaration of truth as a witness statement', which is provided in the Practice Direction to part 27:

This statement (consisting of x pages) is true to the best of my knowledge and belief and I make it knowing that, if it is tendered in evidence, I shall be liable to prosecution if I have stated in it anything which I know to be false, or do not believe to be true.

In contrast to the civil procedure rules, the Criminal Procedure Rules do not require a report in a criminal case to state the substance of the instructions. It may or may not be helpful to do so.

The body of the report

The structure of this broadly follows a standard psychiatric history and examination, with an added section for information about the current alleged offence.

Most experts give discrete sections for different sources of information. Sometimes it is helpful to give a more narrative account. For example, where the collateral history from the defendant's mother ratifies some aspect of self-report, you might decide to include information from both those sources at the same point.

However you choose to organize this, you must clearly distinguish whether information has been gained from:

- the defendant themselves
- your own observations
- other people who know the defendant
- prosecution papers
- past medical records.

There is a very important balance to be achieved between concision and inclusiveness:

- Some reports, particularly from less experienced experts, tend towards over-inclusiveness, perhaps for fear of missing some important issue.
- You must be balanced, and include evidence that both supports and goes against the conclusions you have reached.

The bottom line is that the report should include all the information that is important to your opinion, paragraph 33.3(1) requiring that reports:

- 'contain a statement setting out the substance of all facts given to the expert which are material to the opinions expressed in the report, or upon which those opinions are based' and
- 'make clear which of the facts … are within the expert's own knowledge':
  - For example, observations of mental state may be within the expert's own knowledge, while subjective reports of symptoms are hearsay (which may nevertheless be relied on according to the established rules).

Rule 33.3 also requires a report to:

- give details of any literature or other information on which the expert has relied
- state who carried out any examination, measurement, test or experiment that the expert has used for the report, give that person's qualifications, experience and accreditation, state whether it was carried out under the expert's supervision, and summarize the findings
- summarize the range of opinions that might reasonably be held on any matter, and give reasons for the expert's own opinion
- explain if the expert's opinion is subject to any qualification.

Summary and opinion

Finally rule 33.3 requires every report to 'contain a summary of the conclusions reached'. It is often helpful to give a concise clinical summary of the case, a brief psychiatric formulation perhaps, before going on to give your opinion on how this clinical assessment interfaces with the relevant legal matters.

Box 21.1 Writing psychiatric reports for sentencing

It is helpful if the written reports before the sentencing judge are in tune with each other and refer to each other:

- Always make sure that you see the probation pre-sentence report (PSR) and talk to the probation officer preparing it.
- Make explicit reference to the PSR. Consider whether there are any psychiatric issues that would hinder compliance with a proposed requirement.
- Consider the risk assessment in the PSR. If you think that all the major risk issues have been properly identified and addressed, then say so. If, on the other hand, you think that because of psychiatric issues the group-based actuarial data is not applicable to this individual, then you should explain this.

Always look at the statutory criteria that the court will be considering. Where relevant make sure that:

- your opinion uses the statutory language where possible
- the link between clinical terms and statutory terms is explicit, and that
- all the required elements are present and correct in your report.

Giving Oral Evidence in Court

In most cases oral evidence is not required, unless:

- you have written an unclear or ambiguous report
- there are conflicting opinions available to the court necessitating closer examination
- there is a statutory requirement for oral evidence (e.g. making a restriction order), or
- the psychiatric issues are central to deciding the case (e.g. not guilty by reason of insanity, diminished responsibility).

Criminal trials are difficult to organize and, while courts do their best to work around experts' other professional commitments, you will need to show flexibility.

Prior to the court hearing

It may be some time since you prepared your report:

- Check whether or not there is further evidence available that you did not have at the time.
- Re-read your report, your original handwritten notes, other experts' reports and if necessary the rest of the papers.

You may be asked to attend a conference with the barrister:

- They will want to:
  - ensure that they understand your opinion and clarify any ambiguities
  - discuss any conflicting opinion from other experts
  - satisfy themselves that they know what answers you will give to their questions.
- You should seek an understanding of:
  - the order in which they are going to take your evidence
  - the points that they wish to emphasize.

Consider whether you need to see the defendant again, perhaps at court prior to the hearing; this is essential for fitness to plead.

At court

Dress soberly and smartly, arrive early, know who to inform of your arrival and expect to do some waiting. It is helpful to know how the judge should be addressed (Your Honour most often, sometimes My Lord/Lady):

- For guidance see http://www.judiciary.gov.uk/you-and-the-judiciary/going-to-court/what-do-i-call-judge
- At court, ask the lawyer who has called you, or just wait and see what term the barristers use.

Expect to sit in court prior to giving evidence, to hear other witnesses, expert or otherwise:

- Occasionally you may be asked not to do so, but this is the exception. If in doubt, check with the side who has called you.
- Remember to turn your phone off before going in.

In the witness box

You will be asked whether you wish to be sworn in on a holy book (there are many available) or affirm. You will be asked to give your name, current appointment and qualifications:

- Have a prepared speech to hand, in which you explain your current appointment(s) and your qualifications. For example, MRCPsych might be described as a postgraduate professional qualification in clinical psychiatry.

Understand whom you are trying to persuade of your opinion:

- Never the barristers – they either do or don't agree with you by default.
- Always the judge – even where the issue is for the jury it is helpful to engage with the judge.
- But where a jury is present, it is them that you are trying to persuade.

While a barrister is asking you a question, look at them. But when you are talking, talk to the jury and/or judge:

- Stand facing between the judge and jury, and turn your torso to look at the barrister.
- Make eye contact and try actively to engage with judge/jury.

Speak loudly and more slowly than you would in conversation:

- The judge will be taking notes. Watch their writing hand, pause regularly and wait for them to stop writing before continuing.

Be prepared simply to acknowledge errors and consider the impact of new evidence, which perhaps was heard before you arrived, on your opinions.

Remember that the barrister is there to present a particular case, whereas you are independent:

- You have no emotional investment at all and are entirely non-partisan; your opinion is simply your opinion, given for the benefit of the court, and the court may or may not agree with it.
- You are calm, unbiased, reflective yet robust, and willing to concede a point where necessary.

Your evidence will be split into three parts:

- Examination-in-chief:
  - By the side that has called you.
  - Most barristers will carefully lead you through those parts of your written report that they wish to

adduce. This is fine, though be aware of the possibility that selective use of your evidence might distort the overall picture. Remember that your duty is to give unbiased evidence to the court, and correct this if necessary.

— Your evidence essentially is that contained in your report. That is not to say you cannot explain or expand a little but in the main, you should stick to your report.

— Some barristers will read sections out and simply ask you to confirm that it is your evidence. Others will ask you to read out parts of your report. Sometimes it is difficult to know how much to say and when to stop – keep an eye on the barrister, who will give a sign.

• Cross-examination:
  — By the opposing side.
  — This is a much more flexible affair. Be aware of the strategies commonly used by barristers (Box 21.2).
  — Defend your opinion robustly but where you need to concede a point, do so promptly and without fuss.
  — Always retain your composure. Never become defensive or aggressive.

• Re-examination:
  — By the side that has called you.
  — Usually fairly brief, particularly if the cross-examination has failed to score many points.

Box 21.2 Some strategies used by barristers and how to deal with them

If you are inexperienced then be prepared for a barrister politely to point this out:

• Where they make an accurate factual statement, for example that you are still in training, then simply agree, allowing them to move on as quickly as possible.

• If they extrapolate too far, so as to suggest your opinion is not authoritative, clearly point out that you have all the required qualifications and emphasize the experience that you do have.

Barristers will try to squeeze dimensions into categories and probability into certainty so as to support their case:

• Avoid giving too simple an answer to a complex question, and when a barrister asks whether you agree with a complex statement, take the opportunity to rephrase it in your own words, rather than simply agreeing. Sometimes this leads to a sarcastic response such as 'I thought that was what I just said', but that does not matter.

You know far more than the barrister about psychiatry. So often a barrister will attack your opinion on internal consistencies or inaccuracies in your report:

• Where a typographical error is pointed out, simply acknowledge it.

• Where there is some information which suggests that the history you gained is not accurate, then take time to consider whether it is important in terms of your opinion. In most cases it is not, and it is reasonable to point out that people often give slightly different answers at different times or to different people, so such minor inconsistencies are to be expected; you formulated your opinion with an appropriate tolerance for such things.

Introducing doubt by suggesting alternative explanations for the evidence:

• You may have to concede that a suggested alternative is possible, but ensure that you explain why in your view it is unlikely and why you prefer your stated opinion.

In general barristers are impassive and show little emotion, so as to suggest they are in full control of their case. But they may frown, raise their eyebrows or give quizzical looks of surprise or disbelief, as though to suggest you have said something ridiculous:

• Remember that all such performances are strategic; ignore them and retain your composure.

Less often they show irritation or anger, or accuse you of being pedantic, or of avoiding giving a clear answer:

- Politely assure them that you are just trying to present your evidence accurately for the benefit of the court.

A common strategy is to try to lead you down a cul-de-sac to some conclusion that is helpful to the barrister's case, by asking a series of seemingly innocuous questions, usually requiring just yes or no answers:

- Be aware of this common strategy whenever a cross-examining barrister asks you a yes or no question.
- Be pedantic in your answers and do not give a simple answer unless it is really that simple. Usually in psychiatry it will not be long before you can point out that the issue is rather more complex than the barrister's question implies. This leaves you with a get-out clause, and stymies the barrister's strategy.
- Psychiatrists inevitably rely heavily on the defendant's self-report. Barristers may assert that your whole opinion is solely based on what the defendant told you, and therefore cannot be reliable:
- Point out the other sources of information that you do have, and point to the consistency between sources as being persuasive of veracity.
- Be prepared to explain the syndromal nature of psychiatric diagnosis, and the amount of psychiatric knowledge that the defendant would need in order to feign the disorders that you have diagnosed.
- Be able to explain to the court what features would alert you to feigning.
- Look at the timing of reports of problems, for example if the defendant has complained of the illness in question prior to the offence.
- Look carefully for objective evidence to support your conclusions. This might be straightforward – an abnormal MRI brain scan in dementia, for example, or may be slightly less obvious, such as toleration of high-dose diazepam in alcohol detoxification to support your assertion that they were dependent on alcohol.

References

Coles EM, Veiel HOF. (2001) Expert testimony and pseudoscience: how mental health professionals are taking over the courtroom. *International Journal of Law and Psychiatry* **24**, 607–25

General Medical Council. (2008) *Acting as an Expert Witness*. London: General Medical Council

*Kenny A. (1984) The psychiatric expert in court. *Psychological Medicine* **14**(2), 291–302

O'Grady J. (2002) Psychiatric evidence and sentencing: ethical dilemmas. *Criminal Behaviour and Mental Health* **12**, 179–84

Richardson J. (2011) *Archbold 2011: Criminal Pleading Evidence and Practice*. London: Sweet & Maxwell

Rix KJB. (2008) The psychiatrist as expert witness. Part 1: general principles and civil cases. *Advances in Psychiatric Treatment* **14**, 37–41

Rogers T. (2004) Diagnostic validity and psychiatric expert testimony. *International Journal of Law and Psychiatry* **27**, 281–90

Roscoe A, Rodway C, Mehta H, While D, Amos T, Kapur N, *et al*. (2009) Psychiatric recommendations to the court as regards homicide perpetrators. *Journal of Forensic psychiatry and Psychology* **20**(3), 366–77

*St John-Smith P, Michael A, Davies T. (2009) Coping with a coroner's inquest: a psychiatrist's guide. *Advances in Psychiatric Treatment* **15**, 7–16

Stone A. (1984) The ethical boundaries of forensic psychiatry – a view from the ivory tower. *Bulletin of the American Academy of Psychiatry and the Law* **12**(3), 209–19

Tapper C. (2010) *Cross and Tapper on Evidence*, 12th edn. Oxford: Oxford University Press

Index